The Contradictions of Medical Education

Janet Grant • Leonard Grant
Editors

The Contradictions of Medical Education

A Political View From Practice

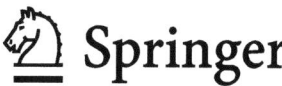 Springer

Editors
Janet Grant
Centre for Medical Education in Context,
CenMEDIC
Hampton, UK

Leonard Grant
School of Medicine
University of Liverpool
Liverpool, UK

ISBN 978-3-031-90393-9   ISBN 978-3-031-90394-6   (eBook)
https://doi.org/10.1007/978-3-031-90394-6

This Springer imprint is published by the registered company Springer Nature Switzerland AG
The registered company address is: Gewerbestrasse 11, 6330 Cham, Switzerland

If disposing of this product, please recycle the paper.

*This book is dedicated to the hope that
everyone involved in medical education will
take a political view, studying their own
conditions, creating their own pathways, not
emulating the solutions of others, but instead
increasing the power of their own context to
affect the future of medical education where
they are.*

Foreword

Among the books I have read on medical education, this collection of perspectives is unique. It is not about how to develop a curriculum, or how to create an assessment of competency, or how to conduct a faculty development workshop. Instead, it is about medical education itself and whether it is a proper discipline as opposed to a practice with a purpose. In my view, the authors correctly conclude the latter but the journey to that answer is what makes the book special.

It is structured around the dialectical method in which a thesis is posited, an antithesis is proposed, and a synthesis is explored. The theses are contributed by 35 individuals engaged in medical education, most of whom are from the Global South. They write on topics of their own choosing and the editors offer their reflections. This produces a rich and authentic mélange of ideas from which several commonalities emerge, three of which are interrelated and speak forcefully to my own experiences.

The first is the lack of evidence for many medical education practices. Ideas are introduced without solid evidence indicating their superiority, or at least their non-inferiority. These become fashionable, dominate health professions education conferences, enter practice through the efforts of a committed group of followers, and generate the beginnings of a body of research. Before there is enough evidence to justify the changes that have already been made, a different idea emerges, and it supplants its predecessor starting the cycle anew. This creates the illusion of progress but not its substance.

The second and related commonality is the dominance, in medical education, of the Global North (i.e. North America, Europe, and Australia). The ideas that feed the fashion frenzy typically start in this part of the world, without reasonable evidence of efficacy. Nonetheless, they are often readily adopted in the Global South. The motivation for this acceptance, to improve the quality of healthcare, is laudable. However, the importance of context in education cannot be understated, and the result is often an ill-fitting 'innovation' utilising precious resources that could be better spent otherwise.

Finally, medical education has become big business. As new medical schools are created, curricula are often purchased, exacerbating the challenges of insufficient evidence and the dominance of the Global North. This, in turn, has created a market for medical educators leading to the proliferation of programmes offering a Master's degree in health professions education. Unfortunately, these programmes are of variable quality, and most are not designed to address the challenges noted throughout this book.

There are two important aspects of the arguments made here that I will take away. First, the power of the dialectical methods is evident, and it can be applied to any aspect of the field to aid in understanding why we do what we do, why we change, how we change it, and what we value. Second, context and culture matter. It makes perfect sense to borrow liberally from others but not to do so without evidence, forethought, and modification.

Honorary Fellow of the Royal College of General   John J. Norcini
Practitioners and the Academy of Medical Educators
London, UK

Research Professor, SUNY Upstate Medical University
Syracuse, NY, USA

Fellow, Presence (a Center at Stanford Medical School)
Stanford, CA, USA

President Emeritus of FAIMER
Philadelphia, PA, USA

About the Book

Medical education is a social and political science. It is also a global undertaking and one that contributes to the export of medical graduates to advantaged countries at the cost of loss to the countries that have invested in their training. This alone makes medical education a political process. But it is a political process from so many other points of view where power, money, and hierarchy operate.

To introduce new methods of teaching and learning, or assessment, or new content and structure for curriculum, or new management and decision-making processes might seem to be neutral acts. But they are not. Each represents a vested idea and a power relationship. These are the essence of politics.

Whether or not to examine the state of the healthcare service and access to care which it does or does not equitably provide, while training medical graduates for that service is a political decision. Whether to equip students to go into training abroad is also a political decision.

In this book, we cannot examine every political element of the field of medical education. But we can start, and hope that others will continue to build the political analysis of medical education and examine all its power and limitations, its actions, decisions, and institutions from that point of view.

Contents

Editors and Contributors

About the Editors

Janet Grant is a chartered educational psychologist who was the first non-clinical lecturer in medical education in the world, appointed at King's College Hospital Medical School in London in 1972. Her PhD in 1980 was on medical students' and doctors' diagnostic thinking processes. Janet is Emerita Professor of Education in Medicine at the UK Open University, and Honorary Professor at University College London Medical School.

For most of her academic life, Janet conducted policy research in medical education for the UK government and professional medical and regulatory bodies. Her interests are in policy research, regulation, educational development, continuing professional development and curriculum. She has worked in many countries and with international organisations around the world, and has written extensively on contextual relevance in these topics.

Janet has been a regulator in both postgraduate medical education and legal education.

Leonard Grant is an early career academic interested in the political economy of work as a determinant of health. Leonard's PhD thesis used a dialectical materialist methodology to consider the workplace as part of the postgraduate General Practice curriculum.

From 2013 to 2024, Leonard was the Academic Course Manager for the FAIMER/Keele MHPE in Assessment and Accreditation where he managed the educational process for hundreds of students, taught Research Methods and wrote on distance and distributed learning.

Leonard has developed and taught a new Public Health MSc at the University of Winchester, and is currently Lecturer in Medical Education in the University of Liverpool School of Medicine where he is also Programme Director for the new PGCert in Clinical Education.

Contributors

Babatunde Ademusire College of Medicine, University of Ibadan, Ibadan, Nigeria

Akinyele Adisa College of Medicine, University of Ibadan, Ibadan, Nigeria

Samar Ahmed Faculty of Medicine, Forensic Medicine Department, Ain Shams University, Cairo, Egypt

Syed Moin Ali Aga Khan University, Karachi, Pakistan

Tonya Arscott-Mills Department of Pediatrics, Levine Children's Hospital, Wake Forest University School of Medicine, Charlotte, NC, USA

Valdes Roberto Bollela University of São Paulo, Ribeirão Preto School of Medicine (FMRP-USP), Ribeirão Preto, Brazil

Megan E. L. Brown School of Medicine, Newcastle University, Newcastle upon Tyne, UK

Vanessa C. Burch Colleges of Medicine of South Africa, Johannesburg, South Africa

Gordon Caldwell Lorn and Islands Hospital, Oban, UK

Aadil S. Chagla Department of Neurosurgery, King Edward Memorial Hospital, and Seth G S Medical College, Mumbai, India

Leena S. Chagla Mersey and West Lancashire Teaching Hospitals NHS Trust, Prescot, UK

Obafunke M. Denloye College of Medicine, University of Ibadan, Ibadan, Nigeria

Kadambari Dharanipragada Jawaharlal Institute of Postgraduate Medical Education and Research (JIPMER), Puducherry, India

Rebecca Gillibrand North Middlesex University Hospital NHS Trust, London, UK

Janet Grant Centre for Medical Education in Context, CenMEDIC, Hampton, UK

Leonard Grant School of Medicine, University of Liverpool, Liverpool, UK

Matthew C. E. Gwee Centre for Medical Education (CenMED), Yong Loo Lin School of Medicine, Singapore, Singapore

Anna Harvey Bluemel Newcastle University, Newcastle upon Tyne, UK
Newcastle United Hospitals Trust, Newcastle upon Tyne, UK

Annabel Heybourne University Hospitals, Southampton, UK

Susan Jamieson School of Medicine, University of Glasgow, Glasgow, UK

Anne Keane Independent Educational Consultant, Edinburgh, UK

Namita Kumar Conference of Postgraduate Medical Deans, London, UK
NHS England, London, UK

Shuh Shing Lee Centre for Medical Education (CenMED), Yong Loo Lin School of Medicine, Singapore, Singapore

Savarra Mantzor Full Circle Health, Pediatrics Residency of Idaho, Boise, ID, USA

Anindya Niyogi King's College Hospital, London, UK

Masayuki Nogi Queen's Medical Center, Honolulu, HI, USA
Kameda Medical Center, Chiba, Japan
John A. Burns School of Medicine, University of Hawaii, Honolulu, HI, USA

Victor A. Odekunle College of Medicine, University of Ibadan, Ibadan, Nigeria

Akintunde A. Odukogbe College of Medicine, University of Ibadan, Ibadan, Nigeria

Adebola O. Ogunbiyi College of Medicine, University of Ibadan, Ibadan, Nigeria

E. Oluwabunmi Olapade-Olaopa College of Medicine, University of Ibadan, Ibadan, Nigeria

Funmilayo E. Olopade College of Medicine, University of Ibadan, Ibadan, Nigeria

M. Ahmed Rashid London School of Hygiene and Tropical Medicine, London, UK

Dujeepa D. Samarasekera Centre for Medical Education (CenMED), Yong Loo Lin School of Medicine, Singapore, Singapore

Evangeline Mary Kiruba Samuel The Institute of Child Health and Hospital for Children, Chennai, India

Muhammad Shahid Shamim Aga Khan University, Karachi, Pakistan

Jillian H. T. Yeo Centre for Medical Education (CenMED), Yong Loo Lin School of Medicine, Singapore, Singapore

Thomas Zilling Department of Surgery, Lund University, Lund, Sweden

INTRODUCTION: PRACTICE—THEORY—PRACTICE: LEARNING FROM THE EXPERIENCE OF MEDICAL EDUCATION

Janet Grant and Leonard Grant

1 How We Constructed This Book

This book collects accounts of the experiences of 35 people working in medical education from around the world. Those authors wrote for themselves, about issues that they chose. We simply asked them to reflect on something that concerned them about medical education where they are. We read each account and then wrote a political dialectical analysis of the issues. This was given to the authors for their comment and approval.

We grouped their accounts into six sections which reflect the general areas of concern. Although the grouping could have been done in many ways, we chose:

- Culture and context
- Globalisation and its problems
- Negotiating identities in medical education and medicine
- Managing the system, the profession and the business of medical education: The neoliberal project
- Medical education and the workplace
- The power and politics of curriculum.

We did not choose the authors according to any sampling framework. We simply gathered together voices of authors whom we already had heard. Lived experience is valid and the basis of political and social understanding. We hope that in future,

J. Grant (✉)
Centre for Medical Education in Context (CenMEDIC), Hampton, UK
e-mail: janet@cenmedic.net

L. Grant
School of Medicine, University of Liverpool, Liverpool, UK
e-mail: Leonard.grant@liverpool.ac.uk

© The Author(s), under exclusive license to Springer Nature Switzerland AG 2026
J. Grant, L. Grant (eds.), *The Contradictions of Medical Education*,
https://doi.org/10.1007/978-3-031-90394-6_1

others will gather further reflections from different places, and deepen the political analysis that we have started here. Such a perspective may tell us much more than educational theory can.

2   The Analysis of Power in Medical Education

Politics is about power relationships.

This book presents a political analysis of the practice of medical education. It is not about theories or frameworks that have been applied to it. It is not about the research that has been published. It is about actual experiences that people have had of medical education, the things that concern them, and a way of looking at those that teases out their contradictions, their individuality, their commonalities and their power relationships.

In doing this, we aim to set out a systematic and generalisable approach to the analysis of medical education. Medical education is often seen, correctly, as a social science. But unless we also apply the concepts and methods of political science, our understanding will be incomplete. 'Medical education' has become a phenomenon, taking many doctors away from practice and moving them into preparing others for the practice that they themselves have often wholly or partially left. Countless journals, departments, conferences, Master's degrees and PhDs now populate this very new area of work. And yet there is no undergraduate degree in the subject. So people can come into the postgraduate degree, and then enter practice as a specialist in medical education, with little relevant academic theoretical background. That is why we have begun our analysis from actual concrete practice.

We cannot address why medicine, which takes in the best learners, might need to examine how to help them to learn. Or whether that examination is producing better doctors than their teachers are. Or whether healthcare services have improved in parallel with the expansion of medical education as an area of specific study and activity. But we can, perhaps, examine a more fundamental question about the political drivers and consequences of the medical education movement, in a world that is, and will continue to be, dominated by power relationships and a one-way flow of ideas, practices, and ideologies. Medical graduates themselves flow in the opposite direction from the flow of medical education ideas. On that basis alone, we could start a political analysis.

2.1   Political Analysis

To achieve this, we describe and apply a dialectical analysis to real examples of medical education practice, to enable us to appreciate the wide variety and determinants of practice and concerns in different contexts, and the ways in which those practices and concerns differ between themselves, and often differ from the theories that are applied to them. These differences are expressions of incompatible tendencies, or contradictions, within medical education. A contradiction, for us, is when there are opposing or incompatible tendencies within the same circumstance. This might be as simple as having the knowledge to make a desired curriculum change but lacking the resources to carry it out, or as complex as the pressure to introduce new teaching methods or accreditations that derive from a completely different culture. The chapters of this book set out a wide variety of contradictions. It is in the resolution of these contradictions that practice develops. These contradictions might become more acute as globalisation of medical education continues (Bleakley et al., 2008; Rao, 2024) and increasing critique is applied to this trend (Rashid et al., 2023; Rashid & Grant, 2024).

The language and idea of dialectics is not new. Plato, Socrates, Hegel and then Marx have all used this approach to set out different and opposing sides of an argument and find their resolution (Maybee, 2020). More recently, dialectical behavioural therapy has been used as a branch of cognitive behavioural therapy to integrate stressful opposing views and experiences of the world (Lynch et al., 2006). It is a widely used analytical method.

3   Applying the Dialectical Method

In our analysis of medical education, we use the dialectical method to identify and describe the contradictions and tensions experienced in the practice of medical education. In doing so, we hope to show that this analytical method, rather than attempts at theory building, might advance medical education appropriately for every context, culture, condition and circumstance.

To explain why we have chosen this analytical pathway, we should introduce our underlying arguments about context, culture and learning, the nature of a discipline, the meaning of theory, and the reasons for adopting dialectical analysis as our method of valuing difference. We will look at each of these before coming back to dialectics as a method.

3.1   Analysis Versus Theory Building

In the study of medical education, specific methods, theories and approaches are often needed that fall under what is generally known as 'the social sciences'. These methods can describe, analyse and explain human behaviour, relationships, their contexts, antecedents and consequences. We would not say that these methods are fundamentally separate or divisible from methods used in the natural sciences. When conducted well and appropriately, they are all compatible examinations of the world, as has been shown in other fields (Richter et al., 2022), and argued for over many decades (Dumain, n.d.; Richter et al., 2022). Bringing together social and natural sciences under the simple heading of 'research methods' seems to resolve an unnecessary contradiction in medical education research, and address current concerns about differentiating between methods (Toomela, 2011).

(Social science)… addresses human behaviour, politics, resources, relationships and values, unlike the analysis of physical phenomena that is the focus of natural science. Although natural science also offers many perspectives, some of which are socially constructed, the intangible complexity of social science means that the choices of ways of generating knowledge must take into account often competing existential and theoretical domains. (Moon & Blackman, 2014) in (Grant & Grant, 2023)

On this basis, a multitude of useful theories can be used or developed that address the same phenomenon from different and competing frames of reference deriving from politics, class, culture (including beliefs about teaching and learning), ethics and values, or simply from fashion. Although the dimensions to be taken into account when building theories are often similar (hierarchy, relationships, culture, power, economics), each expresses itself differently in different contexts. This results in different ways of designing education for different contexts, both specifically in exact teaching and learning methods (Cheng, 2021), and more broadly in curriculum design. For that reason alone, to seek a universal theory of medical education would be a counsel of despair. Instead, a way of supporting the local development of appropriate ways of analysing and framing educational development is needed. We try to build that analysis not to develop an unattainable theory of medical education, but to illuminate the underlying forces that have and do drive this rapidly burgeoning field of activity.

4 Culture and Learning: The Unwarranted Dominance of the Global North

To support our argument that a universal theory of medical education is not possible or desirable, we should look more closely at context, culture and learning.

In terms of context, the actual practice of medicine differs in availability, consultation style, communication, prescribing patterns, treatments, relationship to traditional medicine and much else. It is affected by the patterns of morbidity and mortality, by sources of disease and disorder, by the assumptions and resources of patients and clinicians, by social forces and behaviours, and by the structure of the healthcare service. The literature that reports these differences is considerable and growing. This alone tells us that a local approach to curriculum content and design is needed.

Against this, there are also differences in the ways that teachers and students pursue teaching and learning.

Barbara Lloyd's original work on cross cultural psychology is still seminal. Her anti-racist, academic stance led her to address difficult questions about cognition, coming out of the emerging evidence that '…individuals growing up in different cultures may well learn different rules for processing information from the world around them' (Lloyd, 1972). Given the current unidirectional flow of medical education models from global north to global south, her conclusions are still worryingly relevant:

People in developing countries are demanding a rapid increase in western-type education. Studies reviewed here indicate that children from westernised homes with educated parents will be at a distinct advantage.' (ibid)

At the same time, children from 'non-westernised' environments may be lost to such education. Where medical education exports 'western' ideas, this, therefore, may contribute to inequality and narrow participation, whether at school or at university.

A note on 'the west': Although we sometimes quote authors who refer to 'the west', we do not use this term ourselves, with its unjustified, unstable and historically inaccurate implications of superiority and colonial power over other parts of the world (Mcneil, 1997). Instead, we use the sometimes problematical political/economic terms "global north' and 'global south' which originally were intended to highlight wealth inequalities between nations and regions. Although those inequalities fluctuate, they largely remain intact since these terms were first used in 1980 (Lees, 2021).

Outside medical education, cross-cultural analyses of learning have compared various factors, performances, cognitive features, cultures and contexts. Many relate to aspects of education that are central to learning. For example, the effects of receiving negative feedback vary considerably between European, American and Hong Kong Chinese students, based on their different views of how to pursue their goals (Kung et al., 2016). Related might be differences in levels and effects of self-esteem (Kim et al., 2008) and self-worth (Liu et al., 2017) in North American and East Asian undergraduates, the latter having lower scores in both. Perhaps related to self-esteem, or perhaps to hierarchy or personal relationships, is that teacher emotional affect influences differently the ways in which students in different cultures (this time in Germany, Russia and the United States) respond to negative feedback (Hansen & Mendzheritskaya, 2017). Something as seemingly simple as feedback models are not universally applicable (Chowdhury & Kalu, 2004). We must approach all claims and assertions about globalised education with some critical scepticism.

The reality of different cultural effects on learning is to be found in the comprehensive research that is undertaken, for example, in relation to approaches to learning and teaching in China (Bond, 2012). Such culture-linked approaches tend to be displayed, even when children move abroad (Stevens, 2007). In this case, approaches to focused acquisition of knowledge might not fit with the current educational rhetoric promoted in the global north, but nonetheless show the greatest academic success. There is no universally right way of learning.

The widespread adoption in medical education of often discredited global north ideas such as adult learning, active and passive learning, learner and teacher centredness, or methods such as the flipped classroom, or designs such as competence-based curricula, is rarely supported by evidence, or by an articulated theory, even in their contexts of origin (Didau et al., 2016). They may also be antagonistic to the effective methods of teaching and learning of other cultures. Therefore, the continuing uncriticised ability of the global north to set the agenda might be seen as worrying.

There are many similar discredited examples of ideas used in medical education although largely rejected in their own disciplines, such as 'approaches to learning' and 'learning styles' (Cashdan, 2021; Howie & Bagnall, 2013; Kirschner, 2017; Reynolds, 1997; Riener & Willingham, 2010) or deep, surface and achieving approaches to learning (Watkins, 2011). These concepts were developed in the global north and either do not even apply widely there, or do not apply in other cultures. For that reason alone, we could argue that a unified theory of medical education is an inappropriate aspiration, and that an approach to contextual analysis and illumination of differences might be a more productive and emancipating way forward.

5 Is Medical Education a Discipline or a Practice?

With countless Master's degrees, Professors, university departments and journals, we might imagine that medical education is an academic discipline like any other. But in reality, whether or not medical education is an academic discipline is a contentious issue, based on different views of what a discipline is, and what its components are. For the practice itself, this might not be important, but for the careers of those within it, in establishing offices or training programmes, for example, it might be instrumentally important (Blouin, 2022).

An academic discipline could be said to assume certain components:

> … ontology, what exists in the human world that researchers can acquire knowledge about; epistemology, how knowledge is created; and philosophical perspective, the philosophical orientation of the researcher that guides her or his action. (Moon & Blackman, 2014)

In all this, medical education is still defining itself.

5.1 Ideological Ethnocentrism: The Dominant Global North

Medical education has the additional challenge of being, *de facto*, an international undertaking that is dominated in its ideas by the global north while having most medical schools in the global south. This ethnocentrism of ideologies and practices has been noted in the social sciences for many decades (Stanfield, 1985). It generates contradictions between the dominant group and those who are subject to its ideas, but actually live a different reality.

In medical education, ideas about teaching and learning, management and hierarchy, relationships, values and purposes, generally derive from the global north where individual characteristics, social relationships, and means of influence and power are not necessarily typical even of the whole of that 'north', and certainly not of the variety similarly found in the global south (Wong, 2011; Wong et al., 2021). Even within these areas, we can see the contradictions between what is asserted and what is practised.

This book, therefore, does not attempt to produce a unified view of medical education that will mark it out as its own discipline. Instead, we accept its derivative nature and its many contradictions, and present an analytical approach that values and teases out those differences, whether they are differences between cultures, or between rhetoric and reality, or between theory and practice. The result of this might enable each place and person to identify their own approach, and to be valued for the richness that will bring to the field with a subsequent bi-directional rather than unidirectional flow of ideas.

5.2 Medical Education: A Means-Ends Practice

We argue that, rather than being a discipline, medical education is a practice with a purpose: a means-ends orientated relational (social) practice (Noddings, 2003), the means being the practices of curriculum, teaching and learning, assessment, and educational management, while the ends are defined by the vision of each medical school which will involve the production of medical graduates with qualities defined by that school. If we reflect on the content of Master's degrees in medical (or health professions) education, it is clear that they frequently, and appropriately, address curriculum, assessment and teaching methods, skills and processes, while briefly covering areas such as learning theory in weeks rather than the years such study takes in a psychology degree if a critical perspective is to be mastered. Such medical education degrees do not have the time, or perhaps the inclination, to develop the skills of critique which are fundamental to the social sciences (Tekian & Artino, 2013).

So we argue that medical education is not an academic discipline but a situated practice (O'Brien & Battista, 2020), the betterment of which requires thoroughly understanding local, external and historical factors and relationships. Practice can be evaluated and researched: but that does not make the entity an academic discipline.

For a means-ends relational practice, which is looking to modify education and training to achieve desired outcomes, the instrumental approach we often see is to be expected. But to understand, we need ways of examining that practice, especially in a world where medical education is a topic of global interest, and practitioners and researchers interact from different cultures, contexts and backgrounds. Medical education research tends to be broad-based and iterative rather than additive and theory-building. Since we cannot adduce robust evidence to help us make generalisable judgements about the practices we observe (because such research is rarely based on agreed theory, and the nature of social science often precludes robust evidence and generalisability), we need to apply our own comparative analysis. That comparison might be between theory and practice, or practice and practice.

Knowledge and understanding are accumulated by experience, through relationships, by understanding of culture and context, and may be different and require different research methods in different contexts or for different groups and subgroups. Knowledge is advanced by contextual analysis of practice. In doing so, we can try to explain what we find, but will that lead to the universal theory that underpins a discipline? The ideas that we have mentioned so far, deriving from the global north, do not, and perhaps cannot, have that universal quality.

6   Does Medical Education Have a Theory?

So far, we have argued that medical education is not a discipline, and this is yet another good reason why it has no theories of its own. Medical education tends to import and try to apply parts of theories and ideas from cognitive and educational psychology, and from sociology, anthropology and management, and uses them to frame different areas of research and practice. These ideas are often time-bound, deriving from fading, emerging or dominant social constructs at any one time. The application of sometimes competing imported learning theories is an example of the resultant confusion: medical education adopts, explains, or simply uses, ideas about learning that exist in other domains, although it rarely uses the dominant enduring psychological constructs around learning that focus on memory. The most commonly and uncritically imported ideas, such as adult learning, experiential learning and self-directed learning, do not meet the criteria for a theory at all (Dong et al., 2021; Taylor & Hamdy, 2013). We may question whether the instrumental and uncritical use of ideas from other disciplines serves medical education well. Perhaps in assessment alone, has medical education made a significant original contribution to developing frameworks for conceptualising practice.

6.1   What Is Theory?

The discussion of how to define 'theory' has a long and contentious history (Wacker, 1998). But one common thread is that theory 'provides clear explanations for the pragmatic world' (Wacker, 1998). When that world is characterised by contextual social variation, then a single theory, especially if derived elsewhere, is unlikely to be effective, unless commonalities and differences across contexts are examined. In other words, theory might have to be contextually derived, and be different from context to context. And if that is the case, then we need appropriate methods of analysing and describing the events and qualities of each context, which will enable us to develop our own theories:

> [This] is not a narrowing of focus and the search for one truth, but is a broadening of concepts, theories, reported experience and method, and, we hope, an increasing tendency for each to tell their own truth well. (Grant & Grant, 2023)

So a multiplicity of original local theories might enrich the practice of medical education. From those, commonalities might be derived. Perhaps the skill of theory building is essential to the future of medical education. Or perhaps medical education can remain as a practice, adding a more systematic and contextual analytical approach. To build theory requires the analysis of practice, not once, but repeatedly. The perpetual cycle of knowledge building is practice—theory—practice (Mao, 1937). Although a theory might be defined by many qualities and characteristics (Kivunja, 2018), we would say that, at a minimum, the theories we build should be logical, have defined variables and relationships between them, make testable predictions, and offer explanations for observations. But most importantly, should be grounded in context. And contexts vary.

7 Why Develop Analysis Rather Than Theory?

We have argued that context is all important in understanding how best to design, implement and understand medical education. We have not discussed the evaluation of medical education *per se*, but if we did, we would almost certainly review the social construction of ideas of programme or curriculum evaluation and how those ideas change from era to era depending on dominant economic and social imperatives. Given that ideas, models, purposes and methods change over time, we may conclude that realist, or realistic (Pawson & Tilley, 1997) evaluation which looks at 'What works for whom in what circumstances and in what respects, and how?' is the optimum approach (G. Wong et al., 2012), rather than simply applying an existing approach developed in a different, almost inevitably global north, context, and in a different era for a different purpose (Levine, 2002; Melrose, 1998).

7.1 Analysing the Contradictory Truth of Experience

We are interested in the authentic experience of the authors of the narrative accounts in this book. For us, they are the truth tellers (Grant, 2023).

In all of this, context is the central concern. If context is key, then concrete analysis of context must be the starting place. And given the current problematical relationship between the global north which derives ideas, and the global south which implements them, we argue that the basis of a universally applicable analysis is the examination of contradictions between theory and practice, practice and context, achievement and intention, context and context, culture and culture. While there is no relevant universal theory, or globally applicable practice, there is a method of analysis that applies across all cultures and contexts.

In this book, we set out and apply that analysis of contradictions in medical education to a wide variety of described episodes of practice. That analysis might lead us to see common non-antagonistic contradictions that are amenable to resolution, or antagonistic contradictions that can never be resolved and must be accepted in our own way, wherever we are.

> The fundamental issue is this: If knowledge is socially constructed, relying on the values and experiences of the knowledge generator or summariser, it is therefore limited in its generalisability. How, then, can we confidently make evidence-based quality improvements to our practice? (Grant & Grant, 2022)

The social construction of our knowledge means that any theory or framework is likely to be limited in its applicability. Even theories from cognitive science are limited by the behavioural and social traditions extant in different contexts and times.

Perhaps more importantly, we must recognise that, so far, anything that approaches a theory of any aspect of medical education, be it clinical thinking or simulation, or teaching and learning, or curriculum, or assessment, has derived from a very small portion of the global north, and a particular subset of imported theories that medical education has chosen to espouse. There is no reason to believe that this pattern will change yet, and we do not wish to contribute to it. Stanfield, an African-American Yale sociologist, stated in 1985 (Stanfield, 1985) a position that is still true:

> The social sciences are ethnocultural institutions that … are reflectors and microcosms of the societal hegemony privileges of Euro-Americans.

Relying on the language of social science is, therefore, an exclusionary act, tied only to its own origins. To overcome this, Stanfield called for a new 'multilectic' paradigm, which identifies and then synthesises a multitude of opposites or contradictions. Although he considers dialectical analysis to be inadequate in fulfilling his aspiration, we nonetheless, will begin with that analysis of contradictions and intend to draw them together in the beginning of a final synthesis, presented as our conclusions which might point to a way ahead for medical education that recognises a multiplicity of contexts and contextually appropriate practices.

8   Dialectical Analysis of Medical Education

We have argued that medical education in practice is characterised by contextual differences, and differences between ideas derived in one context and practice applied to another. We wanted to use a method of analysis that is appropriate to this reality. The method that is designed to address such a situation is dialectical analysis which addresses contradictions and conflicting forces and how these might be resolved. It also recognises that it is not always possible to reconcile antagonistically contradictory forces. Sometimes things are just too different to work effectively together. And when that is the case, contextual practice must be the first frame of reference.

Dialectics starts from the analysis of that practice, so we gathered together accounts from many people of issues in their own experience of medical education. We asked that their experience should simply be described without recourse to any theories. So we start purely from practice, and then will apply the dialectical method to the experiences recounted in this book.

Dialectics begins from the world as it exists *in reality*, how it is presented to us and how we experience it. This is the foundation of analysis. We do not begin from what *should* or *could* happen but from what *actually does* and what our contributors feel and think about their experience.

In this method, there is no separation between knowing and doing, of theory and practice. To gain knowledge about something is to take part in it; hence the narrative accounts in this book. We engage, therefore, with those accounts specifically *from practice*. The dialectical method draws connections between the concrete phenomena described in these chapters towards a 'number of determinant, abstract, general relations' (Marx, 1857) and back to a deeper understanding of the whole (Vickers, 2015), since each example represents some fractal of that whole. It is a 'methodological antidote to the subjectivism, idealism, and dualism that inform much of contemporary non-Marxist social science' (Mills et al., 2010).

Dialectics offers a way of thinking about reality that is fundamentally *relational*. In studying an experience, therefore, it cannot be taken in isolation. It is always necessary to consider it as part of a whole, in our case medical education in general, or social and international relations, and especially to look at how it might have been influenced or otherwise affected by those wider phenomena. Dialectics causes us to look at examples of practice, and ask how they were or were not informed by what is said and thought in general about it, in medical education or the economic and political world as a whole. From that, the contradictions can be teased out.

8.1   What Are Contradictions?

Contradictions are opposing or incompatible tendencies *within the same relation*. Because they are contained within the same relation, they are also dependent upon one another. For example, a doctor cannot conduct their profession without the patient but, through this relation, the patient may be alienated from their own care. Resolving this contradiction thus involves removing or transforming the current distinction between doctor and patient. We might see parallels inside medical schools: as medical education experts take more decisions, decide the ways in which the school and teachers should develop, they might simultaneously disempower those who actually provide the education itself. It is through the struggle between these oppositional positions that change occurs. Both the doctor and the patient might negotiate a new relationship. The medical educationalist and the teacher might decide to act collaboratively, each being equally informed by the other. Or the teacher might simply navigate their own path in the light of recommendations, which they can do, given that they are the practitioner. The practice belongs to the practitioner, not to the observer or the planner. In doing this, imported theories might or might not turn out to be relevant or useful. In a dialectal analysis, we seek to observe those contradictions in order to identify a path towards their contextual resolution. The primary frame of reference is practice, not theory.

Dialectics sees everything in a state of continuous movement and change, where something is always developing and something dying away. We can see that easily in the history of medical education where ideas about teaching and learning, and about curriculum, for example, have changed dramatically and often, for at least the last 100 years. Current ideas will also fall away as they are proven or not in practice, or as they reflect dominant social values, and the contradictions are resolved in favour of new ideas. There is a process of constant renewal. Dialectics is therefore a powerful methodology for considering a fluctuating landscape, as it considers change to be inherent. It is not a quest for truth, where there is no universal truth to be found. Dialectics is a philosophy that focusses on movement that permanently exists in society (and in its history) and it is because things are not fixed that there is the possibility of transformation (Silva et al., 2022).

The method we employ is therefore to start from the experience described, to consider the wider context in the literature and theory, to identify contradictions in these, if any, and then to offer a suggestion towards their resolution. In applying this approach, we may find what, if anything, all contexts have in common. And if such commonalities are found, then the elements of a universal theory might be derived. If not, then understanding our own context and building our own theory, or informed practice, is a positive and constructive way forward. The universality might be the method. The politics of that, and power relationships, might underpin every analysis.

References

Bleakley, A., Brice, J., & Bligh, J. (2008). Thinking the post-colonial in medical education. *Medical Education, 42*(3), 266–270. https://doi.org/10.1111/j.1365-2923.2007.02991.x

Blouin, D. (2022). Health professions education as a discipline: Evidence based on Krishnan's framework. *Medical Teacher, 44*(4), 445–449. https://doi.org/10.1080/0142159X.2021.2020233

Bond, M. H. (2012). Oxford handbook of Chinese psychology, January 2010, 1–752. https://doi.org/10.1093/oxfordhb/9780199541850.001.0001

Cashdan, A. (2021, May 13). Learning styles – The myth persists. *The Psychologist*. https://www.bps.org.uk/psychologist/learning-styles-myth-persists

Cheng, Y. (2021). Cross-cultural differences in collaborative learning and relevant factors. In H. Ma, H. W. Lam, & M. Ganapathy (Eds.), Proceedings of the 2021 3rd International Conference on Literature, Art and Human Development (ICLAHD 2021). Springer Nature.

Chowdhury, R. R., & Kalu, G. (2004). Learning to give feedback in medical education. *The Obstetrician & Gynaecologist, 6*(4), 243–247. https://doi.org/10.1576/toag.6.4.243.27023

Didau, D., Bjork, R. A., & Wiliam, D. (2016). *What if everything you knew about education was wrong?* Crown House Publishing.

Dong, H., Lio, J., Sherer, R., & Jiang, I. (2021). Some learning theories for medical educators. *Medical Science Educator, 31*(3), 1157–1172. https://doi.org/10.1007/s40670-021-01270-6

Dumain, R. (n.d.). *'The autodidact project': Quote: Karl Marx on science, Society, & Life.* Retrieved 9 February 2023, from http://www.autodidactproject.org/quote/marxsci1.html

Grant, J. (2023). The scholarship of teaching: Who is the truth teller? *The Asia Pacific Scholar, 8*(2), 83–85. https://doi.org/10.29060/taps.2023-8-2/pv2874

Grant, J., & Grant, L. (2022). Quality and constructed knowledge: Truth, paradigms, and the state of the science. *Medical Education.* https://doi.org/10.1111/medu.14871

Grant, J., & Grant, L. (2023). Quality and constructed knowledge: Truth, paradigms, and the state of the science. *Medical Education, 57*(1), 23–30. https://doi.org/10.1111/medu.14871

Hansen, M., & Mendzheritskaya, J. (2017). How university lecturers' display of emotion affects students' emotions, failure attributions, and behavioral tendencies in Germany, Russia, and the United States. *Journal of Cross-Cultural Psychology, 48*(5), 734–753. https://doi.org/10.1177/0022022117697845

Howie, P., & Bagnall, R. (2013). A critique of the deep and surface approaches to learning model. *Teaching in Higher Education, 18*(4), 389–400. https://doi.org/10.1080/13562517.2012.733689

Kim, Y. H., Peng, S., & Chiu, C. Y. (2008). Explaining self-esteem differences between Chinese and north Americans: Dialectical self (vs. self-consistency) or lack of positive self-regard. *Self and Identity, 7*(2), 113–128. https://doi.org/10.1080/15298860601063437

Kirschner, P. A. (2017). Stop propagating the learning styles myth. *Computers & Education, 106*, 166–171. https://doi.org/10.1016/j.compedu.2016.12.006

Kivunja, C. (2018). Distinguishing between theory, theoretical framework, and conceptual framework: A systematic review of lessons from the field. *International Journal of Higher Education, 7*(6), 44–53. https://doi.org/10.5430/ijhe.v7n6p44

Kung, F. Y. H., Kim, Y. H., Yang, D. Y. J., & Cheng, S. Y. Y. (2016). The role of regulatory fit in framing effective negative feedback across cultures. *Journal of Cross-Cultural Psychology, 47*(5), 696–712. https://doi.org/10.1177/0022022116638172

Lees, N. (2021). The Brandt line after forty years: The more north-south relations change, the more they stay the same? *Review of International Studies, 47*(1), 85–106). s. https://doi.org/10.1017/S026021052000039X

Levine, T. (2002). Educational evaluation: Stability and change in curriculum evaluation. *PERGAMON Studies in Educational Evaluation, 28.* www.elsevier.com/stueduc

Liu, C., Chiu, Y. C., & Chang, J. (2017). Why do Easterners have lower well-being than Westerners? The role of others' approval contingencies of self-worth in the cross cultural differences in subjective well-being *Journal of Cross-Cultural Psychology* https://doi.org/10.1177/0022022116677580

Lloyd, B. B. (1972). *Perception and cognition. A cross-cultural perspective.* Penguin Books Ltd.

Lynch, T. R., Chapman, A. L., Rosenthal, M. Z., Kuo, J. R., & Linehan, M. M. (2006). Mechanisms of change in dialectical behavior therapy: Theoretical and empirical observations. *Journal of Clinical Psychology, 62*(4), 459–480. https://doi.org/10.1002/JCLP.20243

Mao, T. (1937). *On practice.* International Publishers.

Marx, K. (1857). Economic manuscripts: Grundrisse – Introduction [Abstract]. https://www.marxists.org/subject/dialectics/marx-engels/grundisse.htm

Maybee, J. (2020). Hegel's dialectics. *Stanford Encyclopedia of Philosophy.* https://plato.stanford.edu/entries/hegel-dialectics/

Mcneil, W. H. (1997). Western civilisation in world politics. What we mean by the west. *Orbis, 41*(4), 513–524.

Melrose, M. (1998). Exploring paradigms of curriculum evaluation and concepts of quality. *Quality in Higher Education, 4*(1), 37–43. https://doi.org/10.1080/1353832980040105

Mills, A. J., Durepos, G., & Wiebe, E. (Eds.). (2010). *Encyclopedia of case study research.* Sage Publications.

Moon, K., & Blackman, D. (2014). A guide to understanding social science research for natural scientists. *Conservation Biology, 28*(5), 1167–1177. https://doi.org/10.1111/cobi.12326

Noddings, N. (2003). Is teaching a practice? *Journal of Philosophy of Education, 37*(2), 241–251. https://doi.org/10.1111/1467-9752.00323

O'Brien, B. C., & Battista, A. (2020). Situated learning theory in health professions education research: A scoping review. In Advances in health sciences education (Vol. 25, 2, pp. 483–509). Springer. https://doi.org/10.1007/s10459-019-09900-w

Pawson, R., & Tilley, N. (1997). *Realistic Evaluation.* Sage Publications Ltd.

Rao, N. R. (2024). Globalization and medical education in a post-pandemic world. In *The mental health of medical students* (pp. 12–27). Oxford University Press. https://doi.org/10.1093/oso/9780192864871.003.0002

Rashid, M. A., & Grant, J. (2024). Power and place: Uncovering the politics of global medical education. *Medical Education, 58*(8), 930–938. https://doi.org/10.1111/medu.15459

Rashid, M. A., Ali, S. M., & Dharanipragada, K. (2023). Decolonising medical education regulation: A global view. *BMJ Global Health, 8*(6), e011622. https://doi.org/10.1136/bmjgh-2022-011622

Reynolds, M. (1997). Learning styles: A critique. *Management Learning, 28*(2), 115–133. https://doi.org/10.1177/1350507697282002

Richter, I., Roberts, B. R., Sailley, S. F., Sullivan, E., Cheung, V. V., Eales, J., Fortnam, M., Jontila, J. B., Maharja, C., Nguyen, T. H., Pahl, S., Praptiwi, R. A., Sugardjito, J., Sumeldan, J. D. C., Syazwan, W. M., Then, A. Y., & Austen, M. C. (2022). Building bridges between natural and social science disciplines: A standardized methodology to combine data on ecosystem quality trends. *Philosophical Transactions of the Royal Society B, 377*(1854). https://doi.org/10.1098/RSTB.2021.0487

Riener, C., & Willingham, D. (2010). The myth of learning styles. *Change: The Magazine of Higher Learning, 42*(5), 32–35. https://doi.org/10.1080/00091383.2010.503139

Silva, K. L. da, França, B. D., Schreck, R. S. C., Gandra, E. C., & Silva, L. L. F. (2022). Social inequalities for student leaders and professional organizations: Florence nightingale's political legacy. *Revista Brasileira de Enfermagem, 75*(2). https://doi.org/10.1590/0034-7167-2020-0465

Stanfield, J. H. (1985). Chapter 10: The ethnocentric basis of social science knowledge production. *Review of Research in Education, 12*(1), 387–415. https://doi.org/10.3102/0091732X012001387

Stevens, P. A. J. (2007). Researching race/ethnicity and educational inequality in English secondary schools: A critical review of the research literature between 1980 and 2005. *Review of Educational Research, 77*(2), 147–185. https://doi.org/10.3102/003465430301671

Taylor, D. C. M., & Hamdy, H. (2013). Adult learning theories: Implications for learning and teaching in medical education: AMEE guide no. 83. *Medical Teacher, 35*(11). https://doi.org/10.3109/0142159X.2013.828153

Tekian, A., & Artino, A. R. (2013). AM last page. *Academic Medicine, 88*(9), 1399. https://doi.org/10.1097/ACM.0b013e31829decf6

Toomela, A. (2011). Travel into a fairy land: A critique of modern qualitative and mixed methods psychologies. *Integrative Psychological and Behavioral Science, 45*(1), 21–47. https://doi.org/10.1007/s12124-010-9152-5

Vickers, T. (2015). Marxist approaches to social work. In *International encyclopedia of the Social & Behavioral Sciences* (2nd ed., pp. 663–669). Elsevier. https://doi.org/10.1016/B978-0-08-097086-8.28055-0

Wacker, J. G. (1998). A definition of theory: Research guidelines for different theory-building research methods in operations management. In. *Journal of Operations Management, 16.*

Watkins, D. (2011). Correlates of approaches to learning: A cross-cultural meta-analysis. In R. J. Sternberg & L.-F. Zhang (Eds.), *Perspectives on thinking, learning, and cognitive styles.* Routledge.

Wong, A. K. (2011). Culture in medical education: Comparing a Thai and a Canadian residency programme. *Medical Education, 45*(12), 1209–1219. https://doi.org/10.1111/j.1365-2923.2011.04059.x

Wong, G., Greenhalgh, T., Westhorp, G., & Pawson, R. (2012). Realist methods in medical education research: What are they and what can they contribute? *Medical Education, 46*(1), 89–96. https://doi.org/10.1111/j.1365-2923.2011.04045.x

Wong, S., Plowman, C., Puri, D., & Nwibe, I. (2021). Why we have to move beyond the idea of cultural competency. *Medical Education Online, 26*(1). https://doi.org/10.1080/1087298 1.2020.1841398

Part I
Culture and Context

Summary

This book is an analysis of the power and politics of the business and global industry of medical education. Part I presents three statements from Pakistan, Singapore, and the United States and Japan. Through these, we set out the central importance of culture and context and the ways in which forces of cultural imperialism and globalisation attempt to incorporate them into a project of the global north. In turn, we see how that attempt is also resisted or curbed against the dominant power of the global business of medical education.

I.i STATEMENT: Socio-cultural Contexts and Medical Education: Tales from Four Continents

Muhammad Shahid Shamim

1 Introduction

The world is geographically divided into hemispheres, continents and countries. The developed countries of North America, western Europe, Australia, New Zealand and some parts of the Asian continent, where the process of medical education is considered established and standardised, are often referred to as the 'west' in the literature (Ho et al., 2012). In contrast, the 'non-western' countries include most of the Asian, African, South American and central European nations where medical education generally follows western trends and technological progress. However, the acquired (or imposed) educational frameworks from the west may not always align with the local norms and values in the non-western regions. A Dutch social psychologist, Geert Hofstede, well known for his pioneering research on cross-cultural groups and organisations, suggests that in most countries, certain characteristics and ways of life distinguish them from other nations and can be considered their 'national culture or national character' (Hofstede & Bond, 1984). Consequently, it is generally noted that the needs of healthcare students and the roles of educators may differ significantly within these regions due to differing societal norms in diverse national cultures (Kallivayalil & Chadda, 2011). Similarly, Hofstede's work has shown that socio-cultural factors have a strong influence on the mental programming and character of nations, thereby affecting the overall educational process and environment.

This socio-cultural variability raises a critical question in the philosophy of education. John Dewey, one of the most influential educational philosophers of the last century suggests that the ultimate goal of education is to develop the learner as an active member of society (Dewey, 1962). Thereby, the question arises, 'Which

M. S. Shamim (✉)
Aga Khan University, Karachi, Pakistan
e-mail: muhammad.shamim@aku.edu

19

society?': the one where education is being imparted or all the others where the student may later serve as a professional? This dilemma becomes especially relevant in today's globalised context, where graduates often work across cultural and national boundaries.

In this global scenario, I have had the privilege of experiencing four continents as a medical education student, surgeon and educator. In these roles, I worked with people in various socio-cultural contexts across Pakistan, Saudi Arabia, China, Kenya, the United Kingdom (UK), and Australia. I had a great time in each of these places where my professional work was somewhat similar, but the overall experiences have been unique and provided me with valuable lessons about the cultural nuances that exist within medical education systems. Here, I have taken the opportunity to reflect on *my experiences* which allowed me to observe the obvious and subtle differences in various cultural contexts and their implications for the challenges faced by medical education. I have also tried to relate my observations in these places with the challenges I faced (and learned from) as a medical educationist. By sharing *my personal experiences*, I hope to illustrate the impact of diverse socio-cultural contexts on the understanding and delivery of medical education.

2   Understanding Cultural Competence

The goals of education in most Asian contexts are to prepare the learners to care for socio-culturally different people from within their own context. Nevertheless, they are made aware of western norms where they may aspire to practise for further training. Therefore, the term 'cultural competence' is often perceived differently by medical educators in different contexts.

For example, learners (and patients) in largely collectivist cultures, like Pakistan, Saudi Arabia, China and Kenya, belong to a similar, heavily tradition-backed orientation:

> *While taking a clinical ethics session in Kenya, the first question asked by a learner was about the pictures of Caucasian doctors on the power-point slides. She wanted to see more local-looking faces instead.*

I realised that the learners in this part of the world see themselves as an integral segment of the society where they belong, and want to relate physically to the teaching. I observed a similar mindset in Saudi Arabia and some parts of Pakistan, where students (and consultant physicians) would gladly wear a tie-suit to social events or conferences but would wear their national (cultural) dress to the institute (or workplace). Their nationalist or regional appearances are extremely important and perhaps linked to their professional self-identity.

3 Collectivist and Individualistic Societies

In most of these regions, educators or healthcare providers (like most of the population) are often influenced by personal beliefs. These influences on their professional conduct are considered natural, expected and accepted by the majority in their context.

> *One of the internal medicine faculty in Pakistan used to tell medical students that physicians should time dosage of medicines according to the morning, afternoon and evening (Muslim) prayer timings. He and several others used to do the same and were much appreciated by most patients.*

On the other hand, the healthcare institutes in primarily individualistic western societies, like the UK and Australia, usually cater for patients (and learners) from different world regions and cultural backgrounds who need to be seen according to western norms. Cultural competence in this situation often means being conscious of the rights and sensitivities of a diverse group of people and staying secular (not influenced by personal beliefs) in all interactions.

> *An Asian colleague working in Australia thought that the doctor-patient relationship here is extremely mechanical. According to her, interaction with patients (and their families) seemed artificial. She often expressed her feeling that she does not feel really connected with her patients.*

Her feelings were probably due to her upbringing in a collectivist society where 'connecting' with someone is more than a mere display of empathy. Her idea of connecting with people was probably grounded in the cultural norms of her native land. In most Asian cultures, relationships (even professional ones) are developed by inquiring about and sharing personal details, which are often not required in professional relationships elsewhere.

This diversity in the understanding of 'cultural competence' in different regions, may seem trivial, but it can affect every step of educational planning and execution in different regions in creating an educational environment that is conducive for learners from various contexts.

4   Debate on Obligation Versus Responsibility

My medical ethics training was either in the UK or by surgeons trained there. In individualistic cultures, there is a greater emphasis on the autonomy of individuals and one's responsibilities to fulfil the rights of others.

> *On my first day of work in the UK, I was provided with detailed information regarding the rights of others, such as patients, minorities and diverse groups, and my responsibilities to practically ensure them. Similarly, I was also made aware of my rights and was given a list of what I should be expecting from others.*

This was a cultural shock to me. From the collectivist culture I came from, there is a strong emphasis on obligation towards others. Educators, learners and society consider their duties obligatory. Therefore, in countries like Pakistan, Saudi Arabia and China, where professional values have developed from centuries-old traditions and beliefs, inspired by philosophically-influenced cultural concepts and religion, reminding someone of their obligations is generally considered disrespectful and needs to be addressed differently.

> It has been an uphill task to incorporate medical ethics as an explicit part of the curriculum in the countries like Pakistan. A general argument that I often face is that "We don't need to consider ethics; it is something that everybody knows and should be doing anyway".

This shows that in collectivist Asian societies, people are more focused on their obligations towards society, rather than the pressure of the rights of others on their responsibilities.

> *I asked one of my colleagues in China how he felt about the 'one family, one child' policy in the country. He found my concern utterly foolish (and probably selfish). He believed that if it is good for the country then why should he question it? For him, it was an obligation towards 'a greater good' for the nation.*

I observed the same mindset in the provision of patient care where physicians would consider it an obligation to provide the patient with the best care in their opinion, rather than thinking of the right of the patient to decide. Similarly, while conducting a series of workshops in China, I was pleasantly surprised by the timely attendance of students.

> *Over 36 days of workshop sessions in different cities in China, with 20 participants in each session, only one came around ten minutes late in the class. She was repeatedly grilled for her massive mistake not only by the local organisers but also by her fellow students.*

In Chinese culture, people consider it their obligation to be on time. Being late to a commitment is considered a major disrespect.

However, the mindset of putting obligation over rights can also be counterproductive in some scenarios. Therefore, it is important to clearly communicate responsibilities and expectations from people in such cultures.

> *While conducting a faculty development workshop in Saudi Arabia, I heard a basic science professor saying, "My responsibility is to teach the students in my lectures, whether they have understood or not is their problem".*

The 'obligation vs responsibility' debate does not mean that medical professionalism and ethics should not be a part of the curriculum or that faculty should not be made aware of their responsibilities or obligations. However, how we do this needs to be customised for better acceptance in different contexts.

5 Accepting and Questioning Authority

One of the biggest challenges I have faced as a medical educator has been trying to reconcile my understanding of educational theories with the reality of the classroom. In collectivist cultures like Pakistan, Kenya, and Saudi Arabia, students are often more compliant and willing to follow established protocols and societal norms. However, in individualistic cultures like the UK and Australia, students are more likely to question authority and challenge established norms. The problem is that the 'norms' can be very different in various regions.

> *In a multi-disciplinary meeting as a surgical trainee (my first job in the UK), I was sitting in the last row when I saw my chief enter the room. As all the chairs were already taken, he stood by the side wall and the meeting continued. I noticed that all our junior and senior team members acknowledged his presence, but no one offered him a seat. I was totally bewildered! On the other hand, for everybody else, it was business as usual.*

This was perhaps my first exposure to cultural diversity. As I later understood, this was a norm in a western setup. It does not reflect the slightest decrease in respect or any issues with the acceptance of authority for the senior colleague. It is just the way it is. However, in many Asian (and African) traditions, this would have been the highest order of disrespect. In these regions, respect and authority are usually coupled with physical protocols and observable manners. Other such examples may include calling a teacher, or anybody whose position demands respect, by their first names.

My chief of surgery in the UK hospital kept on asking me to call him John, like everyone else in the team. However, even after so many years, when I see him now, I call him Mr Goldsmith. It just does not happen. In my culture, you only call friends or those younger than you in relation or the professional hierarchy by their first names.

The matter becomes more complex if we pitch these views on authority and respect in the clinical scenario. Generally speaking, authoritative and paternalistic attitudes in doctors (and educators) are negatively seen in the west, while they may be the patient's (and learner's) needs in the east. In countries like Pakistan, Saudi Arabia, Kenya and China, people are accustomed to living in community-orientated societies, where extended families reside together and authority for taking important decisions is often given to a respected elder (or the one with the most power) in the family. In addition, the doctor-patient relationship in these regions is hierarchical, with patients less likely to question their doctor's views or seek a second opinion. In contrast, patients in Australia and the UK are encouraged to take an active role in their healthcare decisions and may even seek multiple opinions before making a decision.

While working on my PhD in Australia, it was extremely difficult for my supervisors to comprehend that a patient would want someone else in the family or the treating physician to take the decision for their treatment. Decisions even for sensitive issues like consent for an abortion or high-risk surgery for malignancy are often (willingly) not taken by the patients.

Farhat Moazam, a philosopher and ethics educator in Pakistan, performed an in-depth analysis of cultural influences on healthcare matters within the country (Moazam, 2000). She informs us that the hierarchical structure in these societies gives the doctor an elevated position of power. Patients and their families look up to their doctors and expect them to take decisions in the best interest of the patient. Similar findings are reported from the Arabian Peninsula (Al-Eraky & Chandratilake, 2012) suggesting that in the Arab world, the power balance is tilted towards the physician, and society has given the physician significantly more authority in the clinical decision-making process.

6   The Educational Arena

Such cultural differences are also reflected in the educational arena in different regions. The students in places where collectivism is deeply ingrained in the culture show a strong sense of community. They work together and collaborate on projects even when they are not asked to do so. This was in plain contrast to the individualistic approach I observed in the UK and Australia, where students were more comfortable working independently and taking ownership of their own learning.

> *While waiting for my students to submit their class assignments in Kenya, I noticed that some of the students in the classroom had completed their work. I told them that they can submit their work and leave, however, no one did. Later, when I asked, a student said that they make sure that everyone has completed their work.*

In the Kenyan culture, this is known as 'Harambee' (which means "to pull together") and inspires their approach towards life. The focus is on the community and on working together rather than on individual well-being. Such collective thinking can be effectively used for planning educational endeavours which require collaborative learning and teamwork. This student attribute is also seen in Pakistan and Saudi Arabia, although the social interactions are more conservative from the gender perspective. A close relationship between peers of different genders in these cultures is not considered acceptable by the majority and is looked upon with suspicion. People in these regions generally feel uncomfortable in discussing their issues and problems with colleagues of the opposite gender.

Another striking observation for me was the acceptance of authority. Educators in collectivist cultures are held in high regard, and there is a strong expectation that students would obey them and would not question their authority.

> *While doing sessions in China, Saudi Arabia and several places in Pakistan, it usually took a while to engage students in small group discussions. The students in these regions are culturally programmed to listen to what they are told by the teacher (the supreme leader in the room).*

This was different from the more relaxed and egalitarian approach I encountered in the UK and Australia where the students talk to their teachers freely in the classroom and are encouraged to question and challenge the status quo.

Conversely, learners in the collectivist culture generally expect authoritative or paternalistic behaviour from their educators. They have a high expectation for sincere guidance; to tell them what is good for them. This is contrary to 'learners taking ownership of their learning' concept, often propagated in the west.

The cultural nuances in different regions can guide educators in developing contextually relevant educational strategies that are feasible for the respective educational arenas.

7   Conclusion

My experiences working as a medical education student, surgeon and educator in different socio-cultural contexts on four continents have taught me the importance of being culturally aware and sensitive to cultural conditions. The nuances that I observed have influenced my understanding of medical education in ways that I could not have imagined. In addition, I have realised that professional morality and ethical behaviour are also culture-specific. They are constructed through the interaction of inherited and environmental influences based on obligations and responsibilities between professionals and society.

The experiences that I have shared from different socio-cultural contexts indicate that medical education should not be considered a universally homogenous phenomenon. Instead, the practical implementation of theories in medical education requires modifications to comply with the varying demands of different socio-cultural contexts.

Therefore, as medical educators, we must be mindful of the cultural nuances of our learners, patients and the community at large, to adapt our teaching methods accordingly and modify educational theories to comply with the varying demands of different contexts. By doing so, we may enhance the effectiveness, engagement and cultural appropriateness of medical education around the globe, preparing students for not only the society where education is being imparted but also for all the others where they may later serve as a professional.

References

Al-Eraky, M. M., & Chandratilake, M. (2012). How medical professionalism is conceptualised in Arabian context: A validation study. *Medical Teacher, 34*(sup1), S90–S95.

Dewey, J. F. (1962). The provenance and emplacement of Upper Arenigian Turbidites in Co. Mayo, Eire. *Geological Magazine, 99*(3), 238–252. The Provenance and Emplacement of Upper Arenigian Turbidites in Co. Mayo, Eire.

Ho, M.-J., Lin, C.-W., Chiu, Y.-T., Lingard, L., & Ginsburg, S. (2012). A cross-cultural study of students' approaches to professional dilemmas: Sticks or ripples. *Medical Education, 46*(3), 245–256.

Hofstede, G., & Bond, M. H. (1984). Hofstede's culture dimensions. *Journal of Cross-Cultural Psychology, 15*(4), 417–433.

Kallivayalil, R. A., & Chadda, R. K. (2011). Culture, ethics and medicine in South Asia. *The International Journal of Person Centered Medicine, 1*(1), 56–61.

Moazam, F. (2000). Families, patients, and physicians in medical decision making: A Pakistani perspective. *The Hastings Center Report, 30*(6), 28–37.

I.i COMMENTARY: Cultural Imperialism in Medical Education

Janet Grant and Leonard Grant

Shahid Shamim's illustrated argument is incisive: that 'medical education should not be considered a universally homogenous phenomenon'. But his experiential, observational account, based on his work as a surgeon, as a medical educator, and in bioethics, tells us much more than a story of differences between socio-cultural contexts. It calls into question the current dominant rhetoric in medical education of *globalisation* (universal imposition of one set of values and practices, usually emanating from the global north) and *internationalisation* (expansion of markets by, for example, medical schools establishing replica off-shore branch campuses, or making efforts to attract cross-border students). This, in turn, tells us something important about *cultural imperialism* and the power relationships that underpin that phenomenon, which might explain the author's observation that 'non-western' countries follow 'western' trends, even though the characters of nations, and groups within them, differ so greatly.

The political, ethical and practical problems of globalisation, internationalisation and cross-border standardisation of medical education have been thoroughly discussed elsewhere (Brouwer & Frambach, 2021; Rashid 2022, 2023). The common arguments are that these 'universalist' ideas benefit the already powerful, global north (through enabling medical migration and gaining financial benefit from various forms of selling education and educational services), and that 'transferring solutions across contexts' (Brouwer & Frambach, 2021) is highly risky without detailed local analysis. Shahid Shamim's observations illustrate why this is so by drawing attention to disparate cultural practices and values.

The differences described mean that the content of not only bioethics, but any curriculum, should be tailored to context; the author's major comparators being collectivist vs. individualistic, obligation vs. responsibility, and accepting vs. questioning authority. The author gives examples of where the educational ideas of the global north are not acceptable in other cultures where hierarchy, respect, collectivism, gender roles, and authority require different educational approaches.

Culture and Learning

While it has been shown that the success of curriculum change is limited by organisational and national culture (Jippes et al., 2015), the implementation of new teaching and learning methods is also affected by local cultures of learning. Shahid Shamim's focus on individualist vs. collectivist societies should be an important brake on the globalisation of ideas about teaching and learning. Such methods as problem-based learning (PBL) were exported from North America and have been subject to critique as part of a medical education imperialist agenda, based on western curriculum ideas (Bleakley et al., 2008). PBL was rapidly followed by task-based, team-based, case-based, simulation-based, project-based and peer-assisted learning, situated and self-directed learning, and more recently the flipped classroom, all backed up by often spurious, discredited and bewildering ideas about learning styles (the neuromyth) (Cashdan, 2021; Riener & Willingham, 2010), learning approaches (the doubtful deep and surface levels) (Howie & Bagnall, 2013), and the equally questionable active and passive learning, cognitive styles and adult learning, transformational, experiential and action learning, behaviourist, cognitivist and constructivist learning (Pashler et al., 2008;; May, 2018; Bokhari & Zafar, 2019; Vaishnav & Vaishnav, 2019; Challa et al., 2021; Dong et al., 2021; Newton et al., 2021). The list of methods, their sometimes obscure derivation, and their frequent critiques, often ignored in medical education, is worrying.

Despite so many journals and papers and so much talk of globalisation and internationalisation, what is almost entirely missing from medical education is research in cross-cultural psychology. In other fields, that research shows many differences in culture and leaning, based in social structure, family relationships, the physical environment, and variables such as collectivism and individualism (Harkness & Keefer, 2000; Keith, 2011). We can only assume that the economic predominance of the global north is so powerful, that they remain largely unquestioned inside medical education.

This then, can be seen as a problem of culture, and a process of cultural imperialism.

Cultural Imperialism

'Cultural imperialism', as with almost all social science terms, is open to a number of definitions. Tomlinson's classification is probably the most widely accepted (Tomlinson, 2002):

- *Cultural imperialism* occurs where mass communication and other forms of dissemination of specific ideologies, can influence and support political and social movements.
- *National domination* implies the (conscious or unconscious) efforts of one country to undermine another country's cultural heritage by imposing its own. (Shahid Shamim indicates the identity conflict epitomised in the choice to wear a western suit and tie for formal events, or to wear national dress for the workplace.)
- *The global dominance of capitalism*, the expansion and sometimes global dominance of consumer capitalism whereby culture is used to fuse different societies into one international economic system, thus enabling (western) control of foreign markets and raw materials (and perhaps the production and importation of doctors).
- *The critique of modernity* whereby cultural imperialism is seen as the imposition of modernity, transferring the "lived culture" of the west to other cultures.

A slightly different analysis (Grubbs, 2000) sets out three modes of cultural imperialism:

> *Cultural domination*: whereby an entity recognised as an authority establishes dominance through administrative decree (we might here consider international accreditation of medical education as an instrument of cultural domination).
> *Cultural imposition:* whereby that entity imposes a system on subject groups.
> *Cultural fragmentation:* whereby that entity creates differences between groups which prevents the creation of a critical mass to challenge their authority.

Grubbs (ibid) suggests another option:

> *Cultural emancipation:* whereby democratic coalitions enable the expression of the unique attributes of each member.

Shahid Shamim illustrates the effects of religious belief on prescribing in his country and the lack of any similar framework in western countries where he has worked. He notes the presence of family in the consultation, which is very different in his country and, for example, Australia. Collectivist, religious societies and individualistic, secular societies should have implications not only for medical practice but also for medical education.

Underpinning these ideas, with the exception of cultural emancipation, is one assumption:

> Central to the many definitions of the term 'cultural imperialism' is the idea of the culture of one powerful civilization, country, or institution having great unreciprocated influence on that of another, less powerful, entity to a degree that one may speak of a measure of 'cultural domination'. (Boyd-Barrett, 2018)

In the specific field of medicine, the effects of cultural imperialism on the human right to health, have been thoroughly examined in terms of the argument that human rights are used as an excuse for western countries to intervene in the affairs of other countries that do not share western values, and in terms of the counter argument that no one set of cultural values is superior to another, so no universal standard is justified (Muyskens, 2022). The contrast between individualistic and communitarian cultures and their historical and socio-political roots, has been examined—and it has been noted, as Shahid Shamim also points out, that any analysis that classifies whole countries as having one culture would also be inadequate (Jing-Bao, 2005). Understanding culture demands a constant vigilance and interrogation of the assumptions that any moderniser, standard setter or international regulator might have. It is a vigilance rarely observed or reported.

The Purposes of Cultural Imperialism

To make cultural imperialism work, the more powerful entity must believe that they have a better way of doing things, and the less powerful must accept that (or otherwise be unable to refute it): so international regulators, who almost exclusively come from the global north, and consultants or 'experts' in medical education, who also predominantly come from the global north, must believe that they have something to offer clients in the global south, and those in the global south must agree. At the same time, those who submit themselves to global judgement, or seek advice, must also believe that those who judge them have better ways of doing things.

Shahid Shamim provides vivid examples that allow us to see how these ideas are relevant to medical education, and how they underpin the analyses of other chapters in this book that address the power relations in medical education between global north and global south. He asks what society medical education is preparing its graduates for: *The one where education is being imparted, or all the others where the student will later serve as a professional?* For example, international accreditation and consultancy can be seen as a form of cultural imperialism, asking medical education systems to comply with or adopt what is taken to be 'best practice'. Accordingly, an international consensus on accreditation disappointingly identified 10 qualities of accreditation systems that are the same as those that most established systems in the global north, including systems of global accreditation, already display (Frank et al., 2020).

International Accreditation and Cultural Imperialism

Given this acceptance of the global north as the arbiter of good practice, unsurprisingly, when medical students were asked about the effects of international accreditation such as that provided by the United States' Accreditation Council for Graduate Medical Education—International (ACGME-I), they identified quality improvement, and international opportunities for research and training (Ibrahim et al., 2015). The World Federation for Medical Education programme that evaluates accreditation agencies also had those two same purposes: enhancement of quality and medical migration (World Federation for Medical Education, 2022). Cultural imperialism takes different forms: the 'unreciprocated influence' (Boyd-Barrett, 2018) of requiring evidence that things are done in the way that a powerful 'other' requires is one such manifestation, even when cloaked as quality improvement. This confusion of contradictory purposes is explored in the analysis of the history of an international organisation (the World Federation for Medical Education) and its relation to the nationalist purposes of another organisation (the US Educational Commission for Foreign Medical Graduates) (Rashid, 2023). At the centre of that contradiction are the procedural requirements of one organisation (WFME) demanding the same performance from other organisations (all accreditation agencies worldwide) so that those organisations can satisfy the requirements of a third national organisation (ECFMG).

Exploitation of Markets

Cultural imperialism has been primarily thought about as having both political and economic purposes, for exploitation of markets. The business of medical education, especially in relation to medical migration, has become part of the international trade that has been referred to, both positively and negatively, as 'trade in services' (Hanefeld & Smith, 2019), or being the subject of trade agreements (Martineau et al., 2002).

Savings in educational costs to the receiver country (Ahmad, 2005; Martineau et al., 2002) means that the nearer the education of the provider country is to that of the receiver country, the better that is. Indeed, the idea and purpose of managing variation between medical schools was identified as a driver relating to medical migration specifically to the USA:

> (Managing variation) …. was used as a justification to propel global approaches to medical school regulation by suggesting that this variation needs 'managing', through the notion of 'standardisation' and an idealised, monolithic description of a 'global doctor.' (Rashid, 2023, p. 35)

Educational Neocolonialism and its Effects

Shahid Shamim is concerned that '*the practical implementation of theories in medical education requires modifications to comply with the varying demands of different socio-cultural contexts*'. In this, he recognises that such theories are derived for one culture and are applied to many other cultures. We might wonder why there are not applied theories that derive from those other cultures.

It has been noted (Wu et al., 2022), with regard to the internationalisation of medical education (IoME), that:

> Often, medical curricula are developed in reference to global standards promulgated by the West. (p. 739)

And:

> …although IoME is a global phenomenon, understandings and perspectives of the Global North dominated the medical education literature… (p. 742)

On the basis of these observations, we might call for a process of cultural emancipation (Grubbs, 2000) but consider whether that is ever possible within current economic, political, social, postcolonial, and neoliberal conditions. So we must ask whether education as it is understood in the global north can ever be appropriate in the global south.

In a careful examination of 'educational neocolonialism' (Nguyen et al., 2009), it is argued that 'simplistic transfer' is unlikely to be effective, for all the reasons of values, social relationships, and behaviours that Shahid Shamim illustrates. It is also noted that in situations where educationalists feel pressure to introduce reforms, they are likely to turn to and implement ideas developed in the global north. This is illustrated in many chapters of this book.

In a study of what its author sees as the progressive Americanisation of Spain, it is concluded that although cultural imperialism is now a common phenomenon:

> Cultural imperialism may not be apparent to the population of a culturally colonized country at first, … since propaganda and products are often introduced in such a natural way that we do not stop to think how much of our own culture we are losing or how much is being substituted. …. One may stop and think, of what I have and am today, how much is American? (Tébar, 2021, p. 30)

The most complete discussions of cultural imperialism, and its differentiation from cultural globalisation, are to be found, unsurprisingly, in relation to the analysis of media, where it has been concluded that:

> The world system has long comprised unevenly developed nation-states in a structural hierarchy of asymmetrical and unequal power relations, both coercive and persuasive. This is not likely to change any time soon (Mirrlees, 2013, p. 241).

With the weight of theory and publication in medical education, and now of international regulation, deriving from the global north, we may say the same about medical education. Shahid Shamin exhorts everyone to 'adapt our teaching methods accordingly and modify educational theories to comply with the varying demands of different contexts'. If this happens, both in education and regulation, then cultural specificity will happily replace cultural imperialism.

References

Ahmad, O. B. (2005). Managing medical migration from poor countries. *British Medical Journal, 331*(2 July), 43–45. www.ilo.org/public/english/protection/migrant/download/

Bleakley, A., Brice, J., & Bligh, J. (2008). Thinking the post-colonial in medical education. *Medical Education, 42*(3), 266–270. https://doi.org/10.1111/j.1365-2923.2007.02991.x

Bokhari, N. M., & Zafar, M. (2019). Learning styles and approaches among medical education participants. *Journal of Education Health Promotion, 8*, 1–5. https://doi.org/10.4103/jehp.jehp_95_19

Boyd-Barrett, O. (2018). Cultural imperialism and communication. In *Oxford Research Encyclopedia of Communication.* Oxford University Press. https://doi.org/10.1093/ACREFORE/9780190228613.013.678

Brouwer, E., & Frambach, J. (2021). Solutionism across borders: Sorting out problems, solutions and stakeholders in medical education internationalisation. *Medical Education, 55*(1), 10–12. https://doi.org/10.1111/medu.14384

Cashdan, A. (2021, May 13). Learning styles – The myth persists. *The Psychologist.* https://www.bps.org.uk/psychologist/learning-styles-myth-persists

Challa, K. T., Sayed, A., & Acharya, Y. (2021). Modern techniques of teaching and learning in medical education: A descriptive literature review. *MedEdPublish, 10*(1), 10.15694/mep.2021.000018.1.

Dong, H., Lio, J., Sherer, R., & Jiang, I. (2021). Some learning theories for medical educators. *Medical Science Educator, 31*(3), 1157–1172. https://doi.org/10.1007/s40670-021-01270-6

Frank, J. R., Taber, S., van Zanten, M., Scheele, F., & Blouin, D. (2020). The role of accreditation in 21st century health professions education: Report of an international consensus group. *BMC Medical Education, 20*(S1), 305. https://doi.org/10.1186/s12909-020-02121-5

Grubbs, J. W. (2000). Cultural imperialism. A critical theory of interorganizational change. *Journal of Organizational Change Management, 13*(3), 221–234. https://doi.org/10.1108/09534810010330878

Hanefeld, J., & Smith, R. (2019). The upside of trade in health services. *BMJ, l2208,* l2208. https://doi.org/10.1136/bmj.l2208

Harkness, S., & Keefer, C. H. (2000). Contributions of cross-cultural psychology to research and interventions in education and health. *Journal of Cross-Cultural Psychology, 31*(1), 92–109. https://doi.org/10.1177/0022022100031001008

Howie, P., & Bagnall, R. (2013). A critique of the deep and surface approaches to learning model. *Teaching in Higher Education, 18*(4), 389–400. https://doi.org/10.1080/13562517.2012.733689

Ibrahim, H., Abdel-Razig, S., & Nair, S. C. (2015). Medical students' perceptions of international accreditation. *International Journal of Medical Education, 6*, 121–124. https://doi.org/10.5116/ijme.5610.3116

Jing-Bao, N. (2005). Cultural values embodying universal norms: A critique of a popular assumption about cultures and human rights. *Developing World Bioethics, 5*(3), 251–257. https://doi.org/10.1111/j.1471-8847.2005.00123.x

Jippes, M., Driessen, E. W., Broers, N. J., Majoor, G. D., Gijselaers, W. H., & van der Vleuten, C. P. M. (2015). Culture matters in successful curriculum change. *Academic Medicine, 90*(7), 921–929. https://doi.org/10.1097/ACM.0000000000000687

Keith, K. D. (Ed.). (2011). *Cross-cultural psychology. Contemporary themes and perspectives.* Wiley-Blackwell.

Martineau, T., Decker, K., & Bundred, P. (2002). Briefing note on international migration of health professionals: Levelling the playing field for developing country health systems.

May, C. (2018). *The problem with 'learning styles' – Scientific American.* https://www.scientificamerican.com/article/the-problem-with-learning-styles/

Mirrlees, T. (2013). *Global entertainment media between cultural imperialism and cultural globalization.* Routledge.

Muyskens, K. (2022). Avoiding cultural imperialism in the human right to health. *Asian Bioethics Review, 14*(1), 87–101. https://doi.org/10.1007/s41649-021-00190-2

Newton, P. M., Najabat-Lattif, H. F., Santiago, G., & Salvi, A. (2021). The learning styles neuromyth is still thriving in medical education. *Frontiers in Human Neuroscience, 15.* https://doi.org/10.3389/fnhum.2021.708540

Nguyen, P., Elliott, J. G., Terlouw, C., & Pilot, A. (2009). Neocolonialism in education: Cooperative learning in an Asian context. *Comparative Education, 45*(1), 109–130. https://doi.org/10.1080/03050060802661428

Pashler, H., McDaniel, M., Rohrer, D., & Bjork, R. (2008). Learning styles. *Psychological Science in the Public Interest, 9*(3), 105–119. https://doi.org/10.1111/j.1539-6053.2009.01038.x

Rashid, M. A. (2022). Hyperglobalist, sceptical, and transformationalist perspectives on globalization in medical education. *Medical Teacher, 44*(9), 1023–1031. https://doi.org/10.1080/0142159X.2022.2058384

Rashid, M. A. (2023). Altruism or nationalism? Exploring global discourses of medical school regulation. *Medical Education, 57*(1), 31–39. https://doi.org/10.1111/medu.14804

Riener, C., & Willingham, D. (2010). The myth of learning styles. *Change: The Magazine of Higher Learning, 42*(5), 32–35. https://doi.org/10.1080/00091383.2010.503139

Tébar, A. J. C. (2021). *Beyond Borders: A cultural analysis of American cultural imperialism.* Universidad de Valladolid, Facultad de Filosifía y Letras. https://uvadoc.uva.es/bitstream/handle/10324/51461/TFG_F_2021_055.pdf;jsessionid=E755806BFF682FA91660513BCF0A68FD?sequence=1

Tomlinson, J. (2002). *Cultural imperialism: A critical introduction* (3rd ed.). Continuum.

Vaishnav, B. S., & Vaishnav, S. B. (2019). Cognitive style assessment among medical students: A step towards achieving meta-cognitive integration in medical education. *The National Medical Journal of India, 32*(4), 235–243.

World Federation for Medical Education. (2022). *Benefits of WFME recognition status.* https://wfme.org/accreditation/recognition-programme/

Wu, A., Choi, E., Diderich, M., Shamim, A., Rahhal, Z., Mitchell, M., Leask, B., & DeWit, H. (2022). Internationalization of medical education – Motivations and formats of current practices. *Medical Science Educator, 32*(3), 733–745. https://doi.org/10.1007/s40670-022-01553-6

M. Shahid Shamim is Professor of Health Professionals Education and a surgeon at Aga Khan University, Karachi, where he is also Director for Graduate Studies. He holds a PhD in Medical Education from the University of New South Wales, Australia, and has special interests in curriculum, faculty development, surgical training, bioethics education and collaborative educational research. He has wide international experience of medical education practice and development.

I.ii STATEMENT: Glocalisation of Medical Education: Impact and Challenges

Dujeepa D. Samarasekera, Jillian H. T. Yeo, Shuh Shing Lee, and Matthew C. E. Gwee

1 Introduction to Singapore

The city-state of Singapore is one of the most affluent and developed nations in its region. Home to its population of racially diverse individuals including Chinese, Malays and Indians, Singaporeans have learnt to embrace the diversity of cultures, religions and ideas to coexist in one congenial space. As one nation, it continues to strive to maintain its position as a globally competitive economy by investing in infrastructure, and engaging in innovation and technology. Singapore's achievements are further boosted by its strategic location which encourages global connectivity. The country's small size and hence limited resources makes it imperative to remain open and engaged with global markets. As an open economy which is constantly influenced by the changing tides of global economies, it is ingrained in us to adapt and change swiftly in response to global trends.

2 Globalisation of Medical Education

Globalisation has broken down borders and led to an increasing ease and rapidity of information flow across boundaries. The effect of globalisation is observed even within the field of medical education. Examples include countries expanding the number of recognised international medical schools, cross-border sale of packaged curricula or educational services, and implementing a medical school's business model in a foreign country (Hodges et al., 2009; Rizwan et al., 2018). While

D. D. Samarasekera (✉) · J. H. T. Yeo · S. S. Lee · M. C. E. Gwee
Centre for Medical Education (CenMED), Yong Loo Lin School of Medicine,
Singapore, Singapore
e-mail: dujeepa@nus.edu.sg

J. Grant, L. Grant (eds.), *The Contradictions of Medical Education*,
https://doi.org/10.1007/978-3-031-90394-6_3

medical educators across the globe are keen to learn and apply new tools and pedagogies, the discourse on medical education is often peppered by paradigms conceptualised and applied in the western world (Hodges et al., 2009). As medical educators attempt to adopt new practices by investing time, resources and curriculum changes, they find themselves frustrated when there is a misalignment between the theory and actual practice settings.

3   Globalisation of Medical Education in the National University of Singapore

The need to adapt and evolve is an ethos held by the Yong Loo Lin School of Medicine, National University of Singapore (NUS Medicine). Established in 1905, NUS Medicine has evolved over time from a college to a school, and finally to the academic health centre we have today.

The curriculum has also undergone many changes in an attempt to adopt new pedagogies and 'best practices' as information flow on medical education is made increasingly more accessible. From 1998, the curriculum shifted from a traditional subject-based model to an integrated systems-based model with the intention of improving the student's learning experience (Samarasekera et al., 2015). During that time, NUS Medicine also introduced problem-based learning (PBL) into the curriculum to weave the application of taught biomedical sciences content into clinical scenarios.

4   Problem-Based Learning (PBL) in NUS Medicine

Since McMaster University medical school in Canada created a radical and innovative trend by introducing a PBL curriculum in 1969 to overcome perceived shortcomings of the traditional curriculum, many medical schools globally followed its path (Spaulding, 1969). PBL was highly advocated as a learning design that was described as 'learner-centred', collaborative, contextual, integrated, 'self-directed', and 'reflective'. As PBL represented a major shift in the medical education paradigm, and centres of excellence in countries such as Canada, the Netherlands and the United States began to adopt it as a teaching and learning tool, medical schools globally also felt increasing pressure to incorporate PBL into their curricula.

Swayed by this new trend in medical education, in late 1998 NUS Medicine took swift action to introduce PBL into its curriculum. However, lack of consideration of sociocultural aspects, pedagogical concepts and theories of curriculum within our context, as well as teaching and learning approaches rooted among the students and educators, led to several issues and challenges.

4.1 Clash with the Way Students Learn

The majority of undergraduates in NUS Medicine were educated in junior colleges where didactic teaching was predominant and hence had a more so-called 'passive' approach to learning. They were used to memorising information and reproducing model answers during examinations. Hence, our students struggled with the 'student-centred' approach that demanded a more actively engaged approach, and they grappled with 'self-directed learning'.

Interaction plays an important role in PBL as it requires students to be an active group collaborator and engage in deep interaction during the session, which is said to influence 'deep' or 'surface' learning among students. However, with students coming from a Confucian teaching and learning tradition, they tended to be silent in PBL sessions.

Cultural norms have an impact on how students perceive teaching and learning and the role of teachers. It is ingrained in our students that a correct answer always exists and teachers dispense knowledge and truth. With minimal guidance from the tutor in PBL sessions, our students found it difficult to adapt and learn.

4.2 Problems with Teachers Adapting to the New Method

The abrupt introduction of PBL into the curriculum gave little time for tutors to be trained appropriately to facilitate PBL sessions. Contrary to traditional approaches, tutors now took on the roles of facilitating idea generation, encouraging collaboration and guiding the learning process (Hmelo-Silver, 2004; Hussain et al., 2007). But tutors found themselves giving mini-lectures during the sessions as both tutors and students struggled to appreciate the theories and concepts behind engaging in PBL.

4.3 Lack of Evaluation of PBL in Practice

Given the short period of time in implementing PBL, there was no formal evaluation of PBL incorporated while designing this curriculum. Therefore, the implementation committee was unable to pinpoint areas for improvement or feedback from relevant stakeholders to manage some of the challenges faced.

4.4 Lack of Alignment with Assessment

Blueprinting topics covered during PBL to the curriculum and assessments was not conducted. Hence students found little value in the PBL sessions which took up time which could be spent on revision for 'examinable' topics.

Even though PBL was introduced as a learning format in the curriculum, promoting learning through a problem or case scenario where students discuss and collaborate, the assessments remained the same with a greater focus on content recall. Furthermore, there was no formal assessment of student performance or a structured way of providing feedback to the students at the end of a PBL session. This was mostly left for individual tutors and happened in an *ad hoc* manner.

4.5 Cultural Shifts and Reversion to the Norm

Based on the local hierarchical Confucian culture, students tend to view educators as a source of wisdom and authority. PBL as a 'student-centred' approach which encourages active inquiry and engagement, goes against the grain of traditional Asian educational values. Both students and tutors need to be accustomed to dissolving hierarchical barriers with the introduction of PBL.

The resistance to change due to these challenges and cultural norms rooted among the students and teachers, has consequently seen reversion to the traditional teaching and learning approach. In addition, due to being highly resource intensive, PBL was unsustainable in the long run and slowly phased out in NUS Medicine.

5 A Newly Adapted Teaching and Learning Approach: Collaborative Learning Cases (CLCs)

This experience highlighted the need to ensure that our teaching and learning approach is relevant to the local context. In 2014, NUS Medicine reviewed its curriculum in an attempt to integrate pedagogies which would encourage 'self-directed' and 'deeper' learning. The school incorporated a case-based teaching and learning approach called Collaborative Learning Cases (CLCs) which was adapted from the collaborative pedagogical model used by the Faculty of Education, University of Cambridge, UK (Lee et al., 2018).

The CLCs act as 'capstone' sessions which would tie together lectures, tutorials, simulations and practical sessions. These sessions were designed to encourage novice students to apply knowledge to clinical problems and to develop their own knowledge through collaborative efforts with their peers, guidance from tutors and self-directed learning. CLCs aimed to integrate biomedical sciences with clinical sciences to understand their relevance, to promote 'deeper' learning, to develop relevant skills (e.g. collaboration, communication and leadership) and to encourage self-directed learning.

6   How Were CLCs Introduced?

Learning from our past experiences, NUS Medicine implemented several measures to ensure that CLCs would be integrated smoothly into the curriculum.

6.1   Pilot Testing and Evaluation of Teaching Methods

CLCs underwent many rounds of piloting and re-designing to the current format. Students and tutors who participated in the pilot were surveyed to gather their views on what worked and what did not. The positive responses on CLCs included its ability to foster interactions between students and tutors, and the enjoyable learning experience. Logistics, for example sourcing the venue and determining the optimal tutor-to-student ratio, were raised as potential areas for improvement. The evaluation of this approach is still on-going for there to be further improvement.

6.2   CLC Committee

A CLC committee comprising clinicians, basic scientists and educators was set up to drive the initiative. The committee was responsible for identifying topics and reviewing the cases developed by the case writers. The clearly defined roles and responsibilities of relevant stakeholders ensured smoother integration of CLCs into the curriculum.

6.3   Faculty Development

CLCs cases were written by a group of experienced basic scientists and clinical teachers. Writing sessions were coordinated by administrative staff from the committee to ensure all the relevant experts came together to produce a case. This provided great opportunities for basic scientists and clinical teachers to foster their relationship and collaborate in producing a case with critical guided questions. Prior to case writing, all the case writers were briefed about the theoretical framework that underpinned CLCs and the rationale for this approach. CLC sessions, were facilitated jointly by one basic scientist and one clinical teacher. Facilitators had to attend a workshop to learn how to support the learners and facilitate CLC discussions. They also attended a briefing by the case developers on the content of the case. This ensured that teachers were well trained, understood the pedagogy behind CLCs and enhanced their facilitation skills.

6.4 Relating CLCs to Clinical Practice

Part of the format for the CLCs includes a pre- and post-CLC quiz which would reveal the misconceptions and gaps in knowledge that could be addressed during the discussions. Videos were screened in a sequential manner during the CLCs to strengthen the relevance of a case with the students' clinical reasoning abilities. Under the guidance of both trained facilitators in a session, students are able to relate the CLCs to clinical practice and engage in more contextualised learning, and collaborate and communicate with their team members.

7 Future Plans

While CLCs continue to be part of the curriculum today, we must remain prudent in ensuring its relevance to the current educational climate. Some potential areas for continuous review include updating cases to ensure relevance, moving to online and hybrid formats, focusing on clinical and community management, and evolving CLCs into a virtual ward round.

8 Conclusions

As new educational designs continue to emerge and excite educators globally, it is important to review their applicability in one's own context and make calculated modifications when adopting these tools to ensure that we develop an effective learning environment for our students and residents. Special attention to training and selecting the tutors in facilitating the process as well as taking into consideration available resources (staff, venue and equipment) are crucial in planning a new approach.

References

Hmelo-Silver, C. E. (2004). Problem-based learning: What and how do students learn? *Educational Psychology Review, 16*(3), 235–266. https://doi.org/10.1023/B:EDPR.0000034022.16470.f3

Hodges, B. D., Maniate, J. M., Martimianakis, M. A. (Tina), Alsuwaidan, M., & Segouin, C. (2009). Cracks and crevices: Globalization discourse and medical education. *Medical Teacher, 31*(10), 910–917. https://doi.org/10.3109/01421590802534932.

Hussain, R. M. R., Mamat, W. H. W., Salleh, N., Saat, R. M., & Harland, T. (2007). Problem-based learning in Asian universities. *Studies in Higher Education, 32*(6), 761–772. https://doi.org/10.1080/03075070701685171

Lee, S. S., Hooi, S. C., Pan, T., Fong, C. H. A., & Samarasekera, D. D. (2018). Improving a newly adapted teaching and learning approach: Collaborative learning cases using an action research. *Korean Journal of Medical Education, 30*(4), 295–308. https://doi.org/10.3946/kjme.2018.104

Rizwan, M., Rosson, N. J., Tackett, S., & Hassoun, H. T. (2018). Globalization of medical education: Current trends and opportunities for medical students. *Journal of Medical Education and Training, 2*(1), 35–41.

Samarasekera, D. D., Ooi, S., Yeo, S. P., & Hooi, S. C. (2015). Medical education in Singapore. *Medical Teacher, 37*(8), 707–713. https://doi.org/10.3109/0142159X.2015.1009026

Spaulding, W. B. (1969). The undergraduate medical curriculum (1969 model): McMaster University. *Canadian Medical Association Journal, 100*(14), 659–664.

I.ii COMMENTARY: Cultural and Social Capital, and Globalisation

Janet Grant and Leonard Grant

The authors of this account from Singapore demonstrate the effect of western trends on their own practice, and site that clearly within economic imperatives and the 'global market'. But they also describe the problems of introducing practices from another culture into their own. In other accounts in this book, where authors have reported similar challenges, we explain their wish to adopt others' practices, from the point of view of post-colonial, and neoliberal beliefs, and from a simple wish to export their graduates. The authors of this chapter are clear in giving their conscious rationale for change: to be globally competitive. That, in general, means to comply with practices developed in the global north: the 'information flow' that these authors cite is almost exclusively uni-directional. So globalisation is really about the global south adopting or adapting the practices of the global north. Other authors have referred to this as 'medical education imperialism' (Bleakley et al., 2008, 2011). The authors' account from Singapore demonstrates how they have tackled the problem of introducing such practices from other cultures to the teachers and learners in their own medical school.

A central issue in this chapter is that of 'faculty development' (in other educational contexts known as 'teacher training'), which is a common practice and approach to change in medical education. Although faculty development may be seen as simply a matter of information, induction and training, in this commentary, we look at it from a different perspective.

To analyse the story that these authors have shared, we can turn to the French sociologist of education, Pierre Bourdieu, who was mainly concerned with the 'pedagogic action' role of pre-university schools in reproducing the structural hierarchies of society. We will outline the key relevant aspects of his theorisation and transpose this analysis to our authors' account of the actions taken in their medical school in Singapore, the reactions, the responses, and why. In doing this, we draw on four main texts (Bourdieu, 1977, 1986; Bourdieu & Passeron, 1977; Broadfoot, 1978).

Habitus and Change of Culture

Bourdieu used the term 'habitus' to mean the habits, skills, and dispositions that a person accumulates and develops over their lifetime. He believed that these define a person's position in society and create a sense of shared identity. Bourdieu was concerned with class identity, but that identity could also, for us, refer to cultural or national identity, or even the identity of a medical school.

Habitus is the result of socialised, learned ways of thinking and being. These include, of course, ideas about teaching and learning. If habitus is learned, it can be changed through new socialisation or education, often unconsciously, sometimes consciously. And perhaps that change of habitus is implied by the authors' choice of the term 'glocalisation' which implies the importation of 'global' (usually global north) ways of thinking and being, into other contexts and cultures. It certainly does not imply the imposition of global south habitus on people in the global north.

The most conscious form of trying to change habitus in medical education is seen in the wide adoption of 'faculty development' to support institutional and procedural changes, as described in this chapter (Alhassan, 2022; McLean et al., 2008; Nawab et al., 2021; Proctor et al., 2020; Steinert et al., 2006).

The key issue here is why change of habitus in relation to the limited environment of the medical school, is important, and whether the cultural reference for that change is local or not. Clearly, in relation to the changes discussed, that cultural referential framework is not local, it is from the global north, and the reason for adopting it is to develop, change or maintain the value of the social capital, position or reputation, of the school. Change of habitus is described by the authors' reference to 'changing tides of global economies', and to ideas emerging from North America and the United Kingdom.

The authors' account of trying to bring these practices into their own institution, reports a reliance on faculty development which was conducted differently for the introduction of problem-based learning (PBL), and then of collaborative learning cases (CLCs) (Samarasekera, 2021; Samarasekera et al., 2021): for PBL, faculty development was a training process, while for CLCs, it was conducted as participation in the development of the new teaching method accompanied by training. The second, and more successful, method was more embedded in the local culture, but was still transposing a practice from another culture into their own, and managing that process by trying to change the habitus of the people involved.

Change of habitus, then, involved creation of another culture. More like that of the global north, to place the institution on the global stage. This brings us to two other important ideas that Bourdieu advanced: cultural and social capital.

Cultural Capital and Managing Change

Cultural capital, in Bourdieu's terms, are those things that enable a person to succeed in their given, adopted or aspired to, context. Cultural capital locates a person within a context. It also contributes to economic capital (Bourdieu, 1986), as any medical school that places itself on the global market, might wish. Social and economic capital are inextricably linked (Baum, 2000). The components of anyone's cultural capital might include their knowledge, skills, behaviours, values and beliefs. These will be developed, judged and used in relation to their chosen context. In the NUS Medicine case study, the first attempt to change its cultural capital was seen in the introduction of problem-based learning. The authors describe clearly that this system did not fit with the educational habitus and cultural capital of NUS Medicine. It did not fit with the way in which students learned and teachers taught, nor with the relationships that these groups were bound by. With no change in habitus, and insufficient changes in infrastructure and processes, there would be no change in cultural capital.

The authors describe this as 'resistance to change', siting the problem within the person and their 'cultural norms'. In the literature on managing change in a medical context, a wide variety of reasons are put forward for such 'resistance' including both personal and organisational factors:

> Change is a difficult, stressful process, threatening individual and organizational assumptions about power, role, status, and control (Lane, 2007, p. 90).

It has also been pointed out that:

> ... people do not routinely resist change. Nonetheless, they do resist change if it is not seen as acceptable (Grant & Gale, 1989, p. 256).

So here, 'resistance' implies a considered and behavioural response to something new against a stable cultural background. Raymond Williams sees things differently (Williams, 1980) and argues that society, and people within that, are in a constant state of flux, experiencing a:

> '... struggle between the dominant, residual and emergent cultures. He argues that in any society in any particular period there is a central, effective, and dominant system of meanings and values which are not merely abstract but which are 'organized and lived' (Bryson, 2008, p. 747).

Williams believed that educational institutions are the main agencies of transmission of that dominant culture. But in the case of NUS Medicine, we can see that its own culture of global competitiveness which makes it adopt practices from the dominant global north, might be in opposition to the local dominant social culture that is traditional and has developed over centuries of philosophical practice and thought. Changing habitus and cultural capital under those circumstances will be a challenge. NUS Medicine's second, and more deliberate, attempt to change habitus and social capital with the introduction of collaborative learning cases, seems to have been more successful, but whether and how these isolated changes, encapsulated within an institution, can survive unscathed in the context of a wider society where habitus and social capital retain their identity, is yet to be seen.

Here, we must explore further Bourdieu's idea of social capital.

Social and Symbolic Capital, and Fields

'Social capital' refers to the social networks and contacts that are relevant to advancement and success. Social capital is a characteristic of an individual person, and places them in positions of power relative to others. For Bourdieu, this would normally have been how middle-class people maintain their position in society. In the case of NUS Medicine, however, it is part of its positioning 'to remain open and engaged with global markets'. However, it is not clear whether the graduates of the school will develop more powerful social capital, and therefore have greater social advantage in Singapore, as a result of being educated within a western paradigm. It might be that their social capital has more meaning in another culture.

The authors' arguments for keeping pace with ideas emerging in the global north are not about individual students, but about the global market position of their organisation. Bourdieu did not apply his ideas of social capital to organisations, but others have. We can see the development approach that the authors describe as positioning their school within a global network of similar schools to which both the school and people associated with the school will have easier access, thus increasing the social capital of all parties (Ihlen, 2005). This, in turn, increases the 'symbolic capital' (the prestige, honour, reputation and relative power) of the institution. Social capital is an instrument of public relations (Ihlen, 2005).

It is important to notice, perhaps, that the social and symbolic capital of the authors' institution are increased by adopting, and then adapting, practices from the global north. For Bourdieu, society is divided into several sections called 'fields', each with its own rules, norms, and forms of capital. Fields have their own hierarchies and power struggles. In this, there is a competition to increase their forms of capital.

Medical education is one such field and we see from many chapters in this book that social and cultural capital deriving from the global north and adopted by a process of changing habitus is characteristic of that field in the global south. Of course, faculty development also occurs to a lesser extent in the global north that might also require a change of habitus, or might simply require new ways of working within the same habitus. If a change of habitus is required, then that demands an approach to managing change that recognises the tensions between the habitus required for the new educational process, and the habitus that teachers and students return to in the rest of their cultural lives.

Students, Teachers and Competing Cultures

The authors of this chapter recognise that to use the new systems, students had to change their ideas about learning just as their teachers had to change their ideas about teaching, to relate to new practices from other cultures, while both groups remained firmly within their own unchanged cultures outside the medical school. In terms of habitus, social and cultural capital, there were contradictions to address between the cultures of North America and then the UK, and the culture of the students who come from different backgrounds, likewise the teachers, and then the changing culture of the medical school.

A learning culture is a complex phenomenon made up of the habitus of teachers and of learners, the context and management of the school and its educational processes, the relationships between teachers and learners, the wider academic and professional cultures, and the culture and values of the wider society (Hodkinson et al., 2007). Learning theories in medical education tend to be seen as optional ways of thinking about thinking, or different ways of conceptualising the process of learning (Dong et al., 2021). Ideas that in other circumstances are heavily criticised are still current in medical education (Newton & Salvi, 2020; Opdal, 2022; Sandlin, 2005), yet in this most globalised field of higher education, the effect of culture (and the lack of evidence to support the introduction of almost any educational methods) is often neglected in the theorising, even though, as the authors of this chapter demonstrate, the role of culture, and therefore of habitus, cannot be ignored. This will apply to students as much as to teachers (Ramburuth & Tani, 2009).

Conclusions

The authors of this chapter have provided a careful account of choosing and managing change in their medical school, and have explained their thinking about their choices, partially in terms of the characteristics, the national habitus, of their own country of Singapore. In doing so, they have indicated the interplay of cultural forces that are both within and beyond their school, especially when their mission has been to transpose and tailor with 'calculated modifications', the practice of another culture into their own, and to do this by changing the habitus of the players. But that alone may well set up new contradictions between the school and the society, between local and global north cultures, and between teachers and learners which make necessary their prudence and continuous review.

References

Alhassan, A. I. (2022). Implementing faculty development programs in medical education utilizing Kirkpatrick's model. *Advances in Medical Education and Practice, 13*, 945–954. https://doi.org/10.2147/AMEP.S372652

Baum, F. (2000). Social capital, economic capital and power: Further issues for a public health agenda. *Journal of Epidemiology and Community Health, 54*(6), 409–410. https://doi.org/10.1136/jech.54.6.409

Bleakley, A., Brice, J., & Bligh, J. (2008). Thinking the post-colonial in medical education. *Medical Education, 42*(3), 266–270. https://doi.org/10.1111/j.1365-2923.2007.02991.x

Bleakley, A., Bligh, J., & Browne, J. (2011). Global medical education – A post-colonial dilemma. In *Medical education for the future: Identity, power and location* (p. 171). Springer.

Bourdieu, P. (1977). *Outline of a theory of practice* (Richard Nice, Trans.). Cambridge University Press.

Bourdieu, P. (1986). The forms of capital. In J. Richardson (Ed.), *Handbook of theory and research for the sociology of education* (pp. 241–258). Greenwood.

Bourdieu, P., & Passeron, J.-C. (1977). *Reproduction in education society and culture*. Sage Publications.

Broadfoot. (1978). Reproduction in education, society and culture. *Comparative Education, 14*(1), 75–82.

Bryson, J. (2008). Dominant, emergent, and residual culture: The dynamics of organizational change. *Journal of Organizational Change Management, 21*(6), 743–757. https://doi.org/10.1108/09534810810915754

Dong, H., Lio, J., Sherer, R., & Jiang, I. (2021). Some learning theories for medical educators. *Medical Science Educator, 31*(3), 1157–1172. https://doi.org/10.1007/s40670-021-01270-6

Grant, J., & Gale, R. (1989). Changing medical education. *Medical Education, 23*(3), 252–257. https://doi.org/10.1111/j.1365-2923.1989.tb01540.x

Hodkinson, P., Biesta, G., & James, D. (2007). Understanding learning cultures. *Educational Review, 59*(4), 415–427. https://doi.org/10.1080/00131910701619316

Ihlen, Ø. (2005). The power of social capital: Adapting Bourdieu to the study of public relations. *Public Relations Review, 31*(4), 492–496. https://doi.org/10.1016/j.pubrev.2005.08.007

Lane, I. F. (2007). Change in higher education: Understanding and responding to individual and organizational resistance. *Journal of Veterinary Medical Education, 34*(2), 85–92. https://doi.org/10.3138/jvme.34.2.85

McLean, M., Cilliers, F., & Van Wyk, J. M. (2008). Faculty development: Yesterday, today and tomorrow. *Medical Teacher, 30*(6), 555–584. https://doi.org/10.1080/01421590802109834

Nawab, A., Bissaker, K., & Datoo, A. K. (2021). Contemporary trends in professional development of teachers: Importance of recognising the context. *International Journal of Educational Management, 35*(6), 1176–1190. https://doi.org/10.1108/IJEM-10-2020-0476

Newton, P. M., & Salvi, A. (2020). How common is belief in the learning styles neuromyth, and does it matter? A pragmatic systematic review. *Frontiers in Education, 5.* https://doi.org/10.3389/feduc.2020.602451

Opdal, P. A. (2022). To do or to listen? Student active learning vs. the lecture. *Studies in Philosophy and Education, 41*(1), 71–89. https://doi.org/10.1007/s11217-021-09796-3

Proctor, D., Leeder, D., & Mattick, K. (2020). The case for faculty development: A realist evaluation. *Medical Education, 54*(9), 832–842. https://doi.org/10.1111/medu.14204

Ramburuth, P., & Tani, M. (2009). The impact of culture on learning: Exploring student perceptions. *Multicultural Education & Technology Journal, 3*(3), 182–195. https://doi.org/10.1108/17504970910984862

Samarasekera, D. (2021). Collaborative learning cases: A fresh approach to applied learning | THE campus learn, share, connect. *Times Higher Education.* https://www.timeshighereducation.com/campus/collaborative-learning-cases-fresh-approach-applied-learning

Samarasekera, D., Lieske, B., Aw, D., Lee, S. S., Lim, Y. L., Ang, C. Y., Yeo, S. P., & Koh, D. R. (2021). A new model of teaching and learning approach – collaborative learning cases activities. *The Asia Pacific Scholar, 6*(2), 98–98. https://doi.org/10.29060/TAPS.2021-6-2/MA1602

Sandlin, J. A. (2005). Andragogy and its discontents: An analysis of andragogy from three critical perspectives. *PAACEJournal of Lifelong Learning, 14,* 25–42. https://www.researchgate.net/publication/251338021

Steinert, Y., Mann, K., Centeno, A., Dolmans, D., Spencer, J., Gelula, M., & Prideaux, D. (2006). A systematic review of faculty development initiatives designed to improve teaching effectiveness in medical education: BEME Guide No. 8. *Medical Teacher, 28*(6), 497–526. https://doi.org/10.1080/01421590600902976

Williams, R. (1980). *Culture and materialism.* Verso.

Dujeepa D. Samarasekera is the Head and Senior Director, Centre for Medical Education (CenMED), Yong Loo Lin School of Medicine, National University of Singapore and Adjunct Professor in Medical Education, School of Medicine and Dentistry, Griffith University, Australia. He has been involved in curriculum development, quality assurance and accreditation, and faculty development in health professional courses.

Jillian H.T. Yeo is a medical educationalist in the Centre leading the psychometrics division.

Shuh Shing Lee is a medical educationalist in the Centre leading the research division.

Matthew C.E. Gwee is Emeritus Professor at the Centre for Medical Education of the Yong Loo Lin School of Medicine. He is a pioneer in the field of medical education in Singapore.

I.iii STATEMENT: Exploring the Root Cause of Stagnation in Medical Education

Masayuki Nogi

This is a narrative story of one medical educator living in both the US and Japan, trying to make a change in an apparently rigid, traditional society.

1 Early Influences: From the US to Japan

I grew up in the United States, where educational values emphasised creativity, cultural diversity, and active learning. Moving to Japan introduced me to a vastly different educational environment, one that prized discipline, unity, and tradition. This trend continued even after I entered medical school in Japan, forcing me to adapt to a system focused on rote memorisation and written examinations. Compared to medical students in the UK and US, my peers in Japan were ill prepared to become a clinician right after graduating from medical school. I came to realise this during an eye-opening experience in the United Kingdom, where I did my overseas elective and interacted with younger medical students receiving more comprehensive training. I was devastated. I felt like I was in a bubble. I needed to put myself in a non-traditional Japanese training environment after graduation. That is why I did not select my university's hospital as a postgraduate training site, and instead I chose a community programme that would expose me to a high volume of emergency cases and rural medicine experience in tropical islands in Japan. The result was satisfying. I hyper-charged my clinical experience and became confident. Was

M. Nogi (✉)
Queen's Medical Center, Honolulu, HI, USA

Kameda Medical Center, Chiba, Japan

John A. Burns School of Medicine, University of Hawaii, Honolulu, HI, USA
e-mail: mnogi@hawaii.edu

I competent? I thought so, until I did my observership in the US during my fourth (PGY-4) postgraduate year.

2 Discovering the US Medical Education System

During the observership in the United States, I was exposed to a structured residency programme regulated by the Accreditation Council for Graduate Medical Education (ACGME), which highlighted the benefits of direct supervision, frequent feedback, and well-selected cases. The question of whether accreditation truly enhances the quality of medical education remains unanswered. But at least to my eyes, the US system appeared far superior to what Japan was offering me. This is why I applied for US residency and was fortunate enough to join during my PGY-6 year. While I had more clinical experience than a typical US graduate, I still learned a lot from my teachers and peers. The atmosphere was professional, fostering healthy competition to showcase the best performance to others: one that I wish I had experienced in my Japanese training environment.

I should be careful not to oversimplify a complex system, but from my first-hand experience, I did feel the effectiveness of the outcome-based, competency-based medical education provided in the US. The repetitive assessments were cumbersome, but they helped me realise I was being carefully observed and that I should do the same for others to facilitate deliberate practice. I came to realise that the Japanese training environment was process-based, experience-based medical education. I knew how to handle an electrolyte disorder on the ward, but when questioned about the reason, I did not have a clear logic. The anatomy and pathophysiology were seldom questioned. I had the 'what' and 'how' in my mind but lacked the 'why' in medicine. The side effect of this was variable performance outcomes and a feeling of unfulfillment. Even though I was highly praised and valued in my Japanese workplace, I always felt like 'the grass was greener elsewhere'. However, after training in the US, that feeling disappeared. I felt like my perceived gaps and holes (which we call 'puka' in Hawaii) were finally filled.

3 Embracing Innovation and Leadership

My journey progressed with a deeper exploration of faculty development and a recognition of the critical role of leadership and innovation in medical education. Following my participation in a medical education Fellowship, I had the privilege of enrolling in a relatively new Master's course in health professions education, specialising in accreditation and assessment—an area right down my alley. Engaging in academic rigour and research on this topic prompted me to contemplate deeply about accreditation and its role in medical education. Is it truly the answer for quality assurance?

I was constantly challenged to reconsider the fundamental question, 'What defines quality in medical education?'. Oh, this was a challenging inquiry. After graduation, numerous factors influence a physician's professional development. It is impossible to say that my medical school experience alone shaped who I am as a physician 20 years later. Thus, the safest assertion is that the quality of medical education is contingent upon the extent to which current training adequately prepares individuals to be ready for the next stage of their careers. If this was postgraduate training, that translates to independent practice. And the unique thing is that as the years go by, the goal line changes. Expectations at the next stage change. So, another point that I would expect in a well-designed and executed programme is its adaptability to change. Similar to how a machine becomes rusty and worn, an educational system needs constant monitoring, oiling, and improvement. Just like our body and metabolism, organisational leaders must undergo renewal and succession. Just like computer software, outdated operating systems require updating. Though its imperfections, the US medical education system's adaptability during crises such as the COVID pandemic demonstrated its resilience in evolving.

4 Japan's Path to Change, Déjà-Vu of the 1800s?

Despite my perceptions of slow evolution, Japan embarked on its own journey of reform. In 2007, there was establishment of a non-profit organization: the Japan Council for Evaluation of Postgraduate Clinical Training (JCEP) that initiated the accreditation process of postgraduate training programmes, but it did not have the authority and teeth to change or weed out low-quality programmes. Accreditation bodies for undergraduate medical training were not well established either. Then, in 2017, the Japan Accreditation Council for Medical Education (JACME) was founded to accredit medical schools and drive change. I chose to research this theme, as it seemed to be prompted by an ECFMG announcement (which has since been abandoned) heralding a major change in 2023 whereby if a medical graduate wished to sit USMLE, they should be from a medical school accredited by an agency recognised by the World Federation for Medical Education (WFME). Japan was not a significant exporter of physicians, but international accreditation seemed to be an attractive prize and a compelling external motivator.

This reminded me of the arrival of US ships led by Commodore Perry off the coast of Japan in June 1853. This resulted in the Tokugawa Shogunate signing the Treaty of Kanagawa in 1854 which opened select Japanese ports to American ships, marking the end of Japan's isolationist policy (although they had previously traded with neighbouring countries such as Korea) and the beginning of significant cultural and technological changes. This pivotal event demonstrated that even some long-standing traditions could yield to swift transformation when confronted with external pressures. But it also heralded the demise of the Tokugawa Shogunate and later prompted the restored Meiji government to open the borders and rapidly embrace westernisation to prevent colonisation. Perry's original purpose was to deliver a letter from the US President, requesting assistance for and return of shipwrecked whalers and, perhaps more importantly, seeking trade opportunities to load supplies to support the US whaling fleets. Reaching an accommodation with a more powerful agent can cause a loss of economic and cultural independence, but may have benefits on the international stage.

5   The Limitations of Change

At a recent session at an AMEE conference, the word "neo-colonisation" appeared in the title. Neo-colonisation in medical education refers to the influence or control exerted by Western or developed countries over the medical education systems in developing nations. This often involves exporting educational standards, curricula, accreditation, and regulatory frameworks from wealthier nations or international bodies to lower-income countries. Efforts to standardise medical education globally, often based on models from the US, UK, or other western nations, aim to ensure quality and comparability of medical training across borders. However, critics argue that this leads to cultural imperialism, as these external frameworks may not consider the unique health needs, cultural practices, or socioeconomic conditions of the target countries. Although Japan is not perceived as a lower-income country, when it comes to educational resources or structure, I feel like it is very short. However, unlike the Meiji government in the 1800s, the current medical schools seem motivated to adapt external standards less by fear and more by the desire for recognition on the international stage.

Implementing standards set by JACME posed challenges, yet tangible improvements such as increased resources and counseling systems were documented. Based on my documentary analysis and peer interviews, I sensed minimum resistance to change. Rotation durations were revised, access to electronic resources improved, students were invited to curriculum committees, external educational experts were invited for consultations, self-study rooms were increased, and student well-being was better supported. But through my sceptical lens, surface-level changes documented in official reports raised questions about the actual impact on medical education. Core rotations were still fragmented, lasting two to four weeks in some subjects, likely insufficient to provide an immersive experience. Who would give enough responsibility and autonomy to a student who will come and go in two weeks?

One barrier was the lack of legal support that limited medical students' clinical participation during their clerkship rotations. This was frustrating because active clinical participation is a key component for enhancing our undergraduate training, and a basic right provided to the students I observed in the UK and US. But now there is hope. The recent revision of Japan's Physician Act, which took effect in 2023, explicitly states that medical students can actively participate in clinical practice. This legal recognition finally supports the role of student doctors. However, the fragmented rotations will likely not change because the entrenched mindset is the same. A mindset that believes 'rotating through various subjects adds to a richer experience and cultivates a well-rounded physician'. There is little discussion about the possible hidden agenda of 'each department (or professor) wants a piece of the pie' issue. Some people still believe, rightly or wrongly, that if the student does not rotate through a certain field, they are less likely to choose that specialty. While it may make sense on a personal level, is it a valid reason to compromise every individual's educational experience?

6   Root Causes and Societal Impact

Accreditation standards in Japan aim to enhance the quality of medical education, yet they also risk exacerbating disparities in rural healthcare access, presenting ethical dilemmas. While there is limited evidence suggesting that medical students' rotations affect their future career selection, there appears to be significant resistance from subspecialty societies to relinquish their rotations. Postgraduate training quality assurance may necessitate the closure of subpar training programmes, particularly those in rural areas struggling to retain faculty. In rural Japan, young physicians in training are expected as a stable workforce, despite being in the midst of their training.

Indeed, the underlying issues in medical education reform reveal societal complexities, encompassing historical, political, and economic factors. Communicating these challenges to the public proves challenging. However, the closure of rural clinics due to dwindling training programmes and workforce is more apparent to the public. Policy makers who want to please the public may avoid this situation at all costs.

Japan undeniably boasts one of the world's highest life expectancies. However, does this correlate with the quality of healthcare and education? I doubt it. What concerns me most is Japan's insufficient collection and reporting of data on healthcare quality standards. Consequently, the public lacks information on where to access high-quality and safe healthcare. While healthcare costs are rising, the burden on the public's out-of-pocket expenses remains relatively low. Not all new, expensive, and effective treatments need to be prescribed, but the public is unaware that approximately 30% of new medications or medical technologies utilised in the US are unavailable in Japan. Medical errors often go unnoticed and lack adequate attention. Healthcare workers experience burnout and may overlook the normalisation of numerous errors due to fatigue. I feel that these facts are creating a false perception of medical quality in Japan to be high with a low cost, meaning high value!

Consequently, there is a significant need for social accountability to ensure quality medical care. While acknowledging Japan's achievements in healthcare, I would like to emphasise the necessity of systemic change and a paradigm shift in societal values to drive forward medical education. This may involve embracing external motivators such as international accreditation.

7 Is This My Battle?

Acknowledging similar issues worldwide, I contemplated the balance between idealism and realism in addressing complex healthcare challenges. I advocated for a paradigm shift to drive meaningful change in both medical education and healthcare. However, the more I reflect, the more profound the roots appear. There are finite depths one can delve into in a lifetime. Individual ideas and effort seem powerless in front of the headwind of inertia and preference of the status quo.

Leaders should embody wisdom and altruism, prioritising the welfare of the entire public over exploiting the rural workforce. If a 'leadership timer' existed, mandating that leaders depart if they cannot effect significant change within a specified timeframe, I believe Japan would be a more dynamic nation, fostering continuous innovation and confronting challenges. In my opinion, stagnation in the Japanese medical education system is a consequence of leadership, that has deliberately resisted involving external driving forces, including the public. In addition, the lack of adaptability and reluctance to fully embrace international accreditation further exacerbate the stagnation. Surface compliance will do no justice to the public. Without a concerted effort to adapt to external standards and integrate global best practices, the Japanese medical education system risks falling behind.

I've ventured so far and invested considerable time; it would be unworthy to surrender. Instead, I pledge to dedicate my remaining time to effecting change from the grassroots level, forging networks and alliances, inspiring apprentices, and adopting a global perspective.

But what will the ones who are just starting their educator journey do? If the current leaders fail to afford them a chance to make changes or instill hope, I foresee potential consequences. Disillusioned, they may quietly depart—abandoning their schools, workplaces, regions, and potentially, their country. In my opinion, the best way to prevent an unwanted physician migration is through change. By fostering a supportive environment that values innovation, collaboration, and continuous improvement, we can empower the younger generation.

I am tired of listening to symposiums that aim to 'increase awareness' of the need to change. Everyone around me knows that. Instead of dwelling on awareness campaigns, it's time for action-oriented strategies that mobilise resources to enact transformative changes that drive tangible results. If the most realistic option for moving the needle is to engage in international accreditation, then I am willing to take the chance.

I.iii COMMENTARY: The Cultural Imperialism of Medical Education and Accreditation, and its Limits

Janet Grant and Leonard Grant

In this chapter, Masayuki Nogi reflects on his experience of two very different educational environments: Japan and America. He analyses Japanese medical education through an American lens. He makes a thought-provoking historical parallel between what is happening now in medical education and the arrival of American warships in Japan more than 150 years ago, when the Tokugawa Shogunate of the Edo Period signed the Kanagawa Treaty with the US. The changes that followed during the subsequent Meiji restoration were dramatic, with every aspect of Japanese life being reconstructed along modern (so-called 'western') lines (Starrs, 2011). Yet Masayuki Nogi's experience more than a century later shows that assimilation of the values and processes of another culture has not entirely happened.

In other chapter commentaries, we highlight the tensions between the global north and global south, and the domination of global north ideas over global south practice. We site this in the lens of economics, politics and power, and the unidirectional trade in medical graduates. But in this chapter, we see something different. The tension that Masayuki Nogi discusses is about differences between countries and cultures which are part of the same economic group. Japan is not a global south country. It is a developed, rich nation, a member of G7 (the informal association of seven of the world's most powerful industrialised nations: Canada, France, Germany, Italy, Japan, the UK and the USA) and an International Monetary Fund advanced economy, with better health expectations than any of the other G7 countries (Tsugane, 2021).

There are none of the economic forces of medical education imperialism at work here (Bleakley et al., 2008, 2011). There is no significant export of doctors. For example, in 2023, only 353 UK NHS staff members out of 1.51 million, were Japanese (Baker, 2023). At the same time, 500 overseas nurses (out of 1.3 million in all) were working in Japan (Kaneda & Yamashiro, 2023). There is no desire for control or funding of Japanese medical schools from the US or UK: there are no external material forces exercising power over Japanese medical education. To the outsider, it might seem that Japan is a huge success story in terms of keeping control of its medical education and maintaining the health of the people.

We might wonder why such a country felt the need for external confirmation of its quality.

What Is the Problem?

The author's concerns are not those that are discussed in other chapters. There was 'minimum resistance to change' associated with the JACME application for WFME recognition; there were improvements in resources, student support and participation, and openness to external review. Perhaps clinical rotations could still be improved but are now supported by a legal framework. There might still be the need for students to rotate through all specialties. Rural areas actually need them to provide a service that is visible to the voting population.

Despite all this, Masayuki Nogi feels that a comparison with US medical education is not favourable to Japan. It has not embraced change to the extent that he would like. He attributes the health of the nation to other factors—and is certainly right in doing so. He links this with the social accountability of medical schools and the need to have 'a paradigm shift in societal values to drive forward medical education'. But what problem makes such a shift necessary, is not entirely clear. This seems to be a clash of views based on different experiences. Masayuki Nogi is invested in both US and Japanese medical education by accident of his own history.

No shift in the Japanese view of medical education will happen internally, Masayuki Nogi believes, and so concludes that 'external motivators' such as international accreditation, will be required, even though the effect of this has already been shown to be limited, at best. And as global practices become more publicised, he believes that Japan is at risk of the medical migration that other countries already experience.

The Importance of Culture

We write repeatedly in other commentaries that context and culture are important and to be respected, and that the importation of ephemeral and evidence-free fashions in ideas about education should be treated with caution. Perhaps Masayuki Nogi is now challenging us to think about what that means. Japan has protected its own history and culture, even when it adopted western commercial practices and its industry dominated international trade (Kakiuchi, 2017). Japan has changed many processes and practices of medical education, as the author points out, but in doing so, has also preserved more of its previous ways of being and doing than Masayuki Nogi would like. Perhaps it is simply that Japan is not America, and where there is no force of trade, or economic advantage, it has no need to be.

On the other hand, where there is no economic or political power struggle, this does not mean that there is no hierarchy, even among the equals of the G7. America has by far the strongest economy. The G7 not only is dedicated to trade liberalisation, but also to having 'shared beliefs and shared responsibilities' as industrial democracies, including 'the government of an open democratic society, dedicated to individual liberty and social advancement' (Reland, 2021). In the current world order, as we see in other chapters, this harmonisation of beliefs and practices translates into medical education whereby practices that were invented in North America, the UK or western Europe are transferred to other parts of the world. The combination of being first among equals and the harmonisation of practice means that processes such as international accreditation will see global north countries which are strong economically adopting the essentially cultural practices of even more powerful economies. And so western ideas about medical education spread to other parts of the world, including the global north, because the global north is also subject to a hierarchy of power.

Masayuki Nogi is both Japanese and American, and that brings into focus this complex set of contradictions.

Where the Personal Is Political. A Tale of Two Cultures

In other chapters, we argue that 'the global north' has an oppressive effect on 'the global south' in medical education. We stand by that argument, and although Masayuki Nogi does not address any such effect, he does challenge us to consider the role of people and culture in trying to enact change across borders. People are the agents who enact the issues, and staff the global and international systems that this book discusses. In this chapter, we see that some of these tensions, and so the politics and power that we discuss, are now located within one person who has two cultural perspectives.

The term 'the personal is political' was brought to prominence by the feminist movement of the 1970s, arguing that:

> … many personal experiences (particularly those of women) can be traced to one's location within a system of power relationships (Kelly, 2022).

This is relevant here, simply because the author's dominant opinions about medical education have been acquired in one location and set of relationships that those he would like to convince have not experienced. Trying to apply these ideas to a different location and set of relationships therefore meets with limited success.

There are countless models of opinion formation and opinion change (Helbing, 1995) which show that beliefs about the world are based on a wide variety of influences: free or forced experience, the weight and sources of information, social influence, and much more. Knowledge, experience and social behaviour along with the power of promulgation of views, is common to many models. We might manage to change others' behaviour, but changing the beliefs and opinions that underpin those is an uncertain discipline, even if we mistakenly believe that cognitive dissonance triggered by forcing new behaviours will cause a change of view (McGrath, 2017). The implicit theory underpinning accreditation is exactly that: yet it is hardly surprising, as Masayuki Nogi has observed, that forcing new behaviours is of limited effect, and those forced behaviours do not induce any deeper-level change. Changing behaviour is more easily managed than changing culture (Coulson-Thomas, 2015).

So here we have a tension between the US-acquired view of our author (his new nationalism), and its application to his country of origin which has not shared his experience (his transnationalism) (Conway et al., 2008). This mirrors entirely the premiss of international accreditation, and perhaps even international consultancy: that if we impose our processes, people will change. But they might not, in any meaningful way. The resolution of this tension is almost certainly not in the current fashion for accreditation as a means of externally imposed quality control, since, as he shows, the power of cognitive dissonance and so the effect of changing behaviour in the hope of changing deeply held, socially developed beliefs, is limited.

This view from two worlds is reinforced by analysis of the somewhat contradictory work of medical diaspora organisations which both try to preserve their cultural identity and heritage, and their connections with their countries of origin, at the same time as promoting the educational systems of their adopted countries, perhaps to justify themselves and enable others to migrate (Hussain et al., 2024).

The Instrumental Use of Accreditation

JACME seems to reflect this divergent view. Although Japan does not export or import doctors to any appreciable level, JACME nonetheless responded swiftly and directly to the (now abandoned) ECFMG requirement for medical school accreditation by a WFME recognised agency for medical graduates to sit USMLE:

> JACME is directed not only to provide Japanese faculties of medicine and medical schools with the standards and guidelines they need to ensure that their graduates qualify for application to an ECFMG examination, but also to improve the quality of medical education and to assure the quality of medical education in accordance with international standards (Japan Accreditation Council for Medical Education, 2021).

This rationale of enhancing the possibility of medical migration, is perhaps difficult to understand in the light of the very low migration rate of Japanese medical graduates, and the problems of providing healthcare for an ageing population and the consequent novel importation of healthcare workers from other southeast Asian countries (Asis & Carandang, 2020). Linking this with improving the quality of medical education by reference to 'international' practices is not entirely logical, given lack of robust evidence of effect even within the same cultures of origin, and certainly not for translation of such innovations to different cultures.

Nonetheless, WFME recognition seems to have had an instrumental use, as it must have done for many agencies worried that the US would be closed to their medical graduates. At this level, JACME has done exactly as Masayuki Nogi would have wanted. But his argument is that the effect is only at surface level as it is always likely to be in any country: behaviour change and culture change are different things. Meaningful change does not happen as a result of dislocated edicts from above or elsewhere. It derives from the common recognition of a problem and the common drive to share in addressing that (Gale & Grant, 1997).

Cultural Imperialism and Cultural Preservation

Cultural imperialism can be seen as:

> … the imposition by one usually politically or economically dominant community of various aspects of its own culture onto another nondominant community (Tobin, 2020).

From his perspective, Masayuki Nogi concludes that the culture of Japan is one that is reluctant to embrace such cultural change, despite offering evidence to the contrary both as a country as a whole and in medical education specifically. He does see that international recognition of the Japanese accreditation agency made some differences and that the changes were met with 'minimum resistance', but, to him, these changes were relatively shallow. Perhaps this could be seen in a different way: changes were made that have also preserved aspects of the Japanese medical education culture. And perhaps this is the understandable and important case wherever such changes are made. Enforced changes are not culture-deep.

Culture has been thought of in terms of *organisations* that bind individuals, *identity* whereby an individual locates themselves within a particular culture, and *practice* or the actual activities that typify any one cultural location (Watling et al., 2020). A response to any attempt at cultural change might be at any level in any of these aspects. So the target of Masayuki Nogi's frustrations could be understood as a careful national response, at the level of practice, to improvement of the medical education system in Japan which resisted deference to medical education imperialism by leaving intact organisations (even though JACME was relatively new) and identities (Bleakley et al., 2008, 2011).

There is much debate and analysis around the development and status of Japanese culture. It has been argued that, even during the period of isolation that Masayuki Nogi mentions:

> Japan has followed a cycle of selectively absorbing foreign cultural values and institutions and then adapting these to existing indigenous patterns (Masai et al., 2024).

Despite his sceptical observations, Masayuki Nogi's frustration tells him that if the culture does not facilitate change, then international accreditation might—even though he has shown that such accreditation has actually had limited effect. For this author, the problem is located in the Japanese culture, and the answer is located in the historically western culture of accreditation (Anon, 1980; Brady, 1988). But perhaps we might consider that the opposite is the case.

What Is the Alternative to International Accreditation?

In business schools, it has been shown that:

> … international accreditations, on average, send positive signals to the market…, losing the accreditation status may lead to substantial economic losses ….. However, the effect of the signal is weakened with every cycle (Okulova & Shakina, 2022, p. 624).

There are parallels with medicine. The main driver of international accreditation was the now abandoned US requirements for participation in their market in medical migration (Shiffer et al., 2019). With that driver now diminished, it is hardly surprising that the effect wanes: it is not logically possible that the process of accreditation, which takes place over months of preparation of largely tick-box documentation and then ends with one, possibly performative, site visit, should persist in its effect over the years before the next inspection. Despite all this, no credible or acceptable alternative model has been put forward.

Masayuki Nogi is frustrated that Japan will not behave like another global north culture. He interprets this as stagnation. But Japan has changed and has adopted some western qualities such as individualism, which has created personal and societal tensions (Ogihara, 2017). If we value context, then we must value culture. In the case of Japan, that culture has been actively, if not entirely successfully, protected since 1853 when Japan opened itself to a wider world. Westernisation, unsurprisingly, has had some negative effects (Pike & Borovoy, 2004). The lesson from this must be that, if we really believe in the quality of medical education for its context, the time has come to work with countries on their own terms, within their own cultures and conditions, to assert their own ways of defining, assuring and supporting the quality of what they do (Rashid et al., 2023), based on problems that they identify for themselves. Hoping that one country will adopt the practices of another, or that one culture can become another is likely to result in disappointment.

References

Anon. (1980). Historical development of accreditation. *AAHE-ERIC/Higher Education Research Report, 9*(6), 20–33. https://doi.org/10.1002/aehe.3640090607

Asis, E., & Carandang, R. R. (2020). The plight of migrant care workers in Japan: A qualitative study of their stressors on caregiving. *Journal of Migration and Health, 1–2*, 100001. https://doi.org/10.1016/j.jmh.2020.100001

Baker, C. (2023). *NHS staff from overseas: Statistics*. https://researchbriefings.files.parliament.uk/documents/CBP-7783/CBP-7783.pdf

Bleakley, A., Bligh, J., & Browne, J. (2011). Global medical education—A post-colonial dilemma. In Medical Education for the Future: Identity, Power and Location (p. 171). Springer.

Bleakley, A., Brice, J., & Bligh, J. (2008). Thinking the post-colonial in medical education. *Medical Education, 42*(3), 266–270. https://doi.org/10.1111/j.1365-2923.2007.02991.x

Brady, J. E. (1988). Accreditation: A historical overview. *Hospitality & Tourism Educator, 1*(1), 18–24. https://doi.org/10.1080/23298758.1988.10685362

Conway, D., Potter, R. B., & St Bernard, G. (2008). Dual citizenship or dual identity? Does 'transnationalism' supplant 'nationalism' among returning Trinidadians? *Global Networks, 8*, 373–397.

Coulson-Thomas, C. J. (2015). Learning and behaviour: Addressing the culture change conundrum: Part one. *Industrial and Commercial Training, 47*(3), 109–115. https://doi.org/10.1108/ICT-01-2015-0003

Gale, R., & Grant, J. (1997). AMEE Medical Education Guide No.10: Managing change in a medical context: Guidelines for action. *Medical Teacher, 19*(4), 239–249.

Helbing, D. (1995). Opinion formation models. In *Quantitative sociodynamics* (pp. 159–201). Springer Netherlands. https://doi.org/10.1007/978-94-015-8516-3_9

Hussain, I., Haruna-Cooper, L., Isiramen, S., van der Mark, N., Khan, M., & Rashid, M. A. (2024). Educational priorities of low-and middle-income country medical diaspora organisations: A critical discourse analysis. *PLOS Global Public Health, 4*(7), e0003481. https://doi. org/10.1371/journal.pgph.0003481

Japan Accreditation Council for Medical Education. (2021). *About JACME*. JACME.

Kakiuchi, E. (2017). Cultural heritage protection system in Japan: Current issues and prospects for the future. *Gdańskie Studia Azji Wschodniej, 10*. https://doi.org/10.4467/2353872 4GS.16.013.6170

Kaneda, Y., & Yamashiro, A. (2023). Addressing nursing shortages in Japan: Toward quality and quantity enhancement. *Journal of Public Health and Emergency, 7*, 35–35. https://doi. org/10.21037/jphe-23-63

Kelly, C. J. (2022). The personal is political. Description, origin, and analysis. In *Encyclopedia Britannica*. https://www.britannica.com/topic/the-personal-is-political

Masai, Y., Masamoto, K., Notehelfer, F. G., Toyoda, T., Sakamoto, T., Jansen, M. B., Watanabe, A., Hijino, S., Hurst, G. C., & Latz, Gil. (2024). Japan – Culture, traditions, religion. In *Encyclopedia Britannica*. https://www.britannica.com/place/Japan/Cultural-life

McGrath, A. (2017). Dealing with dissonance: A review of cognitive dissonance reduction. *Social and Personality Psychology Compass, 11*(12). https://doi.org/10.1111/spc3.12362

Ogihara, Y. (2017). Temporal changes in individualism and their ramification in Japan: Rising individualism and conflicts with persisting collectivism. *Frontiers in Psychology, 8*. https://doi. org/10.3389/fpsyg.2017.00695

Okulova, O., & Shakina, E. (2022). Is there value in international accreditation beyond quality? An empirical analysis of the AACSB accredited schools. *Higher Education Quarterly, 76*(3), 612–625. https://doi.org/10.1111/hequ.12331

Pike, K. M., & Borovoy, A. (2004). The rise of eating disorders in Japan: Issues of culture and limitations of the model of westernization. *Culture, Medicine and Psychiatry, 28*(4), 493–531. https://doi.org/10.1007/s11013-004-1066-6

Rashid, M. A., Ali, S. M., & Dharanipragada, K. (2023). Decolonising medical education regulation: A global view. *BMJ Global Health, 8*(6), e011622. https://doi.org/10.1136/ bmjgh-2022-011622

Reland, J. (2021, May 27). *G7 summit: Everything you need to know*. UK in a Changing Europe. https://ukandeu.ac.uk/explainers/g7-summit-everything-you-need-to-know/

Shiffer, C. D., Boulet, J. R., Cover, L. L., & Pinsky, W. W. (2019). Advancing the quality of medical education worldwide: ECFMG's 2023 medical school accreditation requirement. *Journal of Medical Regulation, 105*(4), 8–16. https://doi.org/10.30770/2572-1852-105.4.8

Starrs, R. (2011). Constructing Meiji modernity. In *Modernism and Japanese culture* (pp. 13–36). Palgrave Macmillan UK. https://doi.org/10.1057/9780230353879_2

Tobin T. W. (2020, May 26). Cultural imperialism. In *Encyclopedia Britannica*. https://www.britannica.com/topic/cultural-imperialism

Tsugane, S. (2021). Why has Japan become the world's most long-lived country: Insights from a food and nutrition perspective. *European Journal of Clinical Nutrition, 75*(6), 921–928. https://doi.org/10.1038/s41430-020-0677-5

Watling, C. J., Ajjawi, R., & Bearman, M. (2020). Approaching culture in medical education: Three perspectives. *Medical Education, 54*(4), 289–295. https://doi.org/10.1111/medu.14037

Masayuki Nogi was born in Japan and grew up in the USA, completing his medical degree from Kyoto Prefectural University of Medicine, Japan, and his postgraduate training in acute care in both Japan and the USA. He completed his Medical Education Fellowship at the University of Hawaii, and the UK FAIMER-Keele University Master's in Health Professions Education with Distinction. He is co-founder of the Japan Chief Medical Residents Association (JACRA). He currently has an appointment in Hawaii as an academic hospitalist, associate clinical professor, Division Chief of Hospital Medicine, and Associate Medical Director for Instructional Design and Technology. Since 2023, he also holds a cross-appointment in Japan as the Internal Medicine Residency Programme Director at a renowned training hospital, providing him with a real-time perspective on the two countries from a clinician-educator's viewpoint. He is passionate about international medical education, faculty development, physician migration, and accreditation.

Part II
Globalisation and Its Problems

Summary

The global business of medical education inevitably brings with it the effects of the economic dominance of the global north over the global south, and its imperial and colonial history. That continuing history causes unexamined assumptions of where 'best practice' might be found, and so in which direction the export of ideas should flow. It also brings the continuing exploitation of resources: the flow of trained doctors runs in the opposite direction from the flow of ideas. Export of global north ideas about medical education (sometimes reinforced by international or global accreditation of programmes or practices) enables easier export of doctors from the global south to the global north.

This state of affairs concerns people in medical education in both the global north and the global south. So in Part II, authors explore how the post-colonial habit of easy, uncritical acceptance of global north ideas, along with global standardisation, have inhibited medical schools from focusing on their own communities and contexts. These worries also emerge in the global north itself, where we can ask whether the colonial legacy can possibly be escaped in respectful and friendly global partnerships.

II.i STATEMENT: The 'Fast and Fashionable' Syndrome

Syed Moin Ali

1 The Rise of the Fashion

My association with medical education goes back to 1993, when I started attending workshops on educational planning, assessment and evaluation. In 1995, my employers sent me to the University of Maastricht to learn how the system of problem-based learning (PBL) worked, so that I could 'transfer the technology' back home. By 1996, I and colleagues had developed Pakistan's first integrated medical curriculum with PBL as a major instructional method. Since the mid-nineties, thus, I have been watching institutions and institutional heads follow internationally (read 'western') acclaimed trends without thinking of the impact of these 'innovative' methods in our context. This has prompted me to write about academic fashions or trends that seem to have gripped Pakistan for more than three decades. We are not only eager to adopt western methods; we race to take the lead in doing so! Hence, the title of this chapter. I have attempted to trace the history of how medical education evolved in Pakistan with the sole purpose of linking its evolution with its impact on undergraduate medical education policies and practices. The primary purpose of writing this is to share my reflections, my perspective, about how and why things transpired to be the way they are and what may be done to improve the situation.

S. M. Ali (✉)
Aga Khan University, Karachi, Pakistan
e-mail: syedmoin.ali@aku.edu

© The Author(s), under exclusive license to Springer Nature   67
Switzerland AG 2026
J. Grant, L. Grant (eds.), *The Contradictions of Medical Education*,
https://doi.org/10.1007/978-3-031-90394-6_5

2   Medical Education in Pakistan: A Short History

The world of medical education in Pakistan has been full of adventure and activity. In Pakistan, medical education traces its history to the early 1970s when the WHO Collaborating Centre for Medical Education was established in the College of Physicians and Surgeons (CPSP). The first two to three decades were characterised by sporadic workshops, meant more for sensitisation than skill development. In the early 2000s, with a change in CPSP leadership, the number of faculty development sessions increased exponentially and medical education moved from the élite halls of postgraduate education to that of undergraduate education, solely because the supervisors of postgraduate training were involved in teaching the undergraduate programmes as well. During this time, there were only three or four medical doctors with MHPE qualifications. In 2004, the first diploma level qualification was offered by the CPSP, followed by the first MHPE programme offered by Dow University of Health Sciences, Karachi in 2009.

These qualifications instantly caught the fancy of the medical and dental communities even though they did not provide any associated career path. By 2011, almost two dozen doctors were enrolled in the MHPE programme.

In 2015, the Pakistan Medical and Dental Council (PM&DC), the only accrediting body of Pakistan, officially proclaimed medical education as a basic science discipline and gave it a career structure. Furthermore, it was made mandatory for every medical and dental college to have a Department of Medical/Dental Education headed by a duly qualified faculty member, thereby catapulting the demand for MHPE qualifications. Institutions who had qualified MHPEs or PhDs in medical education clamoured to offer MHPE programmes. In 2023, the number of faculty members with MHPE qualifications must have gone beyond 200, by a conservative estimate.

In 2017, Jinnah Sindh Medical University offered the first blended, 6-month Certificate in Health Professions Education (CHPE) programme with the aim of improving teaching and assessment skills. This trend also caught on mainly because, in 2018, PM&DC made the CHPE one of the mandatory requirements for faculty members for their promotion.

3   The Era of the Fashion

Many institutions have now started offering CHPE programmes, some of which are purely online. There is, as yet, no consensus among the course-offering institutions about the purpose of this course and their targeted skills. Institutions have not been able to decide whether the purpose of the Certificate is to provide updates on the latest teaching and assessment methods and/or to develop skills. The number of nation-wide faculty members with CHPE qualifications must now be approaching 1000.

With this deluge of medical educationists in the market, there has been an explosion of eager ideas and practices advocated by these nouveau specialists. Keeping in mind the varying quality of MHPE graduates, the concepts they advocate to their institutions are based on literature, mainly emanating from the west. Some of this literature presents a social scientist's personal thoughts, supported by scant scientific evidence. The heads of medical and dental colleges get their counsel from these specialists whose concepts are variable and at times based on international trends alone, with little consideration of local realities. Anecdotally speaking, when I asked such leaders about the rationale for their decisions, I frequently got the answer 'because it is expected of us', 'because it is the modern thing to do… just like ABC institution is doing', 'because it is in vogue in the West'! When I dug a little deeper, I found that the idea was implanted by, most commonly, a medical educationist they met either at an international or national conference.

A number of medical educationists have advocated teaching methods, assessment tools or curricular designs that may work in a dynamic and resource-rich environment but may not be suitable in our more traditional and resource-constrained context. In order to make these innovations work, people then have come up with hybrid forms of teaching methods or curricular designs that have weak theoretical foundations. I have not been able to ascertain why this happens. This may be because people think that if an academic activity is believed to be popular in the developed world, it must be generalisable and beneficial for all contexts.

This has made me think of whether we need to sit back and reflect seriously on our MHPE programmes and the quality of graduate entering the workforce from them. A balance between critical thinking and content expertise needs to be explicitly emphasized by MHPE programme directors. Programme standards need to be contextualised and the philosophy of the programme needs to be clearly identified. Such a movement, of analysing MHPE programmes locally, has started but is still in the evolutionary phase.

4   The Advent of the 'Fast Syndrome'

To compound the issue, probably to be at par with the west, an institutional head will declare that an innovation must be adopted, that too within the shortest possible time. Such directives give minimal time for not only evaluating the innovation's suitability and sustainability for the local context but also for preparing for it and pilot-testing it, resulting in the faculty doing whatever it feels best under the circumstances. There are a lot of scurried, chaotic activities to meet the proclaimed deadline; what transpires in reality and ultimately in the classroom may not always be what was intended.

A college I visited in 2022 had problem-based learning, team-based learning, case-based learning, case-based discussions and tutorials shown in their weekly teaching schedules. When I inquired as to why they had so many formats of 'student-centred' activities, the faculty (including some heads of departments) said that they

were told to include as many as possible. Each faculty member had their own definition of the method. The common misconceptions, among these otherwise highly
accomplished medical specialists, was that lectures were 'out' and discussions were
'in'. They were apprehensive and felt unsure as to how they would perform professionally if this rule (of no lectures) came to pass. I assume such institutions intend
to improve the quality of their teaching and of their graduates but lack of rationalisation and critical evaluation of the educational tools being employed seem to be at
the bottom of their decisions. This could be food for thought for the MHPE programmes that are emphasising content coverage without stressing enough on the
core competencies of reasoning and critical thinking.

5   Evidence-Free Innovation

Another fashion that has hit the educational scene in Pakistan is that of the integrated curriculum. Harden's article on the ladder of integration (Harden, 2000),
which makes no claim to be evidence-based, is considered a gospel. The fact that
there is non-existent evidence about integrated curricula producing more competent
doctors or better students than the traditional design has never been debated. The
benefits of integrated curricula are so fixed in the minds of the medical faculty, that
one of the largest medical universities in Pakistan has made it mandatory for all the
medical colleges affiliated with it to implement it with immediate effect. Little
thought has been given to faculty readiness; an important factor to be considered
whenever an innovation is to be implemented (Jippes et al., 2013; Quearry et al.,
2019). The university could have given more time to the colleges to develop their
resources, and their teaching and assessment systems in order to deliver education
that can ensure optimal student learning. More faculty development sessions would
definitely have helped improve the skills of the faculty in developing courses that
are of satisfactory academic quality and in line with the unique strengths and limitations of their institutions.

   The poorly understood constructivist perspective on learning, of which there are
different types in cognitive theory, epitomised by Piaget's and Vygotsky's views
(Huang, 2021), is frequently talked about by many medical educationists. This is
often erroneously presented as learners 'creating' their own knowledge and understanding. It is therefore incorrectly assumed that teaching will get in the way of this
construction, so 'active learning' which avoids direct teaching is the way to go. Of
course, all learning (even rote learning) is constructed, or stored, inside the learner's
head, no matter how it is taught. And the best thing a teacher can do is to offer well-
organised knowledge for the learner to store rationally, based on their previously
stored knowledge (Ausubel et al., 1978). Constructivism does not preclude teaching, in fact, it requires it.

   As a result of medical education's misunderstanding of this key concept in cognitive psychology, 'adult' learning theory, problem-based learning, case-based
learning and team-based learning have been advocated and incorporated as learning

methods, at times in hybrid formats. The reality of what actually transpires in the class, however, is known only to the concerned faculty and the students. The effects of these approaches are largely unknown. If these methods are to be used, then teachers must be appropriately trained and must understand their strengths and weaknesses. In turn, medical educationalists must also understand the background and rationale for these methods. Citing 'constructivism' and adult learning theory is not enough.

It appears that there is now a pattern emerging from these developments; there is an 'expert' who informs the decision-makers of what needs to be added or amended in a curriculum in order to 'improve the educational system'. These 'experts' are believed since they have a high status in the eyes of the decision-makers who then issue directives that the idea needs to be implemented without further ado!

6 What's in a Name?

The functions that medical educationists perform in institutions across Pakistan vary tremendously. They range from being glorified secretaries to the heads of institutions, to having the authority to plan and implement changes. Regardless of the academic clout and influence such medical educationists have, there are others in the institution who proclaim to be medical educationists even though they have no qualifications in this field. According to them, since they have been teaching medical students for decades, they have the right to be called medical educationists. The first time I heard this, I was visibly shocked! A very senior professor of physiology claimed to be a medical educationist. It seems their claim is not without logic! This realisation made me question my own professional identity and initiate a search for it, a quest that is going on!

It must be acknowledged that Medical Education, or Health Professions Education, is not a fully-fledged profession at the moment. To start with, it lacks an official, agreed-upon definition. This gravely affects the development of professional identity and self-efficacy (Chin et al., 2020; Holden et al., 2012). In Pakistan, faculty members whose sole postgraduate qualification is MHPE and who have adopted this as a full-time occupation, suffer because they feel they are in a grey zone. Their roles are ill-defined and are based largely on assumptions made by people with variable understanding of what such professionals are qualified to do. This amorphous professional identity has led to MHPE-qualified, full-time medical educationists following the dictates of administrators and managers resulting in a diminished sense of professional fulfilment. For the neo-profession of medical education to be established, suitable steps will have to be taken whereby the tenets and requirements of a profession are accomplished (Marcus, 1999). It has been shown that professionalisation improves the quality of service (Polat & Benligiray, 2022). This process should start with developing a consensus-based, widely accepted definition, having a code of ethics and an office that looks after the affairs of people with such qualifications (Chambers, 2004; Holtz-Bacha, 2015).

7 Conclusion

Medical education has shown a dramatic rise in Pakistan over recent decades. From infrequent, limited-access faculty development sessions to large-scale, rampant programmes, medical education has become a commodity. Faculty members clamour for certifications, for reasons ranging from merely obtaining eligibility for promotions to thoughtfully improving the academic system around them.

Being a social science, education has the propensity to be interpreted in more than one way. People translate educational theories and principles in languages that they understand best: the languages of their past experiences, motivations, cultural norms, institutional traditions and policy boundaries. What has resulted is an academic vernacular that seems familiar but is being understood differently by different stakeholders. People are eager to speak it fast but are not always sure of the actual, underlying meanings.

In my opinion, purely subjective and based on my observations, our faculty, from the coasts of the south to the mountains of the north, are a little lost where medical education is concerned. They are complying with decisions they had little say in, they are following what the dictates are to retain their positions, they are hopeful that what is happening around them will be of benefit to the students and to the patient community.

Health professions education (HPE) in Pakistan, and indeed around the world, needs to be carefully evaluated, monitored and supported.

We need to take a step back, breathe, relax and question our own actions and decisions. By 'question' I do not mean 'criticise'; I simply mean ask ourselves, introspect! We need to evaluate whether our quick decisions have resulted in graduates today who are better in academic performance than the graduates of a decade back. How much have we been able to enhance their clinical skills by incorporating the trends in teaching and assessing? What benefits are we getting from integrating our content? How much 'programmatic assessment' can be implemented in our unique set-up? Has mandating the Mini-CEX enhanced the clinical competence of our residents and improved outcomes of our patients?

Moving away from the inclusion of innovative strategies, including artificial intelligence, and practices in undergraduate and postgraduate education of the health professionals, I would like to discuss the essential issues of those who practise 'medical education' or 'health professions education' (HPE) as a full-time occupation; such faculty members have at least a Master's-level qualification in HPE. In Pakistan, these educationists are having a great impact on how medical, dental and nursing undergraduate and postgraduate programmes are conceptualised, designed and implemented. Despite a rapid rise in their numbers, and indeed in their influence, health professions educationists, or medical educationists, are, ironically, not part of a recognised profession.

There is no globally accepted definition of 'health professions education' or 'medical education'. Research articles and books use these terms to mean the education of health professionals or, alternatively, for those who learn how education should be imparted to healthcare providers. There is no recognised code of ethics dedicated for these educational practitioners nor is there an officially designated body that regulates their activities. Each of these components must surely be present for an occupation to be known as a profession. Due to lack of formal regulation from a recognised authority, HPE recommended practices proliferate unchecked. This and the hyperplasia of Master's programmes in health professions education has created a set of qualified professionals, with their own set of concepts and misconcepts, guiding institutions, faculty and accrediting bodies towards 'progress'.

It is, therefore, high time that health professions educationists took stock of their own world before attempting to improve those of others!

References

Ausubel, D. P., Novak, J. D., & Hanesian, H. (1978). *Educational psychology. A cognitive view* (2nd ed.). Holt, Rinehart and Winston.

Chambers, D. W. (2004). The professions. *The Journal of the American College of Dentists, 71*(4), 57–64.

Chin, D., Phillips, Y., Woo, M. T., Clemans, A., & Yeong, P. K. (2020). Key components that contribute to professional identity development in internships for Singapore's tertiary institutions: A systematic review. *Asian Journal of the Scholarship of Teaching and Learning Special Issue, 10*(1), 89–113.

Harden, R. M. (2000). The integration ladder: A tool for curriculum planning and evaluation. *Medical Education, 34*(7), 551–557.

Holden, M., Buck, E., Clark, M., Szauter, K., & Trumble, J. (2012). Professional identity formation in medical education: The convergence of multiple domains. *HEC Forum, 24*(4), 245–255.

Holtz-Bacha, C. (2015). Professionalization. In *The international encyclopedia of political communication* (pp. 1–7). John Wiley & Sons, Inc.

Huang, Y.-C. (2021). Comparison and contrast of Piaget and Vygotsky's theories. *Advances in Social Science, Education and Humanities Research, 554*, 28–32.

Jippes, M., Driessen, E. W., Broers, N. J., Majoor, G. D., Gijselaers, W. H., & van der Vleuten, C. P. M. (2013). A medical school's organizational readiness for curriculum change (MORC). *Academic Medicine, 88*(9), 1346–1356.

Marcus, E. R. (1999). Empathy, humanism, and the professionalization process of medical education. *Academic Medicine, 74*(11), 1211–1215.

Polat, G., & Benligiray, S. (2022). The impact of family business professionalization on financial performance: A multidimensional approach. *Journal of Small Business and Enterprise Development, 29*(7), 1149–1175.

Quearry, M., Bonaminio, G., Istas, K., Paolo, A., & Walling, A. (2019). The impact of communication strategies on faculty members' readiness for curricular change. *Medical Science Educator, 29*(1), 51–55.

II.i COMMENTARY: Globalisation, Post-Colonial Habits and Medical Migration

Janet Grant and Leonard Grant

Syed Moin Ali has presented a complex series of concerns about the identity of medical education in his country. The lack of identity of medical education in his country is founded on the instrumental and reactive rapid adoption of 'western' educational practices. It is a casualty or consequence of rapid globalisation. Medical education specialists were needed to support that process before medical education as a profession or specialty itself was defined. That 'fast and furious' adoption of 'western practices' seems to have precluded that definition still.

In his own reflection, the author takes the stance of a person who is focused on the improvement of practice. And he wonders whether the current processes and pathways of medical education serve that purpose in his country. In his analysis, he chooses not to consider the business of medical education and its many ways of making money, nor the role of medical education in preparing its product, the graduates, for export. These are serious but separate issues. For this author, the state and status of medical education in his country, in which he is a leading authority and to which he has devoted his academic life, is the issue at hand. We are reading the words of an authentic, situated, reflective practitioner (Dewey, 1938; Schön, 1984) who worries about the unsituated adoption of medical education practices from elsewhere.

The Issues

Syed Moin Ali is concerned that in his country, ideas in medical education are adopted quickly and uncritically. Those ideas emanate from 'the west'. Such fast implementation of innovations (to keep up with what is believed to be happening in the global north?) seems to preclude proper understanding, reflection, analysis, preparation, piloting and change management. Why might this happen? We can perhaps best understand this firstly, in terms of the current state of globalisation in medical education; secondly, in terms of the relationship between Pakistan (or any previously occupied and colonised country) and the former coloniser; and thirdly, in terms of the medical migration that Syed Moin Ali does not discuss. These three factors are related.

Globalisation

The rhetoric of globalisation pervades medical education. This term has been defined in many ways, rooted in changing economic practices (Scholte, 2007):

- as internationalism based on growing transactions and interdependence between countries
- as liberalisation and neoliberalism with a reduction in national regulatory barriers
- as universalisation, or the dispersal, or imposition of entities and practices across the world.

Although we can see elements of these in the current global rhetoric of medical education, these ideas have largely been rejected in the world of trade and economics. However, a fourth definition might seem more even pertinent, given Syed Moin Ali's concerns:

- globalisation as westernisation, in which the ideas and processes of western 'modernity' are spread across the world.

This reflects, for us, a process whereby western medical practices have been adopted throughout the world, whether productively or not (Horton, 2003), and western medical education that teaches those practices has followed in its footsteps. Adopting what are believed to be current western educational methods is therefore part of the process of adopting western medical practices. This is sometimes done without reflecting on the appropriateness of wholesale adoption of curriculum practices from a very different context and culture (Bleakley et al., 2008). Syed Moin Ali also is concerned about that in terms of the continuing uncritical advocacy for western ideas ('international trends') unsupported by evidence, and learned in qualifying courses for medical educators who are necessary to import and implant educational practices from the global north.

Although these definitions have fallen out of favour beyond medical education, the underlying premiss has not:

> Any analysis of globalisation must ... examine the political aspects involved. On the one hand, these politics involve actors: that is, power relations. (Scholte, 2007, p. 1497)

We might not question the global dominance of western medicine, which seems to be underpinned by science and so is neutral in its application. And yet, anthropological and sociological research suggests that social and cultural factors play an influential role in the western biomedical tradition, and that other cultures have other approaches (Gottweis & Prainsack, 2006; Logan, 1977; Lupton, 2012).

> Despite the objectivity implied by the scientific principles underlying western medicine, it is still underpinned by a host of assumptions and beliefs developed through living in western culture. (Lupton, 2013)

If this is true of medicine itself, it is even more true of the social, conditioned and interpersonal learning process that is medical education. Nonetheless, the process of globalisation sees the global north dominate the global south in economics and politics (Odeh, 2012) and equally in medical education. Even one of the most prominent global organisations for medical education, the World Federation for Medical Education, has been criticised for having 'seemingly given precedence to the values and priorities of countries in the Global North' (Rashid et al., 2023b).

It has also been noted that although globalisation of medical education has become part of the accepted rhetoric, there are few international studies or collaborative research projects in this field, and that such research as there is, tends to reflect a western perspective (Stadler et al., 2019). The challenges of cultural diversity and unequal power relationships are not to be underestimated.

In these terms, where the global north is dominant in all aspects of medicine and medical education, the drive to be fast and fashionable, and so to need medical education specialists, is understandable.

Post-Colonial Medical Education

Just as Syed Moin Ali's reflections are based in the rhetoric of globalisation, they equally problematise post-colonial values. He worries about the lack of critical thinking, contextuality and philosophical analysis in MHPE programmes, and so in the graduates of those programmes. But where there is an unexamined assumption of the superiority of the 'other', perhaps, this is too challenging to overcome. It has been observed that:

> We need to develop greater understanding of the relationship between post-colonial studies and medical education if we are to prevent a new wave of imperialism through the unreflecting dissemination of conceptual frameworks and practices which assume that 'metropolitan West is best.' (Bleakley et al., 2008)

Decolonisation of the curriculum is a relatively recent but unresearched and already criticised phenomenon in higher education (Dhillon, 2021; Sefa Dei & Cacciavillani, 2024; Shahjahan et al., 2022) and medical education (Sefa Dei & Cacciavillani, 2024; Shahjahan et al., 2022). There is a large and long-standing critical literature on this topic in other disciplines, that relates to Syed Moin Ali's concerns. The arguments appear, for example, in relation to the need for 'indigenisation' of the academic discourse (Alatas, 1993; Atalas, 2005), concerns about the 'export' of western ideas (Naidu & Kumagai, 2016), epistemic violence (or the interpretation of social science data using a dominant, normally global north, ideology that dismisses the value of other, normally global south, ideologies) (Brunner, 2021; Jimenez & Roberts, 2019), and the much-debated modernisation (Meinhof, 2018) that implies a superiority of more 'developed' countries' resulting in the dominance of the global north.

Building on this, authors have discussed the need for an inclusive medical education (Gishen & Lokugamage, 2019; Hartland & Larkai, 2020; Nazar et al., 2015), one that contains an expanded understanding of what is medical knowledge (Lokugamage et al., 2020; Wong & See, 2021). However, we share the concerns that the term 'decolonising' is being 'diluted and depoliticised' (Moghli & Kadiwal, 2021) and becoming disconnected from the wider university structures (Ali et al., 2021; Arday et al., 2021; Tudor, 2021), a cosmetic measure that does not disrupt coloniality so much as revamp it (Rossi & Táíwò, 2020). Indeed, decolonising the medical curriculum is sometimes presented as a vehicle for institutional improvement (Bracken et al., 2021; Finn et al., 2022). This itself is a contradiction given that universities in the global north have presently and historically benefitted from colonial and neo-colonial relations (as well as producing the knowledge that upheld them). Medical education generally understands the movement to decolonise the curriculum as one of inclusion or representation within a framework that is not examined nor, usually, visible. It is partly this framework that Syed Moin Ali seeks to make clear and therefore, available to scrutiny.

This leads the author to wonder about the nature and effects of 'expertise', 'experts', and professional identity in his field.

The author worries that this 'expertise' is leading, but not convincing, colleagues who actually do the job of teaching and training the next generation. The question of who is the real 'expert' is therefore a significant one which, in turn, might lead us to redefine the role of the medical educationalist and so the power relations between 'medical education' and 'medicine', just as it might lead to a similar analysis of the power relations between his country and western medical education. Syed Moin Ali believes that this reflection has to begin by having medical educationalists look at their own education.

Medical Migration: The Basis of 'Fast and Furious'?

Although Syed Moin Ali does not discuss it, a final related factor in these concerns is that of medical migration. Where this is the intention of more than half of Pakistani medical graduates (Hossain & Shah, 2016), it is not surprising that the medical schools might wish to align their education with what they believe about the intended destinations of those graduates, so reinforcing a tendency towards orientation to the global north:

> Kwame Nkrumah understood that despite formal independence, the influence of the former coloniser on the former colonies remained, by having their systems and policies directed from the outside. (Rashid et al., 2023a)

The flow of medical migration is largely uni-directional, from global south to global north. This 'imperialist appropriation' has been examined in other areas, showing that the economic arguments of 'unequal exchange theory' (Hickel et al., 2022) apply directly to medical migration. According to this view, unequal exchange involves a 'hidden transfer of value' from the global south to the global north. In the case of medical migration, the commodity is not at all hidden.

This process reinforces the superior economic position of the global north, based on extracting resources from the global south on advantageous and coercive terms.

We can regard medical graduates, or 'embodied labour', as one such commodity, produced at no cost to the global north, while their education is coerced into alignment with global north education through 'medical education imperialism' supported by initiatives that require a substantial fee to ensure that accreditation agencies meet a requirement originally stipulated by the US Educational Commission for Foreign Medical Graduates (Rashid et al., 2023b). Although it might be argued that migrated doctors render remittances to their original homeland (Alsaied & Madueme, 2015), it has been labelled 'ethically deplorable' that medical migration has made a significant contribution to the health workforce crises in developing countries, while strengthening the already stable healthcare provision of destination countries (Nwagwu, 2015). Despite this, medical migration will play a role in creating the concerns that Syed Moin Ali expresses.

The Contradictions

In this chapter, the drive for development of medical education for the purposes of national improvement becomes entwined with the pressures of globalisation, post-colonial habits, and medical migration. These are complex and powerful forces that define the role and identity of medical education, when pitted against the development of professional medical educationalists that the author supports and worries about. For a full critical understanding, the issues discussed here must be thought about, but it may well be too great a challenge to acquire a social science method of critical thinking when the content of a medical educationalist's kit of skills and knowledge, must be mastered in the relatively short time that it takes to gain an MHPE and be in a position to facilitate the adoption of others' practices.

There is a business case for many medical schools around the 'fast' demonstration of education 'fashion', if that means a market advantage and greater likelihood that students aspiring to emigrate will apply for a place. For a person such as the author, who wishes to develop the production of medical graduates for his own country, but trains the medical educationalists who then simply apply what they believe, rightly or wrongly, to be the practices of the global north, this is a painful contradiction.

References

Alatas, S. F. (1993). On the indigenization of academic discourse. *Alternatives: Global, Local, Political, 18*(3), 307–338.

Ali, K., McColl, E., Tredwin, C., Hanks, S., Coelho, C., & Witton, R. (2021). Addressing racial inequalities in dental education: Decolonising the dental curricula. *British Dental Journal, 230*(3), 165–169. https://doi.org/10.1038/s41415-020-2598-z

Alsaied, T., & Madueme, P. C. (2015). International medical graduates in cardiology fellowship. *Journal of the American College of Cardiology, 65*(5), 507–510. https://doi.org/10.1016/j. jacc.2014.12.012

Arday, J., Belluigi, D. Z., & Thomas, D. (2021). Attempting to break the chain: Reimaging inclusive pedagogy and decolonising the curriculum within the academy. *Educational Philosophy and Theory, 53*(3), 298–313. https://doi.org/10.1080/00131857.2020.1773257

Atalas, S. F. (2005). Indigenization: Features and problems. In *Asian anthropology* (1st ed., pp. 227–243). Routledge.

Bleakley, A., Brice, J., & Bligh, J. (2008). Thinking the post-colonial in medical education. *Medical Education, 42*(3), 266–270. https://doi.org/10.1111/j.1365-2923.2007.02991.x

Bracken, P., Fernando, S., Alsaraf, S., Creed, M., Double, D., Gilberthorpe, T., Hassan, R., Jadhav, S., Jeyapaul, P., Kopua, D., Parsons, M., Rodger, J., Summerfield, D., Thomas, P., & Timimi, S. (2021). Decolonising the medical curriculum: Psychiatry faces particular challenges. *Anthropology & Medicine, 28*(4), 420–428. https://doi.org/10.1080/13648470.2021.1949892

Brunner, C. (2021). Conceptualizing epistemic violence: An interdisciplinary assemblage for IR. *International Politics Reviews, 9*(1), 193–212. https://doi.org/10.1057/s41312-021-00086-1

Dewey, J. (1938). *Experience in education*. Macmillan.

Dhillon, S. (2021, September). An immanent critique of decolonisation projects. *Convivial Thinking*. https://convivialthinking.org/index.php/2021/09/25/critique-of-decolonisation-projects/

Finn, G. M., Danquah, A., & Matthan, J. (2022). Colonization, cadavers, and color: Considering decolonization of anatomy curricula. *The Anatomical Record, 305*(4), 938–951. https://doi.org/10.1002/ar.24855

Gishen, F., & Lokugamage, A. (2019). Diversifying the medical curriculum. *BMJ, l300*, l300. https://doi.org/10.1136/bmj.l300

Gottweis, H., & Prainsack, B. (2006). Emotion in political discourse: Contrasting approaches to stem cell governance in the USA, UK, Israel and Germany. *Regenerative Medicine, 1*(6), 823–829. https://doi.org/10.2217/17460751.1.6.823

Hartland, J., & Larkai, E. (2020). Decolonising medical education and exploring white fragility. *BJGP open, 4*(5), BJGPO.2020.0147. https://doi.org/10.3399/BJGPO.2020.0147

Hickel, J., Dorninger, C., Wieland, H., & Suwandi, I. (2022). Imperialist appropriation in the world economy: Drain from the global south through unequal exchange, 1990–2015. *Global Environmental Change, 73*, 1–13. https://doi.org/10.1016/j.gloenvcha.2022.102467

Horton, R. (2003). *Health wars: On the global front lines of modern medicine*. Review Books.

Hossain, N., & Shah, N. (2016). Physicians' migration: Perceptions of Pakistani medical students. *Journal of the College of Physicians and Surgeons–Pakistan, 26*(8), 696–701. https://www.researchgate.net/publication/307887892

Jimenez, A., & Roberts, T. (2019). *Decolonising neo-liberal innovation: Using the Andean philosophy of 'Buen Vivir' to reimagine innovation hubs*. Springer International Publishing. https://doi.org/10.1007/978-3-030-19115-3_15

Logan, M. H. (1977). Part Five: Anthropological research on the hot-cold theory of disease: Some methodological suggestions. *Medical Anthropology, 1*(4), 87–112. https://doi.org/10.1080/01459740.1977.9965830

Lokugamage, A. U., Ahillan, T., & Pathberiya, S. D. C. (2020). Decolonising ideas of healing in medical education. *Journal of Medical Ethics, 46*(4), 265–272. https://doi.org/10.1136/medethics-2019-105866

Lupton, D. (2012). *Medicine as culture: Illness, disease and the body* (3rd revised ed.). Sage.

Lupton, D. (2013). The cultural assumptions behind Western medicine. *The Conversation*. https://theconversation.com/the-cultural-assumptions-behind-western-medicine-7533

Meinhof, M. (2018). Contesting Chinese modernity? Postcoloniality and discourses on modernisation at a Chinese university campus. *Postcolonial Studies, 21*(4), 469–484. https://doi.org/10.1080/13688790.2018.1507620

Moghli, M. A., & Kadiwal, L. (2021). Decolonising the curriculum beyond the surge: Conceptualisation, positionality and conduct. *London Review of Education, 19*(1), 10.14324/LRE.19.1.23.

Naidu, T., & Kumagai, A. K. (2016). Troubling muddy waters. *Academic Medicine, 91*(3), 317–321. https://doi.org/10.1097/ACM.0000000000001019

Nazar, M., Kendall, K., Day, L., & Nazar, H. (2015). Decolonising medical curricula through diversity education: Lessons from students. *Medical Teacher, 37*(4), 385–393. https://doi.org/10.3109/0142159X.2014.947938

Nwagwu, E. O. C. (2015). Migration of international medical graduates: Implications for the brain-drain. *Open Medicine Journal, 2*, 17–24.

Odeh, L. E. (2012). A comparative analysis of global north and south economics. *International Journal of Current Research in the Humanities, 14*, 67–82.

Rashid, M. A., Ali, S. M., & Dharanipragada, K. (2023a). Decolonising medical education regulation: A global view. *BMJ Global Health, 8*(6), e011622. https://doi.org/10.1136/bmjgh-2022-011622

Rashid, M. A., Naidu, T., Wondimagegn, D., & Whitehead, C. (2023b). Reconsidering a global agency for medical education: Back to the drawing board? *Teaching and Learning in Medicine, 1–8*, 676–683. https://doi.org/10.1080/10401334.2023.2259363

Rossi, E., & Táíwò, O. O. (2020). What's new about woke racial capitalism (and what isn't). *SPE Journal*. https://spectrejournal.com/whats-new-about-woke-racial-capitalism-and-what-isnt/

Scholte, J. A. (2007). Defining globalisation. *The World Economy, 3*(11), 1471–1502. https://doi.org/10.1111/j.1467-9701.2007.01019.x

Schön, D. A. (1984). *The reflective practitioner: How professionals think in action*. Basic Books.

Sefa Dei, G. J., & Cacciavillani, A. (2024). Actualizing decolonization: A case for anticolonizing and indigenizing the curriculum. *Journal of Philosophy of Education, 58*(2–3), 209–226. https://doi.org/10.1093/jopedu/qhae036

Shahjahan, R. A., Estera, A. L., Surla, K. L., & Edwards, K. T. (2022). "Decolonizing" curriculum and pedagogy: A comparative review across disciplines and global higher education contexts. *Review of Educational Research, 92*(1), 73–113. https://doi.org/10.3102/00346543211042423

Stadler, D. J., Archuleta, S., Cofrancesco, J., & Ibrahim, H. (2019). Successful international medical education research collaboration. *Journal of Graduate Medical Education, 11*(4s), 187–189. https://doi.org/10.4300/JGME-D-18-01061

Tudor, A. (2021). Decolonizing trans/gender studies? *TSQ: Transgender Studies Quarterly, 8*(2), 238–256. https://doi.org/10.1215/23289252-8890523

Wong, H. Y. C., & See, C. (2021). Curriculum decolonisation in 3…2…1…. *The Clinical Teacher, 18*(5), 497–499. https://doi.org/10.1111/tct.13385

Syed Moin Ali works in the Department of Educational Development, Aga Khan University, Karachi, Pakistan. He is medically qualified and has worked internationally for much of his career. He has held key positions in medical leadership training, and in national and international regulation. He has special interests in teaching and learning, assessment, innovative curricular designs and use of technology for education.

II.ii STATEMENT: Standardisation: The Root of the Flat Curve

Samar Ahmed

Once upon a time in history, there existed medical schools with a beautiful and probably very efficient apprenticeship system where students learned by doing, were supervised, and mentored and had role models. This was long before the world ever knew about 'general and transferable skills'. As time passed, more and more structure was introduced to make sure that all students were given 'equal opportunities' to learn. So, the main fascination was with making sure that students in one class all learned the same things, but very little effort was applied to ensure that the methods of standardisation promised students the same values, quality and mentorship that was given to their ancestors.

Being an educator in the medical field for the past 20 years, I have come to observe progress in the field of medical education and its growth in the world of medical schools. This influence is exponentially growing, but with little evidence of parallel growth in the value added to learning or in the quality of the graduate. This does not mean that there is no improvement in education happening, but it seems to me that the more medical education grows as a discipline, the more isolated the people in this field get from the educational practitioners. This calls for a pause to reflect on the essence of what is being sold to us as good medical education practice over the past two decades.

S. Ahmed (✉)
Faculty of Medicine, Forensic Medicine Department, Ain Shams University, Cairo, Egypt

Rabdan Academy, United Arab Emirates
e-mail: Samarazim@gmail.com

J. Grant, L. Grant (eds.), *The Contradictions of Medical Education*, https://doi.org/10.1007/978-3-031-90394-6_6

1   The Flexner Report, Standardisation and Identity

Ever since the much-criticised Flexner report, there has been a march towards standardisation of medical education (Bailey, 2017). Standardisation is a concept of quality that originates from product quality control and originated in the engineering industry. The Flexner report that was sequentially issued from 1910 to 1940 made the assumption that the quality standards approach applied to product lines will also apply to education. The aftermath of this report is the escalating reliance on standards and structure in education for healthcare professions (Beck, 2004).

The Flexner Report was an ambitious attempt to standardise medical education across North America, based on the philosophy that basic sciences and clinical experience were fundamental to producing effective physicians. Schools all over the world, not just in the United States of America, started 'conforming' to the Flexner recommendations, which themselves owed a lot to the German university system and its values (Bonner, 1997), working their way towards implementing a Flexnerian system (Kirch, 2010). Even though structure is important, it comes with a cost. Innovation and adaptability can be put at risk by too much structure (Martínez-León & Martínez-García, 2011). For years, schools have struggled to keep their own individual professional identity and to identify areas of professional excellence they can promise their candidates. This is something that we have been dealing with and approaching, as others have (Monrad et al., 2019), as you would approach a polarity (two seemingly opposing values that can complement each other when applied in a balanced way) rather than an either-or solution.

2   Mapping and Aligning Curricula, and Its Effects

In response to medical education trends, medical schools started mapping their curricula, identifying their objectives, and aligning them with teaching and assessment methods. But often, it seemed, documentation became a mission in itself. The time consumed in making sure that this alignment fell into place, together with the effort, started to sometimes deduct from time invested in making education a worthwhile experience for students. A statement in our part of the world became very famous: "Quality assurance work is for the quality assurance unit, what goes on paper is what they ask for.... What we do in the classroom is our job!" So, an unfortunate double personality sometimes invaded our schools, which most probably was not there before. This is a negative effect of too much standardised structure or maybe of abuse of standardised structure.

3   Becoming Identical

It seems that the more we progress in time and grow farther away from the standardising Flexner era, we grow more identical, applying common methods, such as integration, that Flexner would not have liked. And when we see that we are not identical enough, we pressure ourselves and others to become identical. Being compliant and identical is obviously a safer choice that many educators, and thus their schools, are reverting to in order, they feel, to gain international acceptance.

The unique face of local medical education started to disappear especially in urban schools that then found it difficult to identify their educational 'competitive advantage', as strategic plan templates called it. Schools sometimes found it hard to identify their area of unique impact to express in their vision, when they had been struggling to 'standardise' education and call things by their 'proper' names that everyone else also uses. It might become difficult to remember what made each of our schools who we were and what identified us before this standardisation.

4   Global Ranking

Many other tools of modern education have added fuel to the fire of standardisation, including global ranking and the obsession that comes with it. Schools are no longer living their mission but rather are in a race to excel. The values of competition and excellence in relation to the ranking race was probably dictated by the need of schools to build their reputation in order to attract international students who are now a major source of income for schools. This is what happens when schools are looked at in terms of return on investment—a concept from industry that was squeezed into the picture of medical education without much thought about the consequences (Davey et al., 2013).

With medical schools on a well-set racing track towards acknowledgement by 'ranking' agencies, conformity became the rule, and it seemed that the priority is not to improve education or educational outcomes but rather to climb the ranking ladder. The need for internationalisation of medical schools was one corollary of this, pushing schools farther and farther away from the original community-orientated mission they once vowed to fulfil.

5   Decreasing Freedom to Teach

Faculty (teachers) in medical schools have long been the most respected group, and granted a large amount of freedom to educate to their own preference. From being totally autonomous for so long, my belief is that the education system started to worry about too much freedom in educational decision making. With the need to monitor, developed the need to standardise faculty practices accompanied by faculty development initiatives, and to give guidelines for getting things done. After these years of 'too much standardisation', I believe we are seeing its limitations.

The main dilemma that is haunting medical schools now is not about structure alone but also the underuse of cumulative expertise and common sense. In an attempt to standardise more and more, faculty seem now to refrain from using any independent, informed decision-making with the understanding that using models from elsewhere is a safer choice. I am not sure how much good this can be for the educational process.

Models were often introduced to faculty in medical education programmes that are common in the world of medical educators at that time. Such training programmes, in my experience, are often content-based and seem to offer very little emphasis on reflection on learning or critical thinking about teaching. This is rather ironic when people are supposed to be learning how to become better educators and how to incorporate more critical thinking into their curricula. Overwhelming participants with educational terminology and definitions is surely not as important as understanding the essence of education in the medical profession and building on the voice of experience, context, and local needs. Some benefit of this medical education literacy cannot be denied, yet the potential harm done by reliance on standardised training that is out of context, cannot be overlooked either, as others have noted (Huang Hoon et al., 2019). One unintended (or perhaps intended) consequence seems to be that our medical schools are becoming replicas of other institutions, sometimes striving to reach excellence by adopting ready-made curricula or models from other contexts.

Perhaps faculty are getting more and more trapped in models of curriculum, and programme evaluation and assessment, and have stopped reflecting independently on value and enquiry. And yet, all teachers can draw on their thinking skills and decision-making capabilities, rather than all being subjugated by the same guidelines and twelve tips for doing their jobs.

6   Conformity and Getting Back on Track

Standardisation is becoming important in the everyday life of medical schools, often being viewed as a necessary hurdle. To me, the unrealistic implementation and felt need to conform are hurting education more than the actual standards, models and guidelines that exist. These are developed to help education and to allow for voluntary local use and interpretation, rather than to constrain innovation. But there is a fine line between overuse of standards, models and guidelines and using them for the good of the educational process. They are not to be used for blindly building a prescribed educational experience but rather for supporting our contextual experience in our medical schools, coming from years of cumulative exposure to health needs, and for evaluating our practice, perhaps, if the standards are appropriate.

We will be back on track when we start thinking again of our students and what they will be able to offer patients rather than the ranking of our schools or modelling them on others' practice or the latest educational fashion.

We will be back on track when we stop treating medical education as a product line and using the exact same set of quality standards and methods that are not designed for improvement in our context. We need to use faculty development to free our teachers to get back in touch with their learners and check on their learning experience.

What needs to be done, in my opinion, is for schools to take a step back and think more about their missions and how they can reach outside their walls into the communities they serve. For years, universities, and specifically medical schools, were considered the centrepiece of the communities that host them. Before falling into the trap of recognition and acceptance, the only agency a medical school had to impress was their community. Although it is not true everywhere, in my experience, this reflected on community health and for a long period of time we did not have to examine schools for social accountability nor was social accountability a part of any medical curriculum, simply because there was no reason for schools not to be socially accountable. They thrived on affecting community health long before there was international recognition, 'global' standards and methods, and ranking agencies on the table.

References

Bailey, M. (2017). The Flexner report: Standardizing medical students through region-, gender-, and race-based hierarchies. *American Journal of Law & Medicine, 43*(2–3), 209–223. https://doi.org/10.1177/0098858817723660

Beck, A. H. (2004). The Flexner report and the standardization of American medical education. *JAMA: The Journal of the American Medical Association, 291*(17), 2139–2140. https://doi.org/10.1001/jama.291.17.2139

Bonner, T. N. (1997). Abraham Flexner and the German university: The progressive as traditionalist. *Paedagogica Historica, 33*(1), 99–116. https://doi.org/10.1080/0030923970330105

Davey, P., Tully, V., Grant, A., Day, R., Ker, J., Marr, C., Mires, G., & Nathwani, D. (2013). Learning from errors: What is the return on investment from training medical students in incident review? *Clinical Risk, 19*(1), 1–5. https://doi.org/10.1177/1356262213476675

Huang Hoon, C., Mighty, J., Roxå, T., Deane Sorcinelli, M., & DiPietro, M. (2019). 'The danger of a single story:' A reflection on institutional change, voices, identities, power, and outcomes. *International Journal for Academic Development, 24*(2), 97–108. https://doi.org/10.1080/1360144X.2019.1594239

Kirch, D. G. (2010). Commentary: The Flexnerian legacy in the 21st century. *Academic Medicine, 85*(2), 190–192. https://doi.org/10.1097/ACM.0b013e3181c9a5d1

Martínez-León, I. M., & Martínez-García, J. A. (2011). The influence of organizational structure on organizational learning. *International Journal of Manpower, 32*(5/6), 537–566. https://doi.org/10.1108/01437721111158198

Monrad, S. U., Mangrulkar, R. S., Woolliscroft, J. O., Daniel, M. M., Hartley, S. E., Gay, T. L., Highet, A., Vijayakumar, N., & Santen, S. A. (2019). Competency committees in undergraduate medical education. *Academic Medicine, 94*(12), 1865–1872. https://doi.org/10.1097/ACM.0000000000002816

II.ii COMMENTARY: Globalisation, Corporatisation, and Alienation in Medical Education

Janet Grant and Leonard Grant

In this narrative, Samar Ahmed makes important personal observations that call into question the mission of medical education and its effects. She identifies medical education as a standardising force, 'selling' practices around the world which derive solely from the global north. She argues that schools prefer to be compliant and identical rather than pursuing their own contextual individuality, and reflecting this, that global ranking is seen as important (implying that proof of meeting global standards is necessary).

What factors weave these issues together?

Standards and Standardisation

The contradictions of standardisation have been widely discussed in the literature beyond medical education. The issues that bother Samar Ahmed have also been of concern in other fields. For example, it has been pointed out that in management, models such Total Quality Management can be fraught with '…'hidden' contradictions in the form of ambiguous strategies and discourses' (Harnesk & Abrahamsson, 2007) around issues such as 'collectivism versus individualism', 'manipulation versus empowerment' and 'standardization versus innovative learning' (Harnesk & Abrahamsson, 2007). These certainly chime with the Samar Ahmed's concerns.

Just as standards and models in education are often a reflection of current dominant values rather than evidence, so are those in management, cycling from a 'social-normative' focus on the hierarchical power relationship between leaders and workers, to the 'rational-instrumental' approach that focuses on 'controlling productivity through surveillance and improvement of methods, to a strategical design of the formal structures' (Harnesk & Abrahamsson, 2007). Each phase is accompanied by appropriate training of leaders and workers. The same cycle can be seen in medical education's thinking and actions about the relationship between international bodies and local systems, teachers and learners, and the design of curricula, and their accompanying 'faculty development'. Regardless of how these ideas change, however, their effect will be limited by material conditions.

Given that such ideas derive, ultimately, from the historical, political, and economic conditions that control society at any one time (Williams, 1977), and that at this stage of history, much of the world is still experiencing the disproportionate political and economic influence of the formerly and currently economic and cultural imperial countries of the global north, it is not surprising that concerns are expressed by an author from the global south. Given this, and the tensions that

Samar Ahmed describes, we should consider what is both constraining medical schools and forcing them towards standardisation.

However, we should first decide whether standards and standardisation are the same thing. An authoritative sociological analysis of this issue is pertinent to the case of medical education (Timmermans & Epstein, 2010). These authors:

> … place standards and standardization in the foreground as ubiquitous but underestimated phenomena that help regulate and calibrate social life by rendering the modern world equivalent across cultures, time, and geography.

For these authors:

> Standards and standardization are thus omnipresent conduits of a modernizing and globalizing world.

They go on to raise 'sharp questions' about the concerns that standardisation raises for democracy, about how to hold standard setters to account, and who those standard setters should be, about who benefits from standards, about what evidence is sufficient or necessary to implement standards, and about the consequences of standardisation in relation to individual and local concerns. And finally:

> … what does it mean to be nonstandard in a world where standards reign.

These questions are all relevant and important for medical education and remain to be addressed, as does the difference between standards and standardisation. Standards can be seen as a statement of what should or could be done or achieved. In education, this is likely to vary across contexts and cultures. In contrast, standardisation, which derives from the nineteenth century development of science and industry, means uniformity of practice and outcomes (Williams, 1985).

No comparative analysis of standards for medical education is available. It might be that local and national standards do often adhere to the global 'popular culture' and stipulate, for example, that some specific curriculum type or currently fashionable teaching and learning methods, or curriculum designs, should be used, but, nonetheless, choosing to follow the latest unproven global trend is not mandatory, but is a local decision. Nonetheless:

> Just as the choice of one standard over another signals a preference for a specific logic and set of priorities, so the choice of standards of any sort implies one way of regulating and coordinating social life at the expense of alternative modes. (Timmermans & Epstein, 2010)

Although Samar Ahmed writes about her own region, we cannot assume that forces for standardisation are not also working in other parts of the global south and the global north. It is for every school to interrogate its own decisions, and the reasons for them, in the light of its own context. A good rule of thumb is that any change process should begin with an identified and agreed problem (Gale & Grant, 1997): and not following others' practices is not a problem!

Samar Ahmed links the attempt at standardisation with a loss of 'freedom to educate to their own preference'. This is where we can see the necessity of unlinking standards and standardisation. Standards, to be meaningful and not oppressive, should be debated, developed and updated by practitioners, within their own educational context. Although taking a universal set of standards may be a useful starting point for any discussion, it cannot be the end nor the idealised endpoint. Standardisation, which has the goal of uniform production, regardless of its context of origin, will undoubtedly produce these feelings of alienation that Samar Ahmed articulates. In social processes such as education, the goal of uniform production could be seen as counter-cultural.

The question we wish to address now is: What are the forces that tend medical schools towards this standardisation, given that it is clearly not serving educators and practitioners, nor the students they teach nor the context they serve?

Corporatisation

The root of the problem could be seen as a form of medical education imperialism (Bleakley et al., 2008) exerted by the global north upon the global south.

Or perhaps it is a form of corporatisation of medical education, just as medicine itself has been corporatised in parts of the global north, causing moral distress whereby practitioners are unable to act according to their own core values (Beck et al., 2022). Corporatisation of higher education has been widely discussed (Burke, 2021; Robertson, 2010), one aspect of which is seen in institutions attempting to situate themselves within a 'marketplace', by applying the standards of that marketplace, and training employees to meet those standards thus giving the institution an advantage in any benchmarking activity. For medical education, given the international market in medical graduates, that marketplace may be thought of as the entire world which in turn, is interpreted as the global north.

Samar Ahmed describes these processes occurring in relation to the global compliance of medical schools in her country, enacted, for example, in faculty development to achieve standardisation and the adoption of alien curriculum models and practices. She thinks that medical schools should be answerable to 'their community', so perhaps the pertinent question is who or what constitutes that community? It would seem that the 'community' that many medical schools now choose to be answerable to is an international community, forged out of a history of ideas derived in one part of the world, not out of local democratic collaboration. Beginning from Flexner is an insightful position: Flexner himself was of the view that the medical workforce in the US should be homogeneous with the archetype a wealthy, white man from the northern states. It is this history upon which medical education is said to rest (Bailey, 2017). The analogy now extends globally.

Alienation

From the author's depiction, we might imagine that there may also be a process of personal alienation occurring. Downgrading teachers' knowledge and experience in favour of an international view, may induce this feeling of powerlessness in relation to their own work, whereby they are trained and constrained to implement systems and methods that are not their own and may be from an incompatible culture. This process has been identified among teachers in other areas of education (Orr, 2012; Tsang, 2018).

It has been powerfully argued elsewhere, following the work of Lawrence Stenhouse (Stenhouse, 1975) that rather than feeling that teachers are in need of 'faculty development', they should be regarded as the primary 'truth teller' when it comes to teaching and learning: so it should be that:

> The medical educationalist is no longer the primary source of knowledge, or the impartial researcher, but is the means of supporting authentic practice development, helping each teacher to find their own truth. (Grant, 2023)

Such a view rejects the risk of alienation.

Or perhaps in Samar Ahmed's account, there are elements of all these problems. In any case, the result is medical schools outside the global north accepting those, perhaps alien, standards, perhaps wanting their graduates to have the option of working in the global north. Or perhaps simply wanting to be able to compete and fit in with the global medical education community in which the global north is dominant. Emulation of the standards imposed, or models promoted, will follow.

What would a medical school look like without these constraints?

Why Comply?

Samar Ahmed's narrative describes concerns about lack of evidence for recommended changes, the gulf between medical education specialists and teachers, standardisation and conformity that ignore local contexts and needs, structure that stifles innovation, internal focus on developing medical education practice and improving global rankings rather than external focus on the community served, disempowerment and decline in the autonomy of teachers to develop their own practice based on their own experience and expertise, and conformity that denies contextual imperatives. Underpinning all this seems to be, in the author's view, globalisation distributed through faculty development.

Despite all these issues, faculty development and accreditation of institutions against externally and sometimes globally, defined standards are common to medical education everywhere. That being so, we might wonder why there is so much compliance with these largely evidence-light practices, given that there are also concerns. Why is there no form of post-colonial resistance (Shahjahan, 2014)?

There is no research in medical education to help us answer this question. The analysis of compliance and lack of resistance remains to be conducted.

Global Rankings

In this account, global rankings are cited as another alien, imposed system which militates for standardisation of practice:

> Higher education development in the global south remains to a large extent tethered to the institutional model spearheaded in the West, reinforcing the intellectual dominance of Euro-America and the subordination of peripheral countries. (Zhou & Wu, 2016)

There is no reason to assume that demonstrating individuality would automatically cause a decline against the criteria for global rankings (Aithal & Kumar, 2020), if that is important. However, those criteria typically address teaching and learning, research and publications, citations, international profile and activity, and externally generated income, guiding development in those directions rather than in the direction of local values, communities and cultures. In relation to these, four contradictions have been identified for universities in the global south which may give rise to the alienation of academic staff:

- research versus teaching, whereby '....as research outputs are prized at a higher premium, the commitment to improving teaching becomes more and more difficult'
- looking outward versus inward, whereby '...the dominance of Western universalism in knowledge production in Asia is underpinned by a deep sense of ambivalence where the West is both an object of desire and resentment, both a source of critique and emulation, an ultimate other against which one's own sense of self is measured'
- quality versus quantity, whereby speed of production (of teaching or research, for example) is more important than quality of the activity
- egalitarianism versus hierarchy, whereby the European intellectual tradition tends towards liberalism while '.....in some settings, hierarchy may be favored over autonomy to achieve significant results in a compressed timeframe (Zhou & Wu, 2016).

All these contradictions, if resolved in favour of global rankings and criteria that were developed in another culture for another reason, may militate against the professional satisfaction of academic staff.

However, we should take a step back and consider, what is the purpose of a global ranking system in medical education? What is the benefit of participating in such a ranking system? On the face of it, the existence of a ranking system must be to compare institutions. There are two relevant consequences to consider. Firstly, a 'global' medical school would be able to offer migration opportunities to its graduates. It is well documented that British and the US healthcare services rely heavily on doctors trained abroad (most often in the global south). Secondly, a 'global' medical school would be able to attract international students and, potentially, international funding which is a very strong incentive, especially in countries historically affected by underdevelopment. The economic context of medical education in the global south is, unfortunately, not only the local context but also the international.

The Principal Contradiction: Global Versus Contextual

In reflecting on the effects of the field of medical education, its global north identity, its standards and standardisation, and the constant concern with global rankings of universities, Samar Ahmed develops an analysis of forces that, to her, are creating a distance between the medical school and its local community, and are disrespecting the autonomy, expertise and experience of teachers in conducting their educational task. The factors in this concern globalisation vs contextualisation, standards vs standardisation, local orientation vs compliance with global ideas in medical education, and the teacher as operative vs the teacher as autonomous, reflective professional.

Samar Ahmed's concerns suggest that the principal contradiction of globalised medical education creates a situation where medical schools cannot be truly local and contextual, where standards cannot be set through democratic process, where local orientation and individual teacher expression are constrained.

These problems are located at different levels: global vs. international, national vs. community, and technical expert vs. individual practitioner. They are all related in the reflection presented in this chapter. How these are tackled could create further contradictions by imposing global and external training or consultancy to address the local issues, or they could be resolved by liberating and empowering teachers and medical schools to focus on their own tasks, aspirations and communities, for themselves, rather than directing their gaze at global medical education.

References

Aithal, P. S., & Kumar, P. M. (2020). Global ranking and its implications in higher education. *SCHOLEDGE International Journal of Business Policy and Governance, 7*(3), 25–47.

Bailey, M. (2017). The Flexner report: Standardizing medical students through region-, gender-, and race-based hierarchies. *American Journal of Law & Medicine, 43*(2–3), 209–223. https://doi.org/10.1177/0098858817723660

Beck, J., Falco, C. N., O'Hara, K. L., Bassett, H. K., Randall, C. L., Cruz, S., Hanson, J. L., Dean, W., & Senturia, K. (2022). The norms and corporatization of medicine influence physician moral distress in the United States. *Teaching and Learning in Medicine, 1–11*. https://doi.org/1 0.1080/10401334.2022.2056740

Bleakley, A., Brice, J., & Bligh, J. (2008). Thinking the post-colonial in medical education. *Medical Education, 42*(3), 266–270. https://doi.org/10.1111/j.1365-2923.2007.02991.x

Burke, P. J. (2021). Gender, neoliberalism, and corporatized higher education. In N. S. Niemi & M. B. Weaver-Hightower (Eds.), *The Wiley handbook of gender equity in higher education* (pp. 69–90). Wiley. https://doi.org/10.1002/9781119257639.ch4

Gale, R., & Grant, J. (1997). AMEE medical education guide no. 10: Managing change in a medical context: Guidelines for action. *Medical Teacher, 19*(4), 11 (239–249).

Grant, J. (2023). The scholarship of teaching: Who is the truth teller? *The Asia Pacific Scholar, 8*(2), 83–85. https://doi.org/10.29060/TAPS.2023-8-2/PV2874

Harnesk, R., & Abrahamsson, L. (2007). TQM: An act of balance between contradictions. *The TQM Magazine, 19*(6), 531–540. https://doi.org/10.1108/09544780710828395

Orr, K. (2012). Coping, confidence and alienation: The early experience of trainee teachers in English further education. *Journal of Education for Teaching, 38*(1), 51–65. https://doi.org/10.1080/02607476.2012.643656

Robertson, S. L. (2010). Corporatisation, competitiveness, commercialisation: New logics in the globalising of UK higher education. *Globalisation, Societies and Education, 8*(2), 191–203. https://doi.org/10.1080/14767721003776320

Shahjahan, R. A. (2014). From 'no' to 'yes': Postcolonial perspectives on resistance to neoliberal higher education. *Discourse: Studies in the Cultural Politics of Education, 35*(2), 219–232. https://doi.org/10.1080/01596306.2012.745732

Stenhouse, L. (1975). *An introduction to curriculum Research and Development.* Heinemann.

Timmermans, S., & Epstein, S. (2010). A world of standards but not a standard world: Toward a sociology of standards and standardization. *Annual Review of Sociology, 36*(1), 69–89. https://doi.org/10.1146/annurev.soc.012809.102629

Tsang, K. K. (2018). Teacher alienation in Hong Kong. *Discourse: Studies in the Cultural Politics of Education, 39*(3), 335–346. https://doi.org/10.1080/01596306.2016.1261084

Williams, R. (1977). *Marxism and literature.* Oxford University Press.

Williams, R. (1985). *Keywords: A vocabulary of culture and society.* Oxford University Press.

Zhou, Y., & Wu, J. (2016). The game plan: Four contradictions in the development of world class universities from the global south. *Education and Science, 41*(184), 75–89.

Samar Ahmed, the author of this personal reflection is a leader in education reform across the Middle East. With over 25 years of experience in academic leadership, she has held multiple senior positions, including Vice President for Quality Assurance and Accreditation at Ain Shams University, and Associate Dean for Academic Affairs at Dubai Medical College for Girls. She is currently Professor and Senior Education Specialist at Rabdan Academy, Abu Dhabi. She is an expert in curriculum design, inclusive education, and aligning reforms with contextual needs. A key contributor to regional and international collaborations, she has played a pivotal role in advancing medical education research and establishing global accreditation standards.

II.iii STATEMENT: Greater Than the Sum: International Partnerships in Medical Education

Mohammed Ahmed Rashid

Aristotle's expression *'The whole is greater than the sum of its parts'* is widely used to emphasise the importance of synergy and partnership. This notion could be seen as central to medical education in a modern and globalised world, as it has become increasingly apparent that collective action between medical schools, universities, hospitals, and other organisations, is critical to achieving impactful outcomes in health and education around the world. 'Co-operation' and 'collaboration' are becoming familiar bywords in the many discussions about global medical education development which increasingly explore how the mechanics of powerful partnerships might influence the future of global development. Over the last decade, I have worked within a wide range of international partnerships in medical education, spanning countries and continents, across the undergraduate-postgraduate-CPD spectrum, working with students and staff, while utilising a variety of partnership models. Here, I will examine what I have observed, experienced and learned through this time.

1 The Nature of Partnership

Although there is no universal definition of 'partnership working', we can understand it as a process in which two or more organisations work together towards shared goals, with the aim of achieving more than they could as individual organisations. Such relationships may emerge around a specific theme or between organisations that already share similar values and goals. Partnerships often develop organically, without a clearly defined vision at their outset.

M. A. Rashid (✉)
London School of Hygiene and Tropical Medicine, London, UK
e-mail: ahmed.rashid@lshtm.ac.uk

© The Author(s), under exclusive license to Springer Nature Switzerland AG 2026
J. Grant, L. Grant (eds.), *The Contradictions of Medical Education*,
https://doi.org/10.1007/978-3-031-90394-6_7

93

Many different models of partnership exist. At the more informal and loosely connected end, co-operations might focus on periodic exchanges of information or people. At the more formal and coordinated end, close collaborations are likely to include a tighter integration of two (or more) organisations, underpinned by contractual and financial agreements. These types of partnerships are likely to include more sophisticated and sizeable governance, management and delivery team structures to ensure the partnership stays on track and that objectives are realised.

2 Partership, Power and Harm in International Collaborations

Medical education straddles the vast and complex fields of healthcare and education, each of which varies considerably around the world because of sociocultural, economic and technical differences. The perennial danger of international partnerships in medical education, therefore, is that policies and practices can be hastily and inappropriately implemented through a 'lift and shift' model that can lead to unintended harm. This creates an imperative for those involved on either side of a partnership to actively counter this possibility by understanding the nuances of their own political and practical context.

So we must consider what matters and what should matter to those seeking partnerships in medical education, the fundamental importance of relational factors in partnership working, and the moral and ethical backdrop in which financial decisions about partnerships should be taken.

For much of the twentieth century, development was the guiding principle for social policy in low- and middle-income countries, with institutions, professionals, and ideas from high-income countries offering support and guidance to achieve economic growth and prosperity. In recent years, though, thinkers from many parts of the world have challenged the assumption that this apparent development is only possible with some outside assistance or intervention. There has also been a recognition that it is impossible to understand the modern world without seeing it through the historical prism of colonialism that has shaped global systems of power and knowledge. Given the realities of previous global exploitation and harm and their enduring effects on the world, an underlying philosophy of meaningful friendship should underpin any international partnership in medical education, and a scholarly interrogation of practice should be embedded in any partnership to shine a critical light on unintended consequences and potential harm.

What does matter, and what should matter?

3   Values

Although medical education journals are filled with articles about egalitarianism, widening participation, social responsibility, and other worthwhile issues, this values-based scholarship is not always mirrored in the real-world practice of medical education. Whilst the work that is taking place to make medical education fairer and more equitable is laudable, the brutal reality is that in some ways, the landscape remains much the same as it was over a century ago when Abraham Flexner lamented the commercialisation of medical schools in North America, but perhaps did little to advance social justice.

Overwhelmingly, values should be the most important motivational factor. An in-depth understanding of the local context of the partner is not crucial at the outset but with a genuine interest, this will develop as the relationship establishes itself by getting to know the politics, religious holidays, cultural practices, culinary highlights, and sporting interests in the partner's local setting.

4   Profit, Philanthropy and Competition

As a career in medicine remains highly desirable and prestigious all around the world, medical education continues to be a lucrative source of profit. Beyond this financial drive though, the prestige of medicine and the worthiness of improving healthcare means that medical schools are also popular avenues of philanthropy for wealthy individuals and families, perhaps pre-occupied with issues of legacy and image. Although many governments have resisted granting licences for private medical schools, the global medical workforce shortage has caused some to reconsider. But for both private and public schools, the realities of regulatory pressures, admissions targets, and rankings metrics create a highly competitive landscape across the world.

This competitive nature of modern medical education is important as it helps to frame what matters to those seeking international partnerships. The motivation of a medical school leader will depend on what they want to achieve. Anyone designing or developing a medical school wants it to be the best version possible but realistically, the specific focus can vary according to the many stakeholders. For example, a medical school that is run like a corporate business that prioritises profit generation might be motivated by student fee income, which could be enhanced by prestigious affiliations and the associated branding rights. A medical school focussed on moving up in national or international ranking tables, on the other hand, may seek strategic review from an experienced partner to help energise and challenge them to create an improvement plan that is likely to focus on high quality and impactful research. Undoubtedly, enhancing reputation is an enormously powerful overarching motivation factor for many institutions.

5   Understanding Partnership and Power

The reality of international education partnerships is often far different from what one expects when imagining or designing them. They are hard, and at times messy, work for all involved parties and require considerable commitment to enable them to flourish. Those seeking to engage in them should therefore question the values and assumptions that underpin their partnership. Inevitably, power dynamics play a critical role. Educators from an ancient university in a global north country that sits high in international league tables may have a self-confidence or arrogance, fed by the metrics of modern higher education, that colours all their interactions with those from a new university in a global south country that may be fighting to establish itself. It is critically important, then, that those designing and working on partnerships understand and are mindful of these issues. Indeed, a genuine interest and curiosity in the partnership itself, I would argue, should be a primary concern to those seeking to engage in them. Why are these people interested in working with us? Do their values align with our own? Can we see ourselves working together? How will we work together? These fundamental questions are valuable to help understand, in simple terms, whether the partnership may be successful.

6   Competence and Authority

A secondarily important issue is competence. Do the individuals working in this institution have the technical expertise, specialised knowledge (for example, of assessment), operational skills, and decision-making capabilities that are required for the partnership? Furthermore, do they have the delegated authority and institutional support to complete this work and put their skills to use?

7   Relational Factors and Celebration of the Partnership

Whilst partnerships are typically formalised between organisations and departments, it is the individuals involved that animate them and determine their success or otherwise. The concept of international work can be glamorous and may appeal to individuals for a variety of different reasons, including opportunities to travel, progress with one's career and portfolio, and developing new or existing areas for research. Ultimately, though, what matters is that individuals from each side can work together effectively to achieve the aims of the partnership in the light of the complex legal, financial, and academic issues that can emerge.

Working in international partnerships can expose individuals' apparent and real shortcomings. Where it is the most senior individuals within an organisation who are vulnerable to this, it can present a challenge to their credibility as leaders.

International partnerships can disjoint academic hierarchies, as more junior staff from one partner may directly interact with more senior counterparts in their partner institution. This may heighten the tension that comes with differing hierarchies across countries and cultures. There is much potential for unintended harm if relational elements of partnerships are not functioning well.

We can ameliorate this by celebrating partnerships at all given opportunities. Although the involvement between senior leaders may be operationally asymmetrical in the partnership, amplifying successes and landmarks ceremonially with joint leadership teams can send powerful messages to stakeholders within and outside the partnership. Important junctures may include the ceremonial initiation and the formal conclusion of a partnership, but also at key moments including graduation ceremonies, the opening of new buildings, or the achievement of other important milestones.

At the outset of a partnership, the tendency can be to focus on key performance indicators or other metrics that help each partner clarify what 'success' looks like. Whilst this kind of planning and management has benefits, it can shift attention to technical outcomes and neglect the importance of relational factors in terms of the process of achieving outcomes, and as outcomes in themselves. So, not only can strong academic links and relationships help to achieve goals, it can also be a goal in itself by creating a more connected, collaborative partnership.

Focusing on relationships can permeate many aspects of a partnership. When considering staff training and development, for example, leadership and change management may be just as important, as technical topics. Considering individuals' reactions, worries and expectations helps to determine the pace of change and set achievable targets that do not cause disillusionment. This needs to happen longitudinally and continuously throughout a partnership, and not just at the outset. Often, the most useful aspects of a long-term partnership can be moral support and a friendly, external recognition of the hard work and progress that are occurring. Reaching this closeness relies on trust that may take months and years of sincere effort to achieve. Above all, international education partnerships require emotional intelligence and flexibility that allows collaborators to have a clear understanding that they are, indeed, working to the same shared goals.

8 Financial Planning

Medical education is big business. This is not always apparent given the honourable intentions that stakeholders profess to be holding. Nobody seeks to establish a new medical school expressly to prioritise profit, even if that might be an important motivation. In reality, motivations are often quite messy, making it impossible to honestly distinguish the relative importance of different motivational factors for investing in or prioritising medical education.

We must recognise that it is impossible for any international education partnership in medicine to be developed on financially neutral terms. There are costs associated with partnership working, related to, for example, staff time, travel, intellectual property, or brand use. A plethora of partnership models exist, each with its own relative merits and weaknesses, each representing different relative risks and rewards for each partner. All partnerships have an economic and commercial dimension and cannot be conceptualised or planned in a vacuum as many educators would perhaps wish to do. The question, therefore, is where do financial and commercial factors rank in the priority list for each partner?

Whilst individual partners must consider their own institutional priorities and resources, they also must recognise that commercial discussions are influenced by many factors external to each partner, including geopolitics, currency exchange rates, tuition fee affordability, and local education funding support mechanisms. Designing a suitable economic model for a partnership is important and challenging work that will determine how fair and successful it will ultimately be.

A single economic model cannot be applied across different partnerships. As such, academics and clinicians must be part of the financial budgeting process, despite their habitual inclination to avoid that. In particular, they must bring a sense of proportion and honesty to the process, advising transparently about what other options might be available, and what the best 'value-for-money' option would be. They also have a duty to lay out in clear terms what they believe realistic outcomes could be. Whilst it can be helpful to have legal and financial experts contribute to the process of designing a financial plan to underpin an international education partnership, academics and clinicians must remain closely engaged throughout, and do so with a close eye on the values that they want to prioritise and embody.

9   A Friendship Model

Aristotle, whose expression provides the title of this chapter, wrote extensively and famously on friendship, as have philosophers, novelists, poets, and writers from all fields throughout history. Definitions of friendship have been countless and given that it is a seemingly universal human phenomenon across all societies, it is crucial that any account should avoid historical and cultural features. I do not, then, identify friendship with any particular patterns of behaviour that are unique to a specific culture or era.

One important tenet of friendship, which seems to apply regardless of the varying fields and worldviews of those that have written about it, is that friends should care about each other. That is to say, friends should be interested in and invested in one another and experience appropriate emotions accordingly. A friend should feel joy in their friends' successes, disappointment in their friends' failures, and importantly, should have an overriding goal of promoting good for their friends for their own sake and not for any ulterior motive. It is this central reality of friendship that I draw on here.

Sincere friendships cannot be forced, nor can they be expected to develop overnight. It requires time, commitment, and an authentic, deep mutual interest for friendships to form and mature organically and endure through challenging times. I am not arguing, therefore, that partnerships should only be established when there are pre-existing friendships. Rather, I suggest that an acid test of any established partnership is that it should be fundamentally driven by a principle of friendship. The absence of this tenet would be deeply worrying and suggest a transactional exchange invariably being driven by other motives such as financial gain or other forms of neo-colonial power grabbing.

At the heart of an international education partnership is an exchange of ideas, advice, support, and encouragement. An intellectual fascination with applying and adapting educational ideas across cultures and contexts, and a genuine interest in the success of those you are working with, should invariably lead to a position of friendship. Approaching all technical and non-technical elements of a partnership through a lens of friendship is, I believe, the single best way to ensure that it inspires mutual benefit and ensures that no single party is exploited or harmed, inadvertently or otherwise.

10   Power, Harm and Mitigating Scholarship

The field of global health has recently recognised the impact of power relations on how partnerships are developed and sustained. That realisation has occurred following a deliberate and determined focus by outstanding researchers on the unintended harms that can arise even in seemingly benevolent partnership projects. In medical education, a similar process of awakening has begun, but not quickly enough. The most dangerous assumption that those engaged in international partnerships can make is that they exclusively cause benefits. They can and do cause material and symbolic harm.

The focus in education on practice and process, rather than on evaluation and research, allows this harm to happen. Given the invariably rich complexity of international partnership working, there is always an opportunity to incorporate scholarship. In whichever way is sensible and practical, such a scholarly approach must always be built into partnerships from the outset. Sharing evaluations of partnerships in the academic literature signals an intent to learn together and to contribute to advancing the field of medical education.

11   More Than the Sum of Its Parts

Is an international medical education partnership more than the sum of the individual medical education institutions and individuals that form it? The answer is that it absolutely should be and must be. Although medical education may be big business in terms of financial investment and return, its impact in human and societal terms is bigger still. As the global medical workforce crisis extends and medical practice gets ever more complex, high quality medical education is important for policymakers around the world.

Producing locally contextualised medical training that draws selectively on ideas and practices from elsewhere is one way to achieve that based on international medical education partnerships, with appropriate will, humility, interest, and commitment by all of those involved. The danger of imposing, accepting, and applying ideas uncritically must be at the forefront of minds throughout. Continuous and critical examination of international medical education partnerships through the lens of a friendship model is, I suggest, the very best way ahead for those of us working in this space.

II.iii COMMENTARY: Escaping Colonial History in International Collaboration and Consultancy

Janet Grant and Leonard Grant

Ahmed Rashid has for long worked in international collaborations in medical education development. In this chapter, he argues that the economic and geopolitical conditions underlying such partnerships and involving the global north and global south have the potential to cause harm and, indeed, often do. These issues are of wide concern (Eichbaum et al., 2021; Matenga et al., 2019; Monette et al., 2021; Voller et al., 2022; Yorke et al., 2023). He argues that these harms can be mitigated by approaching the work through friendship—making this the lens through which to examine all areas of a working partnership.

The problem identified in his context can be seen as an expression of two things: firstly, the enduring under-development of the global south in relation to the global north, and secondly, the profit motive determining such partnerships. The expression of these contradictions can be found in the tension that Ahmed Rashid is exploring between wanting to enact helping intentions and the material reality of international partnerships within entrepreneurial universities.

Can Partnerships Escape the Colonial Legacy?

All this occurs in the context of historical underdevelopment of global south countries (Rodney, 1972), where, if partnerships are constructed as commercial consultancies, the consulting partner (and therefore the one construed to have greater knowledge or experience which is worth buying) will nearly always be from the global north. In such situations, contradictions may emerge (Horner et al., 2018).

Ahmed Rashid acknowledges the effects of colonialism in such relationships and hopes to mitigate this by focusing on developing friendship which seeks to resolve the contradiction that produces the impossibility of equal partnership.

He has reflected on this elsewhere, in relation to regulation:

> …we cannot think meaningfully about international regulation without considering power relations. The inherent power imbalances between regulators and those they regulate are extended and deepened in the global arena (Rashid et al., 2023, p. 3)

We can see that colonial legacies are always already present in knowledge production, a concept advanced by the decolonial theorist Anibal Quijano as 'the coloniality of power' (Quijano & Ennis, 2000). Through this lens, globalisation and therefore global partnerships exist within a framework in which colonialism and colonial logic already exist and cannot be escaped. This coloniality can be seen within the contractual and financial agreements, and concomitant management and governance, that are mentioned as part of the context of the 'consulting' relation-ship. As others have noted, the full potential of international collaborative activity will only be achieved when the contradictions that lead to the disparity between what is aspired to and what is actually the case are addressed (Saffu & Mamman, 2000). Ahmed Rashid reflects on this dilemma.

Varieties of Relationship, Singularity of Values

Ahmed Rashid suggests that beginning with friendship, rather than other motiva-tions, is a way to militate against the potential exploitative harm of international partnerships: '....the single best way to ensure that it inspires mutual benefit'.

Where the author uses the term 'partnership' in this narrative, others might use different terms. The choice of term reflects the underlying aspiration for the rela-tionship. Where contracts and payment are involved, then others might call this 'consultancy'. At the other end of the spectrum, where the relationship is one for mutual strategic benefit, this might be called a strategic alliance, or a collaborative or co-operative relationship. There are many other options (Saffu & Mamman, 2000) and each one indicates the assumptions, purpose and process of the relation-ship. The issue being explored in this narrative, is whether or not the wide variety of purposes and types of relationship which have a main entrepreneurial motivation, can be supported by the characteristics of friendship.

Partnerships in Entrepreneurial Universities

In Ahmed Rashid's discussion of friendship, the purpose of partnerships, rather than their style, lies beneath the surface. The contradiction is expressed between the purposes of the university and the values of academics which could be at odds with each other. That contradiction may be addressed, perhaps, where it is possible to apply personal principles of friendship within the institutional relationship between the partners. To resolve this contradiction, however, the principles of friendship must be applied universally, both between institutions and the individuals.

While universities become increasingly entrepreneurial, looking for sources of income, it is difficult to find relationships that rest on unfettered sharing of the skills, knowledge and resources of the more, perhaps, senior partner. These have increasingly become commodities to be sold. This developing commodification of academic knowledge and experience as an income generator has been thoroughly explored with hints at the contradictions between the business and the people and relationships that the business rests on:

> ...the emerging role of a modern entrepreneurial university is dichotomous, focusing on both innovation and entrepreneurship that contributes to innovation, competitiveness, and economic growth...
> A number of universities are currently in a state of transition because they are expected to develop a wide range of relationships with stakeholders in order to enhance this dichotomous contribution. (Guerrero et al., 2016)

Relationships, then, may mean one thing to the entrepreneurial university, and another to the academics who are involved in building them. However, we should recognise that the institution, made up of people, must thrive in a market that values profit and thus the institution is as constrained as are the people in it.

Strategic Alliances

Some types of relationship are not based on money flowing from one partner to the other, but are based on mutual benefit. Such strategic alliances, clearly, may have some kind of 'financial consequences' (Saffu & Mamman, 2000) in terms of, for example, marketing new courses, developing new projects, or attracting research funding. All such partnerships will involve the potential of some form of capital benefit. If the consequences are in terms of joint publications, these will affect the reputation of the partners and possible research income which, in turn, makes them more valuable. Saffu and Mamman (2000) identify a possible contradiction between two aspects of the motive for strategic alliance: altruistic and commercial. Ahmed Rashid acknowledges both and positions his values at the former pole of that contradiction, wanting the best for his partners, as a key element of friendship, while also generating income for the institution. Nonetheless, this is an expression of a contradiction that has bothered many authors.

Consultancy

The contradictions of the development of consultancy functions and 'creeping commercialism' within the education sector, based on the 'commodification of knowledge', best seen in the export and sale of curricula, perhaps (Waterval et al., 2017), are well-rehearsed in the literature (Gunter & Mills, 2017). In this, consultancy is seen as:

> ...the power relationships within contractual exchanges with the client, regarding the remit, delivery, and key knowledge to be retailed and evaluated.(ibid)

This definition is further developed to suggest that in this power relationship the process 'is actually controlled by those who are external to the school'. Gunter and Mills claim that 'Contractual exchange relationships with a knowledge market gives status to approved-of knowledge actors…' (ibid). Perhaps this uncomfortable observation of inequality is being addressed by Ahmed Rashid and weakened in his determination to develop a model of friendship. There are good reasons why the term 'knowledge economy' with its 'packaging and trading of facts and techniques' (ibid) has crept into our discourse.

Consultancy is a contractual exchange relationship which brings into focus '…the differences and distinctions between 'values' and value" (ibid). For Ahmed Rashid, value is in the contract, values are in the relationship.

Effects of the Entrepreneurial University on Project Partners

The narrative of this chapter presents the view of an academic working inside the contradictions between institution and person, between value and values. Sturdy (1997) considered this when, decades ago, universities set off on the income generation path beginning, not unexpectedly, with schools of management. He considers '…the pressures and anxieties experienced by consultants, particularly as clients become more demanding and sophisticated' (ibid). But equally, he considers the '…. insecurities over their personal career, functional or departmental power…of the clients who might …turn to experts and new ideas in the same way that the Ancient Greeks turned to myths and legends…' (ibid). There are personal issues for everyone about how and why we execute the institutional entrepreneurial imperative. We might speculate about what it would mean for an individual academic or even a centre or group of academics to entirely reject the profit motive of their university. How long would their centre last? What would happen to their careers? Or is part of being an academic now accepted as being employed to bolster the income of the organisation?

When consultancy was beginning to be an important income-generating, and perhaps influencing, route for universities, Sturdy (1997) depicted this within 'capitalist social relations and managerial labour processes' as:

> …an interactive and dialectical process founded on both consultants' and clients' self-defeating concerns to secure a sense of identity and control.

We can add to that the purposes of the project and the processes of interaction towards those purposes, and hope that they align, in Ahmed Rashid's work as friendship, because:

> …"technoeconomic" forces and the "sociopsychological" are not separate, but mutually constituting – they complement, rather than compete with, each other. (ibid)

The author understands that a history of harm associated with colonisation might be interrupted through the personal relationships forged.

The Role and Paradox of Friendship

There is no common definition of friendship or of its positive and negative effects in the workplace, or of what is a friend, even though friendship is 'at the top of the list when people are asked what gives meaning to their life' (Dickie, 2009). Importantly for the work of academics, there are indications, unsurprisingly, that friendship takes on different meanings in different cross cultural settings (ibid).

Unusually, Ahmed Rashid is clear in his description of friendship, which concerns not only what each partner feels, but also what they want for the other. Contracts and finances do not stop those fellow feelings. Indeed, any contract will involve some interpersonal connection and then each party must decide how to frame and characterise that.

Friendship in the workplace has been extensively studied:

Much of this literature focuses on how workplace friendships can be linked to improving organizational outcomes such as productivity and performance. (Rumens, 2017)

The friendship that is an element of project delivery could be seen as simply a social practice (equivalent to good manners), or a form of social relationship (establishing facilitative roles and behaviours), or a personal relationship (with the implication or actually making authentic friends) (Rumens, 2017). The choice of which type might be personal or a function of the project or reflect the relative power status of partners or the cultural overlap.

Ahmed Rashid's frame of reference for adoption of friendship within partnerships, derives from the effects of a history of colonialism (given that institutions in the global north are often commissioned by institutions in the global south), and the harms that were perpetrated, and a concern that those harms should not persist by failure to interrogate the context and the relationship.

The key issue of whether or not friendship can ever entirely create equality between client and consultant, or between global south and global north, or between payer and payee, is something to be studied. Nonetheless, for Ahmed Rashid, it is still the most effective, and perhaps personally satisfying, approach which demonstrates the values of cultural and contextual respect.

Given this, friendship within such formal and institutional partnerships has many possible dimensions, and could, paradoxically, be an effective means of persuasive normative control given that there is a project imperative (Costas, 2012). It has been argued in relation to trading partnerships, that international integration causes an entrenched hierarchy and continuing dependency of developing countries on developed countries. Could this be true in relation to the consultancy partnerships that this chapter has in mind? Might friendship, unintentionally, make that dependency easier to accept and maintain?

…international integration based on comparative advantage was biased against developing countries due to declining terms of trade. Such unequal exchange was even suggested to lead to the underdevelopment of the global South… From this perspective, globalisation was tailor made to maintain and deepen the stark inequalities among differentially endowed countries. (Horner et al., 2018)

Such a view might be supported in relation to the acceptance of development aid which has emphasised:

> ... the need for 'partnerships that mobilize and share knowledge, expertise, technology and financial resources.' (Koch, 2020)

Although partnership is emphasised in this process, it does not always result in the equality that partners might aspire to:

> ...various scholars went on to examine how the partnership discourse manifests itself in practice—and most arrived at the conclusion that the new narrative talks up the agency of Southern 'partners' while masking unchanged power asymmetries. (ibid)

Perhaps, no matter how much effort is put in by the partners, the order of global power cannot be overcome, experts will tend not to come from the global south, or be marginalised because of that, and 'discriminatory epistemic injustice' (ibid) will continue such that knowledge sharing is unidirectional and controlled.

So perhaps what constrains academic partnerships from being based on terms of friendship, is that partnerships have to be financially beneficial to the global north partner.

The Principal Contradiction

The idea of 'Continuous and critical examination of international medical education partnerships through the lens of a friendship model', which Ahmed Rashid advocates, is a powerful idea. We surely could not demur from the notion of being kind and congenial within a purposeful partnership. But it is not so simple, as he indicates. The material condition of the for-profit, neo-colonial partnership will ultimately shape and determine the interaction between individuals. So friendship, where that occurs, will be enacted within the more powerful context of colonial history and fundamental economic and political inequality between the global north and the global south.

Others have considered all these things from many points of view and within many frames of reference including neoliberalism, capitalism, colonialism, business generation, policy, epistemic injustice, and research. This is a complex area of work. But at its heart is the simple contradiction: The business purposes of the entrepreneurial university may be at odds with the academic purposes and personal values of the people who enact the income-generating projects, and where these are transactions between global north and global south, the relationship is further complicated by entrenched historical, colonial power and politics.

As with the example of alienation in Samar Ahmed's chapter, sometimes individuals are not able to shape partnerships as they wish because they are constrained by the financial goals of the institution or indeed by their own career development. The drive is always towards bringing financial and social capital to the partners.

In that undertaking, Ahmed Rashid is proposing that friendship can fundamentally alter the relationship. We do not know, other than experientially, whether that is the case or not. This commentary has tried to explore the issues raised.

Ahmed Rashid attempts to offer a resolution to the contradictions of the enduring under-development of the global south in relation to the global north, and the profit motive determining partnerships—by beginning from friendship. We can see how this might have the desired effect. Would a friend exploit another friend or seek to impose their way of behaving? Friends will seek to work together, sometimes for one to be subordinated to the other, with open and honest communication as to their goals and constraints. We can see why the author suggests such a route.

However, because of the history of underdevelopment identified, a friendship between already unequal partners would necessitate the global north partner redistributing their resources (if not knowledge, which may be unwanted) to the global south partner. Is this likely in this current geopolitical régime? We encourage everyone to consider Ahmed Rashid's wise words and to imagine what is necessary to truly arrive at global partnerships from a position of friendship. We think that this will ultimately be not possible while the global economic system is dependent on the extraction of resources from the global south to the global north. He does not dwell on this point, but it is very telling: partnerships cannot be developed on financially neutral terms—but what if we consider a world in which they could?

References

Costas, J. (2012). We are all friends here. *Journal of Management Inquiry, 21*(4), 377–395. https://doi.org/10.1177/1056492612439104

Dickie, C. (2009). Exploring workplace friendships in business: Cultural variations of employee behaviour. *Research and Practice in Human Resource Management, 17*(1), 128–137.

Eichbaum, Q. G., Adams, L. V., Evert, J., Ho, M.-J., Semali, I. A., & van Schalkwyk, S. C. (2021). Decolonizing global health education: Rethinking institutional partnerships and approaches. *Academic Medicine, 96*(3), 329–335. https://doi.org/10.1097/ACM.0000000000003473

Guerrero, M., Urbano, D., Fayolle, A., Klofsten, M., & Mian, S. (2016). Entrepreneurial universities: Emerging models in the new social and economic landscape. *Small Business Economics, 47*(3), 551–563. https://doi.org/10.1007/s11187-016-9755-4

Gunter, H. M., & Mills, C. (2017). *Consultants and consultancy: The case of education* (Vol. 4). Springer International Publishing. https://doi.org/10.1007/978-3-319-48879-0

Horner, R., Schindler, S., Haberly, D., & Aoyama, Y. (2018). Globalisation, uneven development and the North–South 'big switch'. *Cambridge Journal of Regions, Economy and Society, 11*(1), 17–33. https://doi.org/10.1093/cjres/rsx026

Koch, S. (2020). "The local consultant will not be credible": How epistemic injustice is experienced and practised in development aid. *Social Epistemology, 34*(5), 478–489. https://doi.org/10.1080/02691728.2020.1737749

Matenga, T. F. L., Zulu, J. M., Corbin, J. H., & Mweemba, O. (2019). Contemporary issues in north–south health research partnerships: Perspectives of health research stakeholders in Zambia. *Health Research Policy and Systems, 17*(1), 7. https://doi.org/10.1186/s12961-018-0409-7

Monette, E. M., McHugh, D., Smith, M. J., Canas, E., Jabo, N., Henley, P., & Nouvet, E. (2021). Informing 'good' global health research partnerships: A scoping review of guiding principles. *Global Health Action, 14*(1). https://doi.org/10.1080/16549716.2021.1892308

Quijano, A., & Ennis, M. (2000). Coloniality of power, eurocentrism, and Latin America. *Nepantla: Views from South, 1*(3), 533–580.

Rashid, M. A., Ali, S. M., & Dharanipragada, K. (2023). Decolonising medical education regulation: A global view. *BMJ Global Health, 8*(6), e011622. https://doi.org/10.1136/bmjgh-2022-011622

Rodney, W. (1972). *How Europe underdeveloped Africa*. Bogle-L'Ouverture Publications, London and Tanzanian Publishing House.

Rumens, N. (2017). Researching workplace friendships. *Journal of Social and Personal Relationships, 34*(8), 1149–1167. https://doi.org/10.1177/0265407516670276

Saffu, K., & Mamman, A. (2000). Contradictions in international tertiary strategic alliances: The case from down under. *International Journal of Public Sector Management, 13*(6), 508–518. https://doi.org/10.1108/09513550010356548

Sturdy A. (1997). The dialectics of consultancy. *Critical Perspectives on Accounting, 8*(5), 511–535.

Voller, S., Schellenberg, J., Chi, P., & Thorogood, N. (2022). What makes working together work? A scoping review of the guidance on North–South research partnerships. *Health Policy and Planning, 37*(4), 523–534. https://doi.org/10.1093/heapol/czac008

Waterval, D., Tinnemans-Adriaanse, M., Meziani, M., Driessen, E., Scherpbier, A., Mazrou, A., & Frambach, J. (2017). Exporting a student-centered curriculum: A home institution's perspective. *Journal of Studies in International Education, 21*(3), 278–290. https://doi.org/10.1177/1028315317697542

Yorke, L., Kim, J. H., Hagos Hailu, B., & Ejigu Berhie, C. (2023). Equitable north-south partnerships for ethical and policy relevant research in times of uncertainty: A collaborative autoethnography from Ethiopia. *International Journal of Social Research Methodology*, 1–15. https://doi.org/10.1080/13645579.2023.2173840

Ahmed Rashid is a primary care physician in the UK National Health Service and Professor at the London School of Hygiene and Tropical Medicine, where he is a member of the university executive team as Pro-Director Education. He is also Honorary Professor at University College London and Chief Examiner for the UK General Medical Council. In previous roles as Vice Dean International at University College London Faculty of Medical Sciences, and International Medical Director of the Royal College of General Practitioners, he has led a wide variety of transnational education partnerships in undergraduate and postgraduate medicine.

Part III
Negotiating Identities in Medical Education and Medicine

Summary

Medical education tends not to examine some key issues experienced by those who move into this field. Those issues derive from both medical education itself, and from its wider social context. While context is a widely discussed concept in medical education, that discussion tends to focus on the global south, implying a context different from those of the dominant global north. But the first two remarkable personal accounts offered here tell us that every society has its own context and social forces and forms that can give rise to contradictions.

When others are considering taking up the practices of the global north, the experiences of our first two authors and their colleagues, described here, suggest that education, as a social practice within a contextually structured society, cannot be so easily exported without an examination of the complex personal, psychological, social and professional environments within which people work in medical education. Even in the contexts in which those practices were developed, things do not always run smoothly. Such powerful assumptions are made about the identity of medicine, that developing a new identity in medical education can be problematical. Part III ends with a meditation on why the profession of medicine demands the development of a strong identity. It can be challenging if that professional identity is moved away from.

III.i STATEMENT: The Road Not Taken: Transitioning to Full-Time Medical Education Research From Clinical Practice as a Junior Doctor

Megan E. L. Brown

> *Two roads diverged in a wood, and I –*
> *I took the one less traveled by,*
> *And that has made all the difference.*
>
> The Road Not Taken, Robert Frost (Frost, 1991)

For a medic, a non-clinical career in medical education is the epitome of Frost's less travelled road. The road is even less well travelled if you leave medicine as a junior, who has never enrolled on a formal speciality training pathway. I had been practising medicine for 2 years when I was confronted by two roads diverging ahead of me—one was clinical practice, a well-trodden and familiar path but which, for me, had become untenable after spiralling disillusionment with the profession, and the other was a less well-travelled academic path, but a path which represented a very necessary change.

When I stood at that fork in the path of my own career journey I felt alone, even though many junior doctors leave clinical medicine each year (Lambert et al., 2018) because of lifestyle choices or finding passion for a career elsewhere (Smith et al., 2018). What pervades research in this area is that doctors are vulnerable to stress, anxiety, depression, burnout (Bhugra et al., 2019) and high rates of suicide (Dutheil et al., 2019) because of the nature of the job and poor working conditions (Riley et al., 2021a, b).

I loved medical school and expected to love being a doctor. But the job quickly wore me down. After only two years, I didn't recognise myself. I had aspired to become a compassionate, empathic doctor who was genial in nature but serious in academic ability. I did not feel like this person when I was working.

M. E. L. Brown (✉)
School of Medicine, Newcastle University, Newcastle upon Tyne, UK
e-mail: Megan.Brown@newcastle.ac.uk

© The Author(s), under exclusive license to Springer Nature   111
Switzerland AG 2026
J. Grant, L. Grant (eds.), *The Contradictions of Medical Education*,
https://doi.org/10.1007/978-3-031-90394-6_8

1 Working Conditions

While working out-of-hours as a Foundation Year One doctor, I was the first port of call for over 300 patients and the staff that were concerned about them. My bleep ceaselessly trilled, forcing me to splinter myself into fragments across the various wards of the hospital. The shift was 13 hours, and I did not eat, drink, or use the bathroom in that time. I felt like a failure when I handed over jobs to the night team.

When I spoke to my educational supervisor about the experience, they told me that it was my fault, I had failed to prioritise and delegate. But the hospital was short staffed, and I had not been well-supported in making this transition, or when I was on the job. Thereafter followed a year and a half of similar experiences where I was anonymous, or bullied because of my role as a trade union representative who fought for those working beyond their contracted hours. Reporting bullying achieved nothing. I became known as a troublesome trainee, depicted as not resilient enough for medicine, not dedicated enough to work long hours without recompense, not genial enough to accept mistreatment.

2 Personal Disillusion

I became disillusioned, discouraged that I could not be the doctor I wanted to be. I was burnt out and depressed, and 'in expressing my pain I inflicted it on others' (Compton, 2020), on both colleagues and, I fear, with patients. I had failed at being a doctor and, if I wasn't a doctor, then what was I?

3 Leaving Medicine

I took an extended period of sick leave and, with relief, decided to leave medicine. But what next? Reflecting on my time at medical school and experiences working, I realised that what I enjoyed were learning, writing, and teaching. So, I could now see a path that intrigued me, but one I knew little about—a career in medical education. Though I felt alone in making the decision to pursue a full-time medical education career, I have since come to realise that this is not the case. The following vignettes describe experiences which resonate with my own:

Dr Anna Collini's Story
I have always been interested in people and this, combined with an aptitude for science, led me to study medicine. I enjoyed medical school, but the reality of practising as a doctor hit me hard. I tried to shape work into something that I enjoyed, taking time out of training to do a teaching fellow role. I began a Masters in Education for Clinical Contexts, and knew I wanted my career to

involve education, but I couldn't see a path other than becoming a consultant with education as a small part of my job. I felt trapped. In 2018, after postnatal depression and anxiety, I made the decision to leave training to do what I loved—medical education. While many people were supportive, some indicated that leaving was a mistake. Despite the uncertainty around my career path, I knew it was the right decision for me. After two years working in an educational role within the NHS, I have just taken up a permanent teaching position at a medical school and I could not be happier.

Dr Ayesha Younas's Story

Some time ago, there was a family gathering at our home. I am the only person in my family who puts the prefix 'Dr' before her name which is a source of generalised interest and converted pride for my elder relatives. Someone asked about my speciality and I replied that I had shifted full-time to medical education. Looking perplexed, he said, 'You can't be an educationist if you are a doctor, aren't they two different fields altogether? It means you are not a doctor anymore!' This dramatic statement was followed by utter silence and shock on the part of most people in that room. I felt I had made a major faux pas and tried to explain, that I was still working in medicine, only in a different way. "But you have given up treating patients, so how can you be a doctor?" I was often asked. Similar snide comments and undertones, sometimes even from those who are in healthcare, implied that as I am not a practising clinician, I cannot know the pressures of clinical work! To me these are a common occurrence now and I have given up trying to explain to people, why I chose to leave clinical practice, why I chose lesser money, a cut-throat environment, and hours and hours of sitting at my computer. Why I chose to fall for something different, which doesn't give me the instant gratification that I could get by seeing my patient get better, but where the rewards are greater, deeper and more profound.

Dr Helen Church's Story

To become a fully trained specialist doctor, there is a well-defined pathway followed by most clinicians. By contrast, there is no equivalent pathway to become a fully-fledged medical educationalist: in higher education institutions, their recruitment criteria often favour the more traditional academic pathway (undergraduate degree, followed by higher degree). This disadvantages clinicians who may have not had the time or opportunity to undertake a higher medical education degree. Junior doctors hoping to apply for substantive medical education posts often have to take time out of clinical practice to acquire medical education qualifications, usually at substantial cost to themselves. Although clinical academic jobs, for qualified Consultants, often provide enrolment on a higher education degree, once in post.

Academic medical education jobs are generally categorised as either 'clinical' (for a practising doctor) or 'non-clinical'. Ex-doctors would only be eligible for the 'non-clinical' postings, which not only overlooks the years of training that they completed, but also comes at a cost; the pay disparity between clinical and non-clinical academics is substantial. Therefore, doctors might reluctantly consider working a few clinical hours per week, to retain the pay scale to which they have become accustomed (and maintain the perceived credibility afforded to those who are 'practising what they teach'). As a current clinical academic, this is one of the main barriers preventing my transition to full-time medical education.

Dr Theresa Martin's Story
I started an academic post in 2013, four years after I left clinical practice due to depression, anxiety, burnout, and trauma. Changing job didn't solve the challenges I experienced in clinical practice, I had to work hard to overcome them. The supportive environment of medical education made that possible—I built good relationships with colleagues. I found in pockets, collegiality, and compassion. However, at times the culture of medical practice crept in, intermingled with an unfamiliar academic landscape I tried hard to understand. Leaving medicine early in my career impaired my progress in medical education—I was somehow seen as lesser—my clinical knowledge and experience downplayed, my teaching experience underestimated. It has been hard to know where I fit—I'm clinical when a clinician can't give a lecture at the last minute, non-clinical when I want to apply for a more senior "clinical academic" position. I found that frequently people were unable to see past the labels, scientist, researcher, doctor and see me and what I uniquely bring. Qualitative research was often snubbed by the senior clinicians and scientists making decisions on promotion panels. Those with a track record of scientific publications did much better. But over a decade ago I was busy taking care of patients, a phronesis that suits me to the caring aspects of academic citizenship (mentoring, student support).

The clinician turned academic is so far from "those who can't, teach"—we are Alice stepping through the looking glass, with the ability to travel between worlds—our responsibility is to honestly reflect what we see in each. What I see is that, despite our values-led approaches to work, some of the legacy issues of society, lack of equity and equality, stigma, discrimination and shame, overwork and overwhelm, cause much destruction in both medicine and medical education.

What do we learn from these four stories, and from my own?

4   Medical Education as a Field

Prior to exploring medical education as a career, I did not think of medical education as a distinct field. I was unaware of the work that goes on—I thought medical education was concerned only with the practice of teaching. In pursuing a Postgraduate Certificate in Health Professions Education, I came to learn about qualitative research, and my opinion of what 'counted' as research changed and I saw that 'medical education research is not a poor relation of medical research; it belongs to a different family altogether' (Monrouxe & Rees, 2009). Coming to understand medical education as a social science transformed my perspective on the field and fostered a passion and engagement that endures to this day.

As a field, medical education research characterises itself as interdisciplinary, as drawing from the knowledge and theory of many fields including psychology, sociology and anthropology. A rich and varied landscape of perspectives is a key strength of the field (Ellaway et al., 2020).

5   Stigma About Not Practising Medicine

Though I am happy working in medical education research, getting to where I am today has not been without difficulty. Anna and Ayesha describe experiencing negative attitudes from family and colleagues at their career shift.

I, too, have been 'warned' of the consequences of my decision by several well-respected seniors who informed me that there would be no career for me in medical education if I was not willing to return to clinical practice, just as Ayesha was told that she is no longer a doctor. This discouraged me for a long time. But as I spent time getting to know those within medical education research, I learnt from anatomists, sociologists, psychologists and physiologists: non-clinical researchers who brought great insight to their work. There is a stigma in the field perpetuated by a minority, that clinicians are best placed to conduct medical education research. Others have noted that 'unable to draw upon cultural capital accrued from clinical work, non-clinical educators faced additional challenges' (Hu et al., 2015). This has certainly been my experience and I would suggest that being clinical and leaving at a junior stage of training brings additional stigma. My own experiences of medical school were not particularly interdisciplinary in nature. I had access to no role models who were not clinical within educational spaces. Medical schools fail to provide information on non-clinical career paths to medical students (Kim et al., 2013) and I wonder if this could narrow one's perspective on who has rights to the field of medical education, propagating stigma and stifling interdisciplinary collaboration.

6   Lack of Job Opportunities and Career Path

Another significant barrier I have experienced concerns the lack of non-clinical job opportunities within medical education research. In June 2023, I conducted a UK job search for 'medical education'. There were only three non-clinical posts that a UK medicine graduate (with postgraduate qualifications in medical education research at Master's level and above) would be eligible to apply for. This lack of opportunity sends a tacit message that non-practising clinicians are not valued or welcomed in the field. How can the field develop, if we do not offer employment opportunities to individuals with more varied backgrounds?

Further, if you manage to secure a medical education research job (which I have been fortunate enough to do, but only after completing a 3-year PhD in the area), there is a significant lack of pay parity between clinical and non-clinical academic roles. I suspect this sends further messages regarding the value of each researcher's input. If I had not been supported by my family, my career path would not have been viable. We talk often of widening access within medical education, but less of widening access to academic careers. There is a 'leaky pipeline' within clinical academia, where minoritised individuals are more likely to leave. Dr. Helen Church's experiences also describe these problems.

As Dr. Theresa Martin stresses, we have a responsibility as a field to treat those within the field well, to be actively non-toxic, and to challenge stigma. All medical education careers are diverse and serendipitous. We should embrace a diversity of backgrounds and career paths different from our own. Just because you cannot easily label someone as 'scientist', 'researcher', or 'doctor' does not mean that they do not bring value and richness to the field.

7   The Importance of Challenging Barriers

Given that many junior doctors leave medicine each year, and the expanding nature of the field of medical education, those leaving the clinical workforce could represent a useful pipeline of hardworking and highly skilled professionals to expand research capacity in the field. There is a missed opportunity at present to adequately fund research training in medical education and advertise such opportunities widely, not only to active clinicians. Following completion of an out-of-programme clinical educator role at one institution, 32% of clinicians did not maintain clinical responsibility which suggests that a significant proportion of trained clinicians may be looking to transition to full-time educational or research roles following experience of medical education (Stocker et al., 2020). There is interest in this path, and medical education and educators would do well to encourage and support these individuals in making this transition.

Dr. Theresa Martin's reflective account highlights the importance of challenging barriers. As hybrid professionals, non-practising clinicians in medical education research offer unique insight into the educational system (such as what it is like to sit an OSCE) and of medical practice, but also the full-time space and capacity to develop and share skills in research methodology, theory, and writing.

8   Conclusion

I would like to end this chapter how it began, remembering the quote from Frost's wonderful poem, *The Road Not Taken*. Taking the road less travelled, for me, has made all the difference to my wellbeing, professional satisfaction, and happiness. I am, and I hope will continue to be, happy and healthy. Medical education research careers are serendipitous, but we must strive, as a community, to open our doors more widely, and welcome all inside.

Acknowledgments My heartfelt thanks to Dr. Anna Collini, Dr. Ayesha Younas, Dr. Helen Church, and Dr. Theresa Martin who generously shared their stories and experiences with me to inform and enrich this chapter. Thank you also to the Wandering MedEd WhatsApp group who have supported me throughout the writing of this chapter. And thank you to anyone who ever told me this career path was not possible—I do so like proving people wrong.

References

Bhugra, D., Sauerteig, S. O., Bland, D., Lloyd-Kendall, A., Wijesuriya, J., Singh, G., Kochhar, A., Molodynski, A., & Ventriglio, A. (2019). A descriptive study of mental health and wellbeing of doctors and medical students in the UK. *International Review of Psychiatry, 31*(7–8), 563–568. https://doi.org/10.1080/09540261.2019.1648621

Compton, T. (2020). The times are a changing: Culture (s) of medicine. In J. M. Parsons & A. Chappell (Eds.), *The Palgrave handbook of auto/biography* (pp. 31–46). Palgrave Macmillan.

Dutheil, F., Aubert, C., Pereira, B., Dambrun, M., Moustafa, F., Mermillod, M., Baker, J. S., Trousselard, M., Lesage, F.-X., & Navel, V. (2019). Suicide among physicians and health-care workers: A systematic review and meta-analysis. *PLoS One, 14*(12), e0226361. https://doi.org/10.1371/journal.pone.0226361

Ellaway, R., Tolsgaard, M., & Martimianakis, M. A. (2020). What divides us and what unites us? *Advances in Health Sciences Education, 25*(5), 1019–1023. https://doi.org/10.1007/s10459-020-10016-9

Frost, R. (1991). The road not taken. In R. Frost & L. Untermeyer (Eds.), *The road not taken: A selection of Robert Frost's poems*. H. Holt and Co.

Hu, W. C. Y., Thistlethwaite, J. E., Weller, J., Gallego, G., Monteith, J., & McColl, G. J. (2015). 'It was serendipity': A qualitative study of academic careers in medical education. *Medical Education, 49*(11), 1124–1136. https://doi.org/10.1111/medu.12822

Kim, K.-J., Park, J.-H., Lee, Y.-H., & Choi, K. (2013). What is different about medical students interested in non-clinical careers? *BMC Medical Education, 13*(1), 81. https://doi.org/10.1186/1472-6920-13-81

Lambert, T. W., Smith, F., & Goldacre, M. J. (2018). Why doctors consider leaving UK medicine: Qualitative analysis of comments from questionnaire surveys three years after graduation. Journal of the Royal Society of Medicine, 111(1), 18–30. https://doi.org/10.1177/0141076817738502

Monrouxe, L. V., & Rees, C. E. (2009). Picking up the gauntlet: Constructing medical education as a social science. *Medical Education,* *43*(3), 196–198. https://doi.org/10.1111/j.1365-2923.2008.03272.x

Riley, R., Buszewicz, M., Kokab, F., Teoh, K., Gopfert, A., Taylor, A. K., Van Hove, M., Martin, J., Appleby, L., & Chew-Graham, C. (2021a). Sources of work-related psychological distress experienced by UK-wide foundation and junior doctors: A qualitative study. *BMJ Open, 11*(6), e043521. https://doi.org/10.1136/BMJOPEN-2020-043521

Riley, R., Kokab, F., Buszewicz, M., Gopfert, A., Van Hove, M., Taylor, A. K., Teoh, K., Martin, J., Appleby, L., & Chew-Graham, C. (2021b). Protective factors and sources of support in the workplace as experienced by UK foundation and junior doctors: A qualitative study. *BMJ Open, 11*(6), e045588. https://doi.org/10.1136/BMJOPEN-2020-045588

Smith, S. E., Tallentire, V. R., Pope, L. M., Laidlaw, A. H., & Morrison, J. (2018). Foundation Year 2 doctors' reasons for leaving UK medicine: An in-depth analysis of decision-making using semistructured interviews. *BMJ Open, 8*(3), e019456. https://doi.org/10.1136/BMJOPEN-2017-019456

Stocker, C., McMullan, D., Langlands, K., Thompsett, A. R., Harris, J., & Thomas, P. (2020). Junior doctors undertaking an out-of-programme career break in medical education enhance their subsequent clinical practice skills and opportunities as well as continuing professional development. *MedEdPublish, 9*(1), https://doi.org/10.1569/mep.2020.000276

III.i COMMENTARY: Identity, Status and Uncertainty in Medical Education

Janet Grant and Leonard Grant

In their chapter, five authors have highlighted two key issues for medicine and medical education in the UK: firstly, that medicine is experienced by many people as an inhospitable environment, and secondly, that medical education is still seeking its own identity and place as a planned career.

Workplace Conditions

The five authors of this chapter are happy in medical education, but all had originally wanted to be doctors, before the working, and perhaps cultural, conditions of that profession led to experiences which made it untenable as a job. Reported rates of stress and attrition tell us that these experiences are shared by others. In the UK:

> Most medical students successfully graduate and start their first foundation year … but only 30% of those completing foundation training in 2021/22 continued straight into GP or consultant training posts.
> Fewer than three in five doctors (56%) in 'core training' remained … in NHS hospital and community services in England eight years later, with half (24%) of this attrition seen in the first two years. (Palmer et al., 2023, p. 3)

From this, the working conditions of junior doctors appear to be problematical. Although this has been described as stressful, doctors are still unwilling to take sick leave (Oxtoby, 2015). Rather than tackling the problem, it has been suggested in medicine that the symptoms of the condition can be tackled by organising wellbeing programmes for marginalised groups of trainees, by creating a supportive culture, and asking trainees what they need (Rimmer, 2023). Resilience has been put forward as a quality to be valued in doctors who are struggling (Shiner et al., 2020), but resilience training has been currently criticised as shifting the onus to improve on the individual rather than changing the system within which they work (Huntington, 2019).

Workload, work-life balance, job stress, reward frustration and their relationship to intention to leave medicine, sometimes related to working during the COVID-19 pandemic, are also reported in Switzerland, the UK, Germany, Finland, France, the US, the Netherlands and China (Abbasi, 2022; Bustraan et al., 2019; Degen et al., 2015; Hämmig, 2018; Pathmanathan & Snelling, 2023; Sayburn, 2017; Zhang & Feng, 2011). The same pattern is seen in other professions, including teaching (CooperGibson Research, 2018).

Women in the Medical Workplace

It is not accidental that the five authors of this chapter are representative of women who contend not only with the inhospitable workplace, but also with gender-based oppressions. Education is still mainly women's work at primary and secondary levels, and while women are increasingly represented on the staff of universities, the leadership and higher-level jobs are still dominated by males (Finding, 2013). Gender pay gaps exist at all levels of education. The triple jeopardy of a low-status, lower-paid field, dominated by women and often by part-time work, means that in those circumstances, the gender pay gap is greatest (Francis-Devine, 2023).

Although women are now increasingly represented in medical schools, if less so as careers progress (British Medical Association, 2021), gender inequality is still evident (Brown et al., 2020), and it is still the case that stereotypes represented by men dominate medical culture affecting both women's aspirations and their achievements (Winkel et al., 2021). It has been concluded that:

> The failure to address structures and policies that favour a workforce of men, allowing sexist attitudes and gender bias to remain prevalent, has led to unequal opportunities for women. (British Medical Association, 2021, p. 32)

Combining this with the lesser status of education in relation to medicine, we might understand why the authors of this chapter are women.

The Path into Medical Education

The authors of this chapter also describe the tensions that can occur when transitioning from 'clinical doctor' to 'non-practising medical graduate' in medical education. As Megan Brown notes, their identity was deeply tied to being a doctor, evidenced in the crisis experienced when she asks: 'If I wasn't a doctor, then what was I?' Part of developing as a doctor involves defining oneself by the professional roles to be inhabited. It is easy to see, then, that leaving medicine might trigger an identity crisis and loss of belonging when medical education has a fragile status in terms of its identity and its relationship to medicine itself. This might be exacerbated in ways explored in the case studies: people can face questioning of their value, knowledge, skills and purpose when they shift roles.

The Difficult Identity of a Doctor Working in Medical Education

There is a large, and sometimes critical, literature that addresses and theorises the development of professional identity in medicine (R. L. Cruess et al., 2014; Cruess et al., 2019; Gill, 2013; Rees & Monrouxe, 2018). That literature almost exclusively reviews methods of developing that identity effectively and efficiently (Mount et al.,

2022). It ties the development of professional identity to the acquisition of medical professionalism, and rarely asks whether tying identity and behaviour together so closely might have negative effects on the person. The literature only occasionally identifies the problems of professional identity formation, such as those experienced by minority groups (Volpe et al., 2021), or problems of leaving medicine when 'work identity is synonymous with personal identity' (Silver, 2016, p. 783). Leaving medicine becomes leaving self.

So the transition to medical education can be challenging, as these authors describe, leaving them with the problem of not being able to describe their identity. This is a problem of medical education itself.

The Unlisted Identity of Medical Education

In a relatively short period of time, medical education has become a major area of activity, with more than 130 journals (Mendeley Data, 2022), and a bewildering number of national and international conferences and professional organisations: in the UK alone, there are the Academy of Medical Educators, the Association for the Study of Medical Education, Medical Education Leaders UK, the Conference of Postgraduate Medical Deans, AMEE, and many others associated with clinical specialties and functions such as CReME which focuses on teaching clinical reasoning (Cooper et al., 2021). There has been a mushrooming of Master's degrees in health professions education from seven in 1996 to 76 in 2012 (Tekian & Harris, 2012) to 158 in 2023 (Schermerhorn et al., 2023), and innumerable medical education departments in medical schools (but almost none in the United Kingdom, as our authors discovered) which might have any of 40 functions (AlSheikh et al., 2022). The number of medically qualified and other people who have chosen medical education as a temporary, full-time, part-time or permanent career, and the associated loss to clinical practice, is unknown. Conference attendances tell us that it is large (Osmosis Team, 2023). The overall effect of all this activity, either on the medical workforce and health care, or on the practice of medical education, is largely unknown.

Although medical education has given rise to the interest bodies described above, the statutory UK national endorsing bodies for science, engineering, humanities, social science and medicine do not recognise medical education as a discipline (Gov UK, 2021). The British Psychological Society does not list medical education as a branch of educational psychology (British Psychological Society, 2024). Medical education is not a specialty listed by the UK General Medical Council (GMC), so no-one in the UK can be registered with the GMC (or any other regulator) as a medical educationalist, simply because, according to the 1983 Medical Act, the GMC is statutorily concerned with regulating the education, training and *current* medical practice of doctors. The UK medical Royal Colleges are likewise primarily concerned with the practice of their specialties, even though some might also be involved in offering Master's degrees in medical education (more often confusingly called 'Master's in Health Professions Education'), not for purposes of a career in that field, but for 'doctors who are intending to have a significant role in medical education' (Royal College of Physicians of London, n.d.). There is, therefore, a contradiction between the primary training of our authors, which set them on the path towards medical practice, and their eventual careers, which took them off that path, with no other path to join. It is not so much a path less travelled, it is a path that had to be cut and then cleaved to differently for each person, as the opportunity arises, and determination allows.

Unsurprisingly, the language of business has slowly entered medical education: profit, entrepreneurship, income-generation, business models, consultancy (which Ahmed Rashid worried about in chapter "Greater Than The Sum: International Partnerships in Medical Education—Statement"), competition, cost, cost-effectiveness and value (Beck Dallaghan et al., 2022; Calvert & Freemantle, 2009; Drolet, 2017; Mahat, 2019; Sepahvand & Hozni, 2018; Walsh, 2010, 2013, 2015, 2016), and the 'commodification and trade of medical education 'goods and services" (Hodges et al., 2009, p. 916) have now entered the lexicon. The business of medical education is addressed further in Part IV of this book.

Despite this, and reading the accounts of the authors' experiences in this chapter, the identity of medical education is still unclear, as is the nature of careers within that, and how these fit into this partly academic, partly practice-based, partly commercial landscape.

Making a Career and Belonging in Medical Education

The author of the next chapter, Anna Harvey Bluemel, has researched careers in clinical education research and highlights two main challenges in forging a career in medical education:

> (1) A cultural challenge from clinical norms. Challenges included differences between the epistemological assumptions of biomedical and clinical research, and the underlying philosophy of education research, which is more closely aligned with the knowledge generation of the social sciences. This led to difficulty communicating the impact of education research to patient care… (2) Structures, systems and relationships for career progression. Practical considerations included time and funding (or lack thereof), the opportunity to undertake formal training, networking and role models. (Harvey Bluemel et al., 2024)

Careers in academia tend to occur in two ways: either a person creates their own career path, such as Holly Tessler has created Beatles Studies through a convoluted personal academic path (University of Liverpool, n.d.); or there is an established academic pathway to join (jobs.ac.uk, n.d.). In the United Kingdom and many other countries, there is no such established pathway in medical education, possibly reflecting its uncertain, unlisted identity. Ways of entering this rather unformed field occur such that '…a pathway into medical education can be as varied and flexible as you want it to be' (Medic Footprints, n.d.).

It is unlikely that anyone leaves school or enters university with a career ambition to enter medical education. If we assume that applicants to medical school intend to practise medicine, it is worrying that in the UK about one third of students intend to leave the NHS within 2 years of graduating while 60% express dissatisfaction with the prospect of working in the NHS. This figure differs between medical schools, but it is not possible to firmly attribute this to any particular variables in the medical school experience (Ferreira et al., 2023, 2024). As with the authors of this chapter, the reasons for leaving medicine are related to what happens after medical school. Improving medical education seems unlikely to affect this exodus, but may, perhaps ironically, provide more medical graduates who consider medical education, or other pathways outside medicine, as an alternative career.

We can see, then, that medical education careers tend to happen serendipitously. But, having left medicine, what is this field that the authors have entered and eventually settled into happily? And what is their new identity?

Given the difficulty of forging a career in medical education, nonetheless in the United Kingdom alone, despite its lack of GMC recognition, lack of medical education departments, lack of statutory recognition, and no formal career structures, in 2018 within the 35 medical schools, the highest proportion of women at Lecturer grade were in medical education (79%) which is 10% more than in obstetrics and gynaecology, and general practice. Medical education also had the highest proportion of clinical academic staff working less than full time. At the same time, medical education had the highest vacancy rate (8%) (Watson, 2018).

It is likely that every UK medical school has a least one professor of medical education, possibly alongside another medical discipline. That title usually comes through a personal, not a structural route. It would be interesting to know whether, if asked, those professors would describe themselves as a member of their original professional group, as our authors describe themselves as doctors, even though the GMC might take a different view. The Academy of Medical Educators defines standards for people working in medical, veterinary and dental education, against which people can voluntarily apply to become a Fellow. This organisation is not a statutory regulator and has no legal powers, but a professional interest body whose influence has been achieved through custom and practice (Academy of Medical Educators, 2021). It is the nearest that a person working in medical education has as a professional 'home'.

In their narratives, the five authors of this chapter find themselves moving into the study of medical education and development of medical education practice. They see this as a field in its own right, functionally and organisationally separate from the field of medicine. Its separateness, which seems to place it outside the field that it studies, relies perhaps on the medical qualifications, and perhaps the current clinical practice of medical educationalists, for its credibility, even though medical education also appoints academics with non-medical backgrounds. There are no particular qualifications for the field.

Overall, the accounts presented in this chapter link professionalisation in medicine with the dominant discourses that prescribe narrow roles. Medicine has paid a lot of attention to professionalisation, but this also brings boundaries that suggest that only doctors can have those professional characteristics, in turn implying, perhaps correctly, that only doctors can fully understand medical education. This is problematical when moving into medical education also moves the doctor away from the practice of medicine and into the domains of other disciplines: psychology, sociology and social science constructs and methods which they will not understand as well as they understand medicine. 'Belonging' in medical education, may therefore hold tensions both for doctors who are not trained in social science, and for social scientists who are not trained in medicine.

Medical Education: An Applied Discipline?

The variety of terms that might be applied to the person working in medical education reflects the variety of definitions of medical education itself. Some might see it as the rational design and delivery of educational programmes (Scheele, 2012), others might see it as a field of applied research and scholarship (Brand et al., 2022; Mann, 2011), while others argue that it is an academic discipline in its own right (Blouin, 2022). We would argue, however, that medical education does not meet all of Krishnan's five criteria for an academic discipline (Krishnan, 2009): it does have an object of study, but generally does not have its own specialised knowledge outside of medicine itself, neither does it have its own theories and concepts, nor specific terminology or research methods linked to medical education alone, but it does, in some countries, have departments or academic appointments, and postgraduate level courses (although no undergraduate level qualifying courses). Therefore, we argue that:

> …medical education is not an academic discipline, but is simply a means-ends orientated relational (social) practice (Noddings, 2003) supported by knowledge, and contextual judgement…. We would also argue that medical education takes strength from being an applied discipline, not a pure one (Hansson, 2007), harvesting its theories and ideas from a wide variety of social science, philosophical and methodological disciplines (Norman, 2011) and from experience. (Grant & Grant, 2023, p. 24)

An applied discipline is one which has strong elements of both practice and theory, which means that:

> …where matters of both theory and practice are of great concern, the range of perspectives widens … in an effort to satisfy the demands of both scholars and practitioners. (Swanson, 2007, p. 321)

This need to respond to the imperatives of both practice and theory, along with no original theories of its own but many borrowed, often in partial form, from elsewhere, places medical education in a challenging place in terms of academic identity. It uses partial ideas from psychology and psychological sub-specialties, from sociology, and anthropology; its research methods are both qualitative and quantitative. Medicine is its context but not its discipline.

There is a tension between the extensive practice of medical education and its actual speciality identity within and in relation to medicine.

What Is to be Done? A Field of Contradictions

A contradiction is an incompatible tendency within the same relation. The relation here is medical training which, as the authors describe, produces both professional identity as a doctor, and the desire to leave the profession, but then also the experience of exclusion from the field, followed by inclusion within a field that does not have a similar strong identity. The clear contradiction in medical education between activity on the one hand, and recognition, organisation and structure on the other hand, is a problem in need of resolution.

The issue of workplace conditions has been a benefit to recruitment to medical education, but what would need to change to make medicine sustainable for everyone, even though the feed into medical education might suffer? Could the collective power of doctors to take their working conditions into their own hands achieve such changes?

The problems identified in this chapter, suggest a number of paths forward which, ultimately, are for the professionals and academics to determine collectively. These might include a more analytical review of the status of medical education, its career structures for medical graduates and non-medical graduates, required qualifications, and professional organisations, and a more critical view of its theoretical base. How medical education is viewed by doctors and teachers who are not part of that field would be an important area of study, to move towards medical education as integral to and integrated with the practice of medicine for the good of a local context, so that all those managing and delivering medical training actually feel supported both by the research and their academic community to fulfil their role.

In terms of the working conditions that caused our five authors to enter medical education, these are part of the context and landscape of education and training, of learning, teaching and assessment, and should be a key issue for all medical educationalists. As we have seen, without that intervention, the changes that medical educationalists make to medical training will not improve the retention of their graduates and postgraduates to apply their knowledge and skills to the care of patients.

References

Abbasi, J. (2022). Pushed to their limits, 1 in 5 physicians intends to leave practice. *JAMA, 327*(15), 1435. https://doi.org/10.1001/jama.2022.5074

Academy of Medical Educators. (2021). *Professional standards for medical, dental and veterinary educators*. https://medicaleducators.org/Professional-Standards

AlSheikh, M. H., Zaini, R., Abdalla, M. E., & Magzoub, M. E. (2022). The wicked role of the medical education department. *Health Professions Education, 8*(1), 3–8. https://doi.org/10.55890/2452-3011.1014

Beck Dallaghan, G. L., Lomis, K., Crow, S., & Coplit, L. (2022). Bridging educational innovation and financial offices: using the Business Model Canvas modified for medical educators to communicate need. *Journal of Communication in Healthcare, 15*(2), 131–136. https://doi.org/10.1080/17538068.2021.1993691

Blouin, D. (2022). Health professions education as a discipline: Evidence based on Krishnan's framework. *Medical Teacher, 44*(4), 445–449. https://doi.org/10.1080/0142159X.2021.2020233

Brand, P. L. P., Leroy, P. L., & de Winter, J. P. (2022). The art and science of clinical pediatric education. *European Journal of Pediatrics, 181*(2), 427–428. https://doi.org/10.1007/s00431-021-03991-7

British Medical Association. (2021). *Sexism in medicine*. https://www.bma.org.uk/media/4487/sexism-in-medicine-bma-report.pdf

British Psychological Society. (2024). *Educational psychologist job profile | BPS*. https://www.bps.org.uk/educational-psychologist-job-profile

Brown, J. V. E., Crampton, P. E. S., Finn, G. M., & Morgan, J. E. (2020). From the sticky floor to the glass ceiling and everything in between: protocol for a systematic review of barriers and facilitators to clinical academic careers and interventions to address these, with a focus on gender inequality. *Systematic Reviews, 9*(1), 26. https://doi.org/10.1186/s13643-020-1286-z

Bustraan, J., Dijkhuizen, K., Velthuis, S., van der Post, R., Driessen, E., van Lith, J. M. M., & de Beaufort, A. J. (2019). Why do trainees leave hospital-based specialty training? A nationwide survey study investigating factors involved in attrition and subsequent career choices in the Netherlands. *BMJ Open, 9*(6), e028631. https://doi.org/10.1136/bmjopen-2018-028631

Calvert, M. J., & Freemantle, N. (2009). Cost-effective undergraduate medical education? *Journal of the Royal Society of Medicine, 102*(2), 46–48. https://doi.org/10.1258/jrsm.2008.080353

Cooper, N., Bartlett, M., Gay, S., Hammond, A., Lillicrap, M., Matthan, J., & Singh, M. (2021). Consensus statement on the content of clinical reasoning curricula in undergraduate medical education. *Medical Teacher, 43*(2), 152–159. https://doi.org/10.1080/0142159X.2020.1842343

CooperGibson Research. (2018). *Factors affecting teacher retention: Qualitative investigation*. www.gov.uk/government/publications

Cruess, R. L., Cruess, S. R., Boudreau, J. D., Snell, L., & Steinert, Y. (2014). Reframing medical education to support professional identity formation. *Academic Medicine, 89*(11), 1446–1451. https://doi.org/10.1097/ACM.0000000000000427

Cruess, S. R., Cruess, R. L., & Steinert, Y. (2019). Supporting the development of a professional identity: General principles. *Medical Teacher, 41*(6), 641–649. https://doi.org/10.1080/0142159X.2018.1536260

Degen, C., Li, J., & Angerer, P. (2015). Physicians' intention to leave direct patient care: an integrative review. *Human Resources for Health, 13*(1), 74. https://doi.org/10.1186/s12960-015-0068-5

Drolet, B. C. (2017). For-profit medical education. *JAMA, 318*(3), 301. https://doi.org/10.1001/jama.2017.7829

Ferreira, T., Collins, A. M., Feng, O., Samworth, R. J., & Horvath, R. (2023). Career intentions of medical students in the UK: A national, cross-sectional study (AIMS study). *BMJ Open, 13*(9), e075598. https://doi.org/10.1136/bmjopen-2023-075598

Ferreira, T., Collins, A. M., Handscomb, A., Al-Hashimi, D., Ferreira, T., Collins, A. M., Horvath, R., Feng, O., Samworth, R. J., Teo, M. K., Wigfield, C. C., Mulchrone, M. K., Pervaiz, A., Lewis, H. A., Wong, A., Gilks, B., Casteleyn, C., Kidher, S., Fitzsimons-West, E., … Dosani, S. (2024). The role of medical schools in UK students' career intentions: Findings from the AIMS study. *BMC Medical Education, 24*(1), 604. https://doi.org/10.1186/s12909-024-05366-6.

Finding, S. (2013). Gender, education and employment in education in Britain. *Observatoire de La Société Britannique, 14*, 173–204. https://doi.org/10.4000/osb.1563

Francis-Devine, B. (2023). *The gender pay gap*.

Gill, D. (2013). *Becoming doctors: The formation of professional identity in newly qualified doctors*. London University. https://discovery.ucl.ac.uk/id/eprint/10020735/1/__d6_Shared$_SUPP_Library_User%20Services_Circulation_Inter-Library%20Loans_IOE%20ETHOS_ETHOS%20digitised%20by%20ILL_GILL,%20D.pdf

Gov UK. (2021). *Disciplines covered by the endorsing bodies for science, engineering, humanities, social science and medicine – GOV.UK*. https://www.gov.uk/government/publications/global-talent-endorsing-bodies/disciplines-covered-by-the-endorsing-bodies-for-science-engineering-humanities-and-medicine

Grant, J., & Grant, L. (2023). Quality and constructed knowledge: Truth, paradigms, and the state of the science. *Medical Education, 57*(1), 23–30. https://doi.org/10.1111/medu.14871

Hämmig, O. (2018). Explaining burnout and the intention to leave the profession among health professionals – A cross-sectional study in a hospital setting in Switzerland. *BMC Health Services Research, 18*(1), 785. https://doi.org/10.1186/s12913-018-3556-1

Hansson, S. O. (2007). Values in pure and applied science. *Foundations of Science, 12*(3), 257–268. https://doi.org/10.1007/S10699-007-9107-6

Harvey Bluemel, A., Burton, O. E., Burford, B., Ellis, J., Finn, G., Bala, L., Byrne, M. H. V., Vance, G., & Alao, A. (2024). Barriers and facilitators to establishing a clinical academic career in clinical education research in the UK: A focus group study. *Medical Teacher, 46*(10), 1369–1377. https://doi.org/10.1080/0142159X.2024.2308783

Hodges, B. D., Maniate, J. M., Martimianakis, M. A., Alsuwaidan, M., & Segouin, C. (2009). Cracks and crevices: Globalization discourse and medical education. *Medical Teacher, 31*(10), 910–917. https://doi.org/10.3109/01421590802534932

Huntington, G. R. (2019). Resilience training is a slap in the face. *BMJ, l4176.* https://doi.org/10.1136/bmj.l4176

jobs.ac.uk. (n.d.). *The essential guide to moving up the academic career ladder.* Retrieved 16 November 2023, from https://www.jobs.ac.uk/media/pdf/careers/resources/the-essential-guide-to-moving-up-the-academic-career-ladder.pdf

Krishnan, A. (2009). *What are academic disciplines? Some observations on the disciplinary vs. interdisciplinary debate.* https://eprints.ncrm.ac.uk/id/eprint/783/

Mahat, M. (2019). The competitive forces that shape Australian medical education. *International Journal of Educational Management, 33*(5), 1082–1093. https://doi.org/10.1108/IJEM-01-2018-0015

Mann, K. V. (2011). Theoretical perspectives in medical education: past experience and future possibilities. *Medical Education, 45*(1), 60–68. https://doi.org/10.1111/j.1365-2923.2010.03757.x

Medic Footprints. (n.d.). *A career in medical education: What you need to know.* Retrieved 13 November 2023, from https://medicfootprints.org/a-guide-to-a-career-in-medical-education/

Mendeley Data. (2022). *Journal options to publish health professions education articles.* https://data.mendeley.com/datasets/rf29ym3bpw/1/files/663c77ad-b1c5-433b-badf-b4bb3685d0a5

Mount, G. R., Kahlke, R., Melton, J., & Varpio, L. (2022). A critical review of professional identity formation interventions in medical education. *Academic Medicine, 97*(11S), S96–S106. https://doi.org/10.1097/ACM.0000000000004904

Noddings, N. (2003). Is teaching a practice? *Journal of Philosophy of Education, 37*(2), 241–251. https://doi.org/10.1111/1467-9752.00323

Norman, G. (2011). Fifty years of medical education research: Waves of migration. *Medical Education, 45*(8), 785–791. https://doi.org/10.1111/j.1365-2923.2010.03921.x

Osmosis Team. (2023). HealthEd: A comprehensive list of major medical education conferences in 2023. In *osmosis.org.* https://www.osmosis.org/blog/2023/02/20/a-comprehensive-list-of-major-medical-education-conferences-in-2023#.

Oxtoby, K. (2015). Why doctors don't take sick leave. *BMJ, h6719.* https://doi.org/10.1136/bmj.h6719

Palmer, W., Rolewicz, L., & Dodsworth, E. (2023). *Strategies to improve the supply of clinical staff to the NHS.* https://www.nuffieldtrust.org.uk/sites/default/files/2023-09/Nuffield%20Trust%20-%20Waste%20not%20want%20not_WEB_FINAL.pdf

Pathmanathan, A., & Snelling, I. (2023). Exploring reasons behind UK doctors leaving the medical profession: A series of qualitative interviews with former UK doctors. *BMJ Open, 13*(9), e068202. https://doi.org/10.1136/bmjopen-2022-068202

Rees, C. E., & Monrouxe, L. V. (2018). Who are you and who do you want to be? Key considerations in developing professional identities in medicine. *Medical Journal of Australia, 209*(5), 202–203. https://doi.org/10.5694/mja18.00118

Rimmer, A. (2023). How can we make life better for doctors in postgraduate training? *BMJ (Clinical Research Ed.), 382,* 1783. https://doi.org/10.1136/bmj.p1783

Royal College of Physicians of London. (n.d.). MSc in medical education. Retrieved 11 November 2023, from https://www.rcplondon.ac.uk/education-practice/courses/msc-medical-education#

Sayburn, A. (2017). Why would a doctor leave medicine? *The Bulletin of the Royal College of Surgeons of England, 99*(1), 16–18. https://doi.org/10.1308/rcsbull.2017.16

Scheele, F. (2012). The art of medical education. *Facts, Views & Vision in ObGyn, 4*(4), 266–269.

Schermerhorn, J., Wilcox, S., Durning, S., Costello, J., Norton, C., & Meyer, H. (2023). Graduate health professions education programs as they choose to represent themselves: A website review. *MedEdPublish, 13*, 13. 10.12688/mep.19498.1.

Sepahvand, R., & Hozni, A. (2018). Megatrens of medical education and health entrepreneurship in the 21st century. *Strides in Development of Medical Education, In Press* (In Press). https://doi.org/10.5812/sdme.79867

Shiner, A., Watson, J., Doohan, N., & Howe, A. (2020). Learning or leaving? An international qualitative study of factors affecting the resilience of female family doctors. *BJGP Open, 4*(1), bjgpopen20X101017. https://doi.org/10.3399/bjgpopen20X101017

Silver, M. P. (2016). Critical reflection on physician retirement work identity, personal identity, and physician health. *Canadian Family Physician, 62*, 783–784.

Swanson, R. A. (2007). Theory framework for applied disciplines: Boundaries, contributing, core, useful, novel, and irrelevant components. *Human Resource Development Review, 6*(3), 321–339. https://doi.org/10.1177/1534484307303770

Tekian, A., & Harris, I. (2012). Preparing health professions education leaders worldwide: A description of masters-level programs. *Medical Teacher, 34*(1), 52–58. https://doi.org/10.310 9/0142159X.2011.599895

University of Liverpool. (n.d.). *Holly Tessler.* Retrieved 13 November 2023, from https://www. liverpool.ac.uk/music/staff/holly-s-tessler/

Volpe, R. L., Hopkins, M., Geathers, J., Watts Smith, C., & Cuffee, Y. (2021). Negotiating professional identity formation in medicine as an 'outsider': The experience of professionalization for minoritized medical students. *SSM – Qualitative Research in Health, 1*, 100017. https://doi.org/10.1016/j.ssmqr.2021.100017

Walsh, K. (Ed.). (2010). *Cost effectiveness in medical education.* Radcliffe Publishing Ltd. https://books.google.co.uk/books?hl=en&lr=&id=xBZTipzw7yUC&oi=fnd&pg=PR1&dq=cost+effe ctiveness+of+medical+education&ots=nfdhOmMQ9w&sig=XFq8wg21L_tSvLK9ycsYa6Gm Z_Q#v=onepage&q=cost%20effectiveness%20of%20medical%20education&f=false

Walsh, K. (Ed.). (2013). *Cost and value in medical education* (pp. 601–611). Oxford University Press.

Walsh, K. (2015). Editorial: Medical schools for profit? *Annals of Medical and Health Sciences Research, 5*(3), 155–156. https://www.ajol.info/index.php/amhsr/article/view/117527

Walsh, K. (2016). The cost bubble in medical education: Will it burst and when? *Annals of Medical and Health Sciences Research, 6*(4), 257–259. https://doi.org/10.4103/amhsr.amhsr_18_16

Watson, N. (2018). *Survey of medical clinical academic staffing levels 2018.* www.med-schools.ac.uk

Winkel, A. F., Telzak, B., Shaw, J., Hollond, C., Magro, J., Nicholson, J., & Quinn, G. (2021). The role of gender in careers in medicine: A systematic review and thematic synthesis of qualitative literature. *Journal of General Internal Medicine, 36*(8), 2392–2399. https://doi.org/10.1007/ s11606-021-06836-z

Zhang, Y., & Feng, X. (2011). The relationship between job satisfaction, burnout, and turnover intention among physicians from urban state-owned medical institutions in Hubei, China: A cross-sectional study. *BMC Health Services Research, 11*. https://doi.org/10.1186/1472-6963-11-235

Megan Brown is a Senior Research Associate in Medical Education in the School of Medicine at Newcastle University in the UK. She has a background in clinical medicine but has transitioned full-time to academia. She is Director of Communications and Social Media for the Association for the Study of Medical Education, and Assistant Editor for the journal *Academic Medicine*. She has a wide range of research interests, including qualitative methodologies, educational theory, retention of healthcare professionals within the workforce, and disability inclusion.

III.ii STATEMENT: Finding the Centre of My Venn: Navigating Experiences of Identity Challenge as a Medical Student

Anna Harvey Bluemel

My first three years at medical school, which encompassed two years of medical studies and one intercalated BSc in the History of Medicine, were more tumultuous than I had hoped when I left my small coastal home to study to be a doctor in London. When I think back to this time, I recognise that much of my discomfort was because of my inability to match up my new identity as a medical student with the myriad other identities that made up my life. Who was I, and how was this affected by what I do? How did my medical education help me gain not just the knowledge and skills needed to practise safely, but also help me 'be' a doctor and feel like 'part of the club'?

1 Social and Academic Life

In many ways I was a 'traditional' medical student when I first entered medical school, coming from a small secondary school in the south east of England. Whilst there was some nervous anticipation as I headed into my medical school career, mostly I was excited. My school did not have a large number of medical applicants and I was assured that medical school would be an opportunity to be in a cohort of people like me, who would be not just colleagues, but friends. Perhaps naively, I assumed that whilst I might find the academic work a challenge, the social side would be manageable—and certainly the patient-facing elements I was very much looking forward to.

A. Harvey Bluemel (✉)
Newcastle University, Newcastle upon Tyne, UK

Newcastle United Hospitals Trust, Newcastle upon Tyne, UK
e-mail: Anna.harvey@newcastle.ac.uk

129

My early experiences were almost the exact opposite of what I had expected. It was not the easy transition I had envisioned. I was surprised that many of my medical school peers didn't seem to be that like me at all. I was just one face in a large student crowd, and my peers were very different and sometimes difficult for me to understand. Many of them came from medical families and large fee-paying public schools, and I struggled to connect with any of my new colleagues, some of whom seemed to have formed tight cliques within hours of arriving on the first day! One of my new peers described me as 'quirky.' This gave me pause—it was certainly not how I would describe myself!

I hadn't realised how important the social aspect of medical school would be. Social connections often allow you to thrive academically at medical school: with peers who share notes, information and support in the run-up to exams, especially practical ones, and with more senior students and postgraduate doctors who can facilitate extracurriculars and share nuggets of information on the eccentricities of the particular medical school exams.

2   Becoming a Doctor, Fitting the Template

I also felt at odds with my learning outcomes, and how I was being taught to 'be' a doctor. 'Professionalism' was presented to me as a fixed point, which I should aspire to, for which I must change aspects of my personality and erase any individuality. In communication sessions during my early years at medical school, I struggled to grasp the secret template that was seemingly needed to gain positive feedback from trainers.

Comments on my clinical performance in my first few years often focused on my informality and sometime lack of structure, though I always collected the correct amount of clinical detail. I was confused by this: I viewed the process of taking a history as a conversation between two people, rather than a doctor (or doctor in training) and patient. I understood the importance of learning a structure to ensure I gathered the information needed, but once I had grasped this, I didn't see why I couldn't keep my communication more natural, aligning with my personality and instincts. Though I generally received good feedback from patients (and simulated patients), I didn't see how, with this immovable aspiration to professionalism, and the curiosity with which some of my peers treated me, I could make myself fit in medicine.

As a young person who had spent much of their time at secondary school performing in amateur dramatics, I was used to playing a character, and I thought this confidence and experience would easily translate into putting on the mask of medicine, until slowly the mask became a part of who I was. But my experiences taught me that even my mask wasn't good enough—that I needed one that didn't look like me at all! I felt as though instead of building on my natural personality, I was being encouraged to wipe clean any of my previous experience and start again, in a very specific way as dictated by my medical school, which didn't align well with my personal identity.

3 Who Am I?

So, I also struggled with amalgating my new medical identity with my other identities. The stereotypes around medical students often made me embarrassed to admit my choice of university course, and the implication of subsequent profession. Doctors hold a place in popular imagination, and assumptions are made by others when you identify yourself as a medical student or doctor. I found this uncomfortable. I didn't fit in anywhere: not medical enough for medical school, but too medical for other groups.

There was also a feeling of guilt at my own distress and failure: I am privileged in so many ways. As a white, educated, able-bodied woman in the UK, there was no reason for me to feel so out of place and dislocated from my peers. But I almost felt a fraud—on the surface I should have been able to easily integrate.

On reflection, I am sure many of my peers spent those fragile, formative years of medical school embroiled in a battle with some inner demon or another of their own. But as a characteristically arrogant 18, 19, 20 year old, I was totally unaware of this, lost and isolated in my own world of feeling the odd one out. There are many reasons why medical training in the UK lasts for 5 or 6 years, but one of them is surely to allow those who come to medical school as 18 year olds, straight from secondary school, the time to mature, to form adult neuronal connections and to deal with the experiences of early adult life that shape peoples' identities.

4 Coming Back to Medicine, Through Humanities

By the end of my second year of medical school, I had had enough. My attendance at lectures and seminars plummeted and I barely scraped a pass in my written examinations, failing my practical exam and having to resit: further proof, in my eyes, that I was inherently not cut out for the profession. I decided to complete my planned intercalated year and then leave medical school with at least a degree. To do, maybe, a Master's before I made any decisions.

There was no sudden realisation that I should continue with medical school. But in many ways my intercalated year, which I spent in the university History department with third year History undergraduates, saved my medical career. Studying humanities was so different from medicine. Students were encouraged to discuss and debate; feedback was given organically rather than a round-the-room discussion of flaws in your performance. Through this experience, I also became more confident receiving and evaluating feedback; using that which was useful, rejecting that which did not align with my personal morals and values, without allowing it to deeply affect or define me. I gained confidence, first in academic discussion, then in social aspects of the group and then, slowly, in my own personality. During my intercalated year, I was part of a much smaller cohort and was treated as an individual, where my seniors took the time to get to know me, not just professionally, but personally. Research has suggested that engagement with the humanities is positive for medical students' wellbeing generally, so my experience isn't a unique one! My humanities tutors openly supported me when I experienced issues relating to my identities outside of the academic space, whereas in medicine these were merely whispered about unless they became a fitness to practise issue.

I also began to quietly participate in the wider medical community, outside of my immediate peer group of students. Finding a community beyond my immediate medical school peers on social media was a real turning point in gaining the confidence to bring my whole self to my learning and developing clinical practice. Seeking out a diverse set of role models, and later, mentors, assisted by social media, helped me to learn that medicine is a place where I can not only survive by changing myself, but also thrive as me.

5   Widening Access

There is clearly still more work to be done to open medicine up to a greater diversity of students, but critically appraising the concept of professionalism (which has continued with little change) makes me hopeful that widening access will begin to not just serve those in the process of applying to medical school, but also students from more deprived backgrounds as they continue their journey into their careers as doctors. Whilst ensuring that a diverse range of students are able to access opportunities to gain a place at medical school, this is not the end of these students' widening access or participation journey: they need to be supported throughout medical school and beyond, with their unique needs recognised and adjusted for.

6   The Hidden Curriculum

Between my penultimate and final year of medical school I took a year out to work at *The BMJ* as head of the student section. As part of this role, I was tasked with hosting and developing the Sharp Scratch podcast, episodes of which are themed around aspects of the hidden curriculum. Learning the term 'the hidden curriculum' was in many ways revelatory, and helped me reframe some of the issues I had had with medical education and my burgeoning clinical and professional identity. Suddenly, here was a term for all the things I had been missing—and me missing them wasn't necessarily an internal failure of my own, but potentially related to an impenetrable education system that expected more learning than teaching, where kernels of professional knowledge were gleaned from doctor parents, siblings and cousins, putting you at a disadvantage if you had no such relations.

One Sharp Scratch episode of which I was particularly proud was themed around shame. In planning this episode, I was able to explore my own shame, and read and listen to accounts of others about shame in medicine and how it affects patients and clinicians alike. In many ways, shame had kept me in medicine when I wanted to leave—fear of the shame of admitting that I had got it wrong, that I had failed, that medicine wasn't for me and all the work I had put into getting to medical school had been wasted. In other ways, shame was what hindered me in medicine: I was ashamed to have a personality that I was told didn't fit, ashamed of not having the gravitas of a doctor, ashamed of taking up space and carving a professional identity that was my own, not projected onto me by other people. Through my experiences with my intercalated degree, finding role models on social media, and working outside of clinical practice, I realised I didn't need to make myself fit the professionalism template, but could mould a version of professionalism that allowed me to integrate my existing identities with the identity of student doctor and future healthcare professional.

I now see 'professionalism' in a different way: not as an immovable point to which everyone should aspire in the same way, but as a spectrum: my clinical persona falls more onto the informal side of this spectrum, which I have accepted is just as valid as any other clinical style. Through my reading, research and interactions with other students and clinicians, I have also learnt that the demographic that shaped our perception of professionalism in medicine is a demographic that no longer best represents the medical community, particularly students and junior doctors.

7 Becoming Me

As I write this piece, I have a new professional identity to navigate: no longer student doctor, but postgraduate doctor, fully qualified (though not yet fully registered). This has its own new facets: time management, system navigation and real responsibility to progress the patient journey rather than spend hours gathering information. I know what I admire in senior doctors I observe, and I hope to continue my journey of development by incorporating these skills into my own practice. Along the way, I have collected some other identities in my personal life: wife, aunt, sister of six. My clinical and professional identities are shaped by the ability to understand what I have learnt and gained from each of them—and transfer this learning and skills to other areas of life, pulling together all my varied identities to form my whole self, unashamedly. I appreciate these different facets of my identity as circles in the Venn diagram that make up who I am.

Although nervous, I feel much better equipped to face the challenges of this transition period than I was during my transition from school student to medical student. This is because I feel at ease with my other identities, and confident that I will be able to integrate them into my future ones as they develop and grow.

In many ways, identity has provided a lens through which I can frame my life, learning to integrate and prioritise my various and varied identities at different times. Sometimes it is more important to be a sister, partner or friend than a doctor. Educators should recognise this in their students and facilitate the development of a professional identity that integrates students' existing identities with their burgeoning professional identity, understanding the multiple roles and identities that students might have outside academic or clinical spaces, where sometimes identities complement one another, and sometimes come into conflict. One task of an educator should be to support students to explore their identities and find congruence within them. It is from this congruence that students can ultimately develop a professional identity that complements the other identities they value and prevent identity dissonance, which can cause intense discomfort for students and trainees.

Ultimately, I believe, it must be acknowledged that being a doctor is not, as much as some might like it to be, 'just a job like any other.' Medical training itself, and the experiences and emotions that we are exposed to through medical training, is a process of lifelong learning and development that naturally will irrevocably shape a person's identity, shifting perceptions of many other aspects of their lives outside of their clinical work.

Medical education, especially in the formative early stages, should encourage students to develop an understanding of their own personal and developing professional identities and find congruence and balance between them.

III.ii COMMENTARY: Social Mobility and the Profession: Lessons on Widening Participation

Janet Grant and Leonard Grant

The literature on the development of professional identity in medicine is vast in terms of how this state is attained. It is clearly an important issue. Yet it does not analyse sources of identity, or why developing a new identity might be necessary, or might be the problematical experience that Anna Harvey Bluemel describes, with the potential psychological cost of upward social mobility that has been discussed elsewhere (Kim et al., 2023).

In a strong, class-based society such as the United Kingdom, moving between those classes is not as easy as simply reserving places in higher education for disadvantaged groups. What this author so clearly describes for medicine, demonstrates that:

> …just bringing different students to a university does not magically make for a wonderful experience. In fact, it comes with a whole new set of problems. Students who differ from the main demographics of an institution often feel marginalised … (Nave, 2022)

That difference might be in terms of ethnicity, gender and sexuality, disability, or, as in our author's case, class. The corollary might be in terms of exclusion and discrimination, or, as in the experience here, identity and belonging.

In the United Kingdom, which is defined by its rigid class structure, a student's social background is perhaps the most significant factor, as Anna Harvey Bluemel describes. Accordingly, in the UK, there have been politically-driven policies to bring more working-class people into higher education, including medical school. These have not necessarily been enough (Apampa et al., 2019) or successful:

> … even after admission, mismatching social, economic and cultural capital continue to make the transition and progression on the course more challenging for WP *(widening participation)* students. Background and, specifically, the social 'class' of prospective students affect not only access but the attainment of even those WP students that do successfully gain admission to medical school. (Sartania et al., 2021)

The concept of social mobility is itself problematical, of course, given that capitalism requires a working class (and middle class) to sell their labour power, to generate profit for members of higher classes. So although widening participation might support increasing the workforce, and can be presented as a social good, the evidence of uptake and effect is unclear (Baines et al., 2022), and *de facto* it cannot achieve any wider social goals and remains largely symbolic since the problems are structural and relational.

Widening Participation and Moving into Another Class

Widening participation in higher education has been a long-standing political imperative in the UK, based on arguments of social justice, equal opportunities and economic development (Taylor et al., 2009). Despite this, social inequality continues to increase (Try, 2023). In medicine, the policy also hopes to produce doctors who will work in deprived areas. Initial results suggest that, for immediate post-graduation at least, this hope is not unreasonable, although the pattern may change with higher specialty training:

> …distance may be a deterrent factor for trainees from low social classes in choosing foundation training posts that are far away from parental home. (Kumwenda et al., 2018)

The story that Anna Harvey Bluemel tells, would be confirmed by very many other 'survivors of meritocracy' (Reay, 2021) who have also trodden her path. The experience of upward mobility in the United Kingdom has been carefully studied: it is an important idea for a society which is primarily structured by social class. While there is praise for the slight increase in working-class or under-privileged students in UK higher education:

> …what has been overlooked is that often social mobility has not led to them being socially and culturally assimilated into a higher social class. (Reay, 2021, p. 54)

Our author describes her experience of being characterised as 'quirky' and not like her peers, feeling that she should erase her own identity to fit in with her new status. Every detail of her experience is reported in the literature: not feeling good enough, thinking of leaving, feeling isolated, not 'belonging', culture shock, not being socially in line, feeling intimidated by more privileged students, working hard to counter this (Ikhlaq et al., 2023; Krstić et al., 2021) but is still inadequately researched, and as the author's experience suggests, inadequately catered for:

> …the psychological literature shows that working-class students suffer from negative stereotypes in regard to both their intellectual and academic competences, and that this affects their interactions with more privileged students (Reay, 2021, p. 55)

Alienation and Social Mobility

These feelings have recently been theorised in terms of the Marxist concept of alienation, where workers have control over their work increasingly removed. This concept has been applied to society, whereby more powerful groups create their own culture (around, for example, ideas of professionalism) which excludes others, resulting in experiences of powerlessness and loneliness (Øversveen, 2022). We might see a parallel in the territory of a profession and who 'belongs'.

Social class is a relational and defining characteristic where those who are either upwardly or downwardly mobile find it difficult to embed themselves into their adopted class. Bourdieu's research with upwardly mobile working-class students describes Anna Harvey Bluemel's experience, where students combined a commitment to academic learning and development of their academic capital with a more ambivalent view of social activities and interactions, and consequently had limited success in developing social capital of their own (Bourdieu, 2007).

This problem is not only experienced in the rigid class structure of the United Kingdom, even though many would be reluctant to claim membership of the working class in particular, known as a process of dis-identification (Savage et al., 2010), it has been reported throughout Europe where access to university is still characterised by social inequality (Nairz-Wirth et al., 2017). Other groups inside medicine also experience similar problems. A sense of shame that clinical skills are not sufficient, feelings of anxiety, lack of confidence, imposter syndrome and a need for psychological support is reported elsewhere by doctors of all grades, but especially those who are returning from a career break (Community Research, 2020).

Continuing Inequality in Medicine

Despite widening participation policies, it is still the case that poorer applicants are far less likely to receive an offer for medicine than their wealthier counterparts. Eighty per cent of medical students come from professional households and more than a quarter from private schools (Steven et al., 2016). As has been the case for a long time (Lentz & Laband, 1989), the advantage in human and social capital that derives from growing up with parents who are doctors still ensures that their children will feel that medical school is for them, while children who are the first in their family to consider university are still likely to feel that medical school is not for them (Moore, 2021).

Medicine remains one of the most closed-off professions to those from lower socio-economic classes (Friedman & Laurison, 2019). The class position of professions is a contested area (Engels & Marx, 1848; Halliday, 1983), but this does not really matter when the educational system itself cannot change the class structure of society from which inequality emanates, and does not fundamentally alter social mobility (Goldthorpe, 2016). That being so, students who could be identified as having widened participation, experience the cultural dislocation, and subsequent challenges of identity, that Anna Harvey Bluemel describes. Those challenges have been characterised in terms of 'the stickiness of working-class habitus' in contradiction with the logic of practice of the élite field they have striven to be part of, yielding:

…the lack of symmetry between the two that generates discomfort, intimidation, withdrawal, lack of confidence, even terror, pain and isolation for some of the working-class students. (Reay, 2021, p.61)

Widening access and participation currently seems to focus rather than decrease this problem, leaving its solution in the hands of the individual, as Anna Harvey Bluemel recounts. Not everyone is sure of the goodness of the idea of individual social mobility which might cause us to ignore the plight of the poor, and to imagine that anyone can benefit from that directional social movement, which clearly, they cannot:

> With upward mobility, society needs a better myth. The current one is dysfunctional—individualistic, unrealistic, and prone to promise more than it can deliver. (Delgado, 2007, p. 913)

It is not enough to accept widening participation as a social good without thinking this through further either in relation to the individual, the actions of the school, the career that follows, or the effects on society as a whole.

The Problem of Identity

Anne Harvey Bluemel reminds us that it is a person with an existing identity who enters medicine, and is faced with the task of becoming identified with a new group. The distance between the existing and the intended identity will influence the nature and success of the journey. How personal identity is 'pulled' into professional identity, or pushed away from that burgeoning identity, and how those processes contribute to feelings of self-doubt and isolation is well-documented (Volpe et al., 2021), and supports the picture painted by our author.

What Is Professional Identity?

The literature on professional identity shows a very wide range of definitions and factors, and no definitional agreement (Fitzgerald, 2020; Li et al., 2020). There seems to be no satisfactory way of measuring such identity (Matthews et al., 2019), although why that measurement might be important is unclear. Likewise, it has been concluded that professional identity is not a topic for regulation (Professional Standards Authority for Health and Social Care, 2016).

There is a considerable body of research about professional identity in the healthcare professions, which addresses the issues that are important for Anna Harvey Bluemel: belonging, the lived experience, working and professional contexts, the individual, and learning and qualifications. Nonetheless, it has been concluded that:

> Professional identity research is under-represented in many health professions and is poorly theorised ... Critical perspectives of professional identity in the health professions literature is lacking, particularly with respect to race and indigeneity, socioeconomic status and gender. (Cornett et al., 2023)

Professional Identity and Professionalism

For Anna Harvey Bluemel, professional identity seems to be defined by the idea of professionalism as taught in the curriculum, and of group membership based on that shared idea. The concatenation of professionalism and professional identity has been advocated since the first sociological study of medicine was conducted (Merton et al., 1957) and has subsequently often been taken for granted (Chandran et al., 2019; Krishnasamy et al., 2022), but perhaps deserves further analysis since socialisation, a developmental perspective, and a variety of enablers and barriers are also at play (Findyartini et al., 2022; Sarraf-Yazdi et al., 2021). These 'professional codes' are problematical and 'may or may not reflect reality' and may, as our author shows, be constructed by the individual for themselves, amalgamating many aspects of their experience, including the formula taught in the curriculum (Lane, 2018). This requires crucial and conscious reflection.

Indeed, the idea that 'Professional identity is different from professionalism' has been well-argued (Cruess & Cruess, 2017). Developing professional identity might also involve participation in a community of practice and developing a shared culture (which might or might not display the qualities of 'professionalism'). It has been noted that students who enter medicine via a widening participation route bring 'different cultural assets' (Garlick & Brown, 2008), so, as Anna Harvey Bluemel explores, as well as individual and professional identity, a person will also have their own cultural identity:

> …cultural identity can be understood as the experience, enactment, and negotiation of dynamic social identifications by group members within particular settings. (Chen & Lin, 2016)

Social Identity

Cultural identity links a person to their group (Hofstede et al., 2010). In the case of widening participation, that group will most probably be social class and ethnicity. What happens in practice when such an existing cultural identity varies from that of another group that must be joined, is described by Anna Harvey Bluemel.

Although the literature tends to focus on the loss of cultural identity linked to globalisation and migration, it can happen, as we see in this chapter, at a much more local level. As we move from one context to another, we can also move between a variety of such identities. Anna Harvey Bluemel has chosen to adopt a medical identity while retaining what she can of her own existing social, personal and cultural identities. An important question might concern choice of primary identity, and membership of the primary group, and what of other identities is shared with each group.

Social identity theory and research have examined the ways in which individuals construct their self-identity from their membership of social (and, in our case, professional) groups. Considerable pride, purpose and self-worth can be derived from such belonging, accompanied by the prejudice, bias and discrimination that characterises inter-group behaviours (Tajfel & Turner, 1979, 1986). Anna Harvey Bleumel's account demonstrates all of these.

Professional identity formation is a much more challenging process than simply teaching 'professionalism'. It is both individual and social-contextual (Monrouxe & Rees, 2015). If those aspects do not align, then the journey is difficult. The resolution of role confusion, as Anna Harvey Bleumel seems to suggest, might be as relevant to this stage, as it was during adolescence (Block, 2011).

The volume of publications on this topic suggests that it is generally accepted that a person cannot easily practise as a doctor unless they feel like a doctor, and situate themselves as a doctor (Mount et al., 2022), even though what that means might not be entirely clear. The consequences of that for people who experience, or perhaps resist, the upward social mobility that might accompany being a doctor, may be profound—not least because the class structure and the individual's identity with it, remain.

References

Apampa, A., Kubacki, A., Ojha, U., & Xiang, J. (2019). Challenges in widening participation outreach: Is enough being done to tackle the under-representation of low-income students in medicine? *Advances in Medical Education and Practice, 10*, 917–923. https://doi.org/10.2147/AMEP.S211895

Baines, L., Gooch, D., & Ng-Knight, T. (2022). Do widening participation interventions change university attitudes in UK school children? A systematic review of the efficacy of UK programmes, and quality of evaluation evidence. *Educational Review*, 1–20. https://doi.org/10.1080/00131911.2022.2077703

Block, M. (2011). Identity versus role confusion. In *Encyclopedia of child behavior and development* (pp. 785–786). Springer. https://doi.org/10.1007/978-0-387-79061-9_1447

Bourdieu, P. (2007). *Sketch for a self-analysis*. University of Chicago Press.

Chandran, L., Iuli, R. J., Strano-Paul, L., & Post, S. G. (2019). Developing "a way of being": Deliberate approaches to professional identity formation in medical education. *Academic Psychiatry, 43*(5), 521–527. https://doi.org/10.1007/s40596-019-01048-4

Chen, Y.-W., & Lin, H. (2016). Cultural identities. In *Oxford Research Encyclopedia of Communication*. Oxford University Press. https://doi.org/10.1093/acrefore/9780190228613.013.20

Community Research. (2020). *Understanding the nature and scale of the issues associated with doctors' induction (including those returning to practice)*. https://www.gmc-uk.org/about/what-we-do-and-why/data-and-research/research-and-insight-archive/understanding-the-nature-and-scale-of-the-issues-associated-with-doctors-induction

Cornett, M., Palermo, C., & Ash, S. (2023). Professional identity research in the health professions—A scoping review. *Advances in Health Sciences Education, 28*(2), 589–642. https://doi.org/10.1007/s10459-022-10171-1

Cruess, S. R., & Cruess, R. L. (2017). From teaching professionalism to supporting professional identity formation: Lessons from medicine. *Mercer Law Review, 68*(3) https://digitalcommons.law.mercer.edu/jour_mlr/vol68/iss3/8

Delgado, R. (2007). The myth of upward mobility. *University of Pittsburgh Law Review, 68*(4), 879–913.

Engels, F., & Marx, K. (1848). *The communist manifesto*. Workers' Educational Association.

Findyartini, A., Greviana, N., Felaza, E., Faruqi, M., Zahratul Afifah, T., & Auliya Firdausy, M. (2022). Professional identity formation of medical students: A mixed-methods study in a hierarchical and collectivist culture. *BMC Medical Education, 22*(1), 443. https://doi.org/10.1186/s12909-022-03393-9

Fitzgerald, A. (2020). Professional identity: A concept analysis. *Nursing Forum, 55*(3), 447–472. https://doi.org/10.1111/nuf.12450

Friedman, S., & Laurison, D. (2019). *The class ceiling. Why it pays to be Privileged*. Policy Press.

Garlick, P. B., & Brown, G. (2008). Widening participation in medicine. *BMJ, 336*(7653), 1111–1113. https://doi.org/10.1136/bmj.39508.606157.BE

Goldthorpe, J. H. (2016). Social class mobility in modern Britain: Changing structure, constant process. *Journal of the British Academy, 4*, 89–111. https://doi.org/10.5871/jba/004.089

Halliday, T. C. (1983). Professions, class and capitalism. *European Journal of Sociology, 24*(2), 321–346. https://doi.org/10.1017/S0003975600004094

Hofstede, G., Hofstede, G. J., & Minkov, M. (2010). *Cultures and organisations: Software of the mind. Intercultural cooperation and Its importance for survival*. McGraw-Hill.

Ikhlaq, H., Agarwal, S., Kwok, C., Golamgouse, H., Derby, S., McRae, N., Brown, M. E. L., Collin, V., Parekh, R., & Kumar, S. (2023). Medical students impacted by discrimination: A qualitative study into their experiences of belonging and support systems at medical schools in the UK. *BMJ Open, 13*(12), e078314. https://doi.org/10.1136/bmjopen-2023-078314

Kim, T., Shein, B., Joy, E. E., Murphy, P. K., & Allan, B. A. (2023). The myth of social mobility: Subjective social mobility and mental health. *The Counseling Psychologist, 51*(3), 395–421. https://doi.org/10.1177/00110000221148671

Krishnasamy, N., Hasamnis, A., & Patil, S. (2022). Developing professional identity among undergraduate medical students in a competency-based curriculum: Educators' perspective. *Journal of Education Health Promotion, 11*(1), 361. https://doi.org/10.4103/jehp.jehp_329_22

Krstić, C., Krstić, L., Tulloch, A., Agius, S., Warren, A., & Doody, G. A. (2021). The experience of widening participation students in undergraduate medical education in the UK: A qualitative systematic review. *Medical Teacher, 43*(9), 1044–1053. https://doi.org/10.1080/0142159X.2021.1908976

Kumwenda, B., Cleland, J. A., Prescott, G. J., Walker, K. A., & Johnston, P. W. (2018). Geographical mobility of UK trainee doctors, from family home to first job: A national cohort study. *BMC Medical Education, 18*(1), 314. https://doi.org/10.1186/s12909-018-1414-9

Lane, S. (2018). Professionalism and professional identity: What are they, and what are they to you? *Australian Medical Student Journal*. https://www.amsj.org/archives/6294#:~:text=This%20conveniently%20for%20me%20encompasses,the%20delivery%20of%20open%20disclosure

Lentz, B. F., & Laband, D. N. (1989). Why so many children of doctors become doctors: Nepotism vs. human capital transfers. *The Journal of Human Resources, 24*(3), 396–413.

Li, L., Gan, Y., Yang, Y., Jiang, H., Lu, K., Zhou, X., Nie, Z., Opoku, S., Zheng, Y., Yu, F., & Lu, Z. (2020). Analysis on professional identity and related factors among Chinese general practitioners: A National Cross-sectional Study. *BMC Family Practice, 21*(1), 80. https://doi.org/10.1186/s12875-020-01155-4

Matthews, J., Bialocerkowski, A., & Molineux, M. (2019). Professional identity measures for student health professionals – A systematic review of psychometric properties. *BMC Medical Education, 19*(1), 308. https://doi.org/10.1186/s12909-019-1660-5

Merton, R. K., Reader, G. G., & Kendall, P. L. (1957). *The student-physician: Introductory studies in the sociology of medical education*. Harvard University Press.

Monrouxe, L. V., & Rees, C. E. (2015). Theoretical perspectives on identity: Researching identities in healthcare education. In J. Cleland & S. J. Durning (Eds.), *Researching medical education* (pp. 129–140). Wiley Blackwell.

Moore, L. (2021, March 11). 'Not for people like me': The class ceiling within the health sector workforce – Hospital times. *Hospital Times*. https://www.hospitaltimes.co.uk/not-for-people-like-me-the-class-ceiling-within-the-health-sector-workforce/

Mount, G. R., Kahlke, R., Melton, J., & Varpio, L. (2022). A critical review of professional identity formation interventions in medical education. *Academic Medicine, 97*(11S), S96–S106. https://doi.org/10.1097/ACM.0000000000004904

Nairz-Wirth, E., Feldmann, K., & Spiegl, J. (2017). Habitus conflicts and experiences of symbolic violence as obstacles for non-traditional students. *European Educational Research Journal, 16*(1), 12–29. https://doi.org/10.1177/1474904116673644

Nave, L. (2022, October 10). Universities must do better at bridging the gap between diversity and belonging. *Times Higher Education.*

Øversveen, E. (2022). Capitalism and alienation: Towards a Marxist theory of alienation for the 21st century. *European Journal of Social Theory, 25*(3), 440–457. https://doi.org/10.1177/13684310211021579

Professional Standards Authority for Health and Social Care. (2016). *Professional identities and regulation: A literature review.*

Reay, D. (2021). The working classes and higher education: Meritocratic fallacies of upward mobility in the United Kingdom. *European Journal of Education, 56*(1), 53–64. https://doi.org/10.1111/ejed.12438

Sarraf-Yazdi, S., Teo, Y. N., How, A. E. H., Teo, Y. H., Goh, S., Kow, C. S., Lam, W. Y., Wong, R. S. M., Ghazali, H. Z. B., Lauw, S.-K., Tan, J. R. M., Lee, R. B. Q., Ong, Y. T., Chan, N. P. X., Cheong, C. W. S., Kamal, N. H. A., Lee, A. S. I., Tan, L. H. E., Chin, A. M. C., … Krishna, L. K. R. (2021). A scoping review of professional identity formation in undergraduate medical education. *Journal of General Internal Medicine, 36*(11), 3511–3521. http://extra.shu.ac.uk/alac/text/Article The Politics of Widening Participation.doc.

Sartania, N., Alldridge, L., & Ray, C. (2021). Barriers to access, transition and progression of widening participation students in UK medical schools: The students' perspective. *MedEdPublish, 10*(1), 10.15694/mep.2021.000132.1.

Savage, M., Silva, E., & Warde, A. (2010). Dis-identification and class identity. In E. Silva & A. Warde (Eds.), *Cultural analysis and Bourdieu's legacy: Settling accounts and developing alternatives. Culture, economy and the social* (pp. 60–74). Routledge.

Steven, K., Dowell, J., Jackson, C., & Guthrie, B. (2016). Fair access to medicine? Retrospective analysis of UK medical schools application data 2009-2012 using three measures of socioeconomic status. *BMC Medical Education, 16*(1), 11. https://doi.org/10.1186/s12909-016-0536-1

Tajfel, H., & Turner, J. C. (1979). An integrative theory of intergroup conflict. In W. G. Austin & S. Worchel (Eds.), *The social psychology of intergroup relations* (pp. 33–47). Brooks/Cole.

Tajfel, H., & Turner, J. C. (1986). The social identity theory of intergroup behaviour. In S. Worchel & W. G. Austin (Eds.), *Psychology of intergroup relations* (pp. 7–24). Nelson-Hall.

Taylor, G., Mellor, L., & Walton, L. (2009). *The politics of widening participation: A review of the literature.* http://extra.shu.ac.uk/alac/text/Article The Politics of Widening Participation.doc

Try, L. (2023). *Growing inequality across Britain has left millions of families exposed to the cost-of-living crisis.* The Resolution Foundation. https://www.resolutionfoundation.org/comment/growing-inequality-across-britain-has-left-millions-of-families-exposed-to-the-cost-of-living-crisis/

Volpe, R. L., Hopkins, M., Geathers, J., Watts Smith, C., & Cuffee, Y. (2021). Negotiating professional identity formation in medicine as an 'outsider': The experience of professionalization for minoritized medical students. *SSM – Qualitative Research in Health, 1*, 100017. https://doi.org/10.1016/j.ssmqr.2021.100017

Anna Harvey Bluemel is an NIHR Academic Clinical Fellow training in obstetrics and gynaecology and researching clinical education in Newcastle. She is a former BMJ Editorial Scholar (2019/20) and sits on the Committee of Trainees in the UK Association for the Study of Medical Education. Outside of work she is a sister, wife and current Mum to one.

III.iii STATEMENT: Medical Education: What Should We Be Teaching Future Generations?

Aadil S. Chagla and Leena S. Chagla

Medicine is a profession that deals with all aspects of health and healing. Four goals of medicine were set out for the Hastings Center Goals of Medicine project in 1999. These are applicable today and for the foreseeable future:

(1) Prevention of disease and injury, and the promotion and maintenance of health.
(2) Relief from pain and suffering caused by illness.
(3) To care and cure those with an illness, and to care for those who cannot be cured.
(4) To prevent premature death and to aim for a peaceful death for all.
 (Hanson & Callahan, 1999)

Science is moving at a fast pace (nano-technology, the microchip …), and as we dive into this new and exciting world of minutiae, we must not miss the bigger picture. It is so important to have a strong foundation in a good education, and to learn to heal humans and not just particular medical conditions.

A. S. Chagla
King Edward Memorial Hospital, Mumbai, India

Seth G S Medical College, Mumbai, India

L. S. Chagla (✉)
Mersey and West Lancashire Teaching Hospitals NHS Trust, Prescot, UK
e-mail: Leena.Chagla@merseywestlancs.nhs.uk

© The Author(s), under exclusive license to Springer Nature
Switzerland AG 2026
J. Grant, L. Grant (eds.), *The Contradictions of Medical Education*,
https://doi.org/10.1007/978-3-031-90394-6_10

1   Putting Patients First

In this era of subspecialisation, we learn more and more about less and less, with the aim of becoming masters in our field. Sometimes pursuing personal milestones in one's career can be at the cost of service delivery and patient care. But as physicians, it is imperative that we put our patients first.

Medical schools should have a mission and a vision to teach their students not only to cure, but to care for patients, so both their physical and emotional needs are met.

Take, for example, the mission of Oxford Medical College, Hospital and Research Centre in Bangalore, India:

> To impart learner centered education for excellence in knowledge, skills and attitude in providing holistic health care services to the society with compassion, commitment, confidence and conviction. (The Oxford Medical College, 2025)

This institution seeks to combine the science and social mission of medicine. This sort of mission could be replicated in all medical schools globally.

2   Learning from Practice

In the development of the discipline, fundamental learning from practice (professional experiential knowledge) is often downgraded with emphasis laid on evidence-based medicine and set protocols. We sometimes forget that our own experience, local knowledge and personal outcomes may be necessary and more beneficial to help our own local patient population. We must have the conviction to share our experience with others and not be afraid to be trend setters rather than mere followers.

Students should be taught that medicine is a profession and professional judgement comes with experience. Clinical bedside teaching should be part of every consultant's job plan. Books are important but you cannot learn without seeing patients, as every case is different. In the words written on Sir William Osler's bookplates:

> He who studies medicine without books sails an uncharted sea, but he who studies medicine without patients does not to go to sea at all. (Duncan, 1980)

3   Experience and Judgement: The Identity of a Profession

As educators, we also need to look at the economics of health care. We need to stop practising defensive medicine. To do this there must be almost little or no litigation, and for this we need the help of the public, the media and the politicians. Today in medicine, especially with access to the internet, everyone thinks they are experts. A profession is not defined by acquisition of knowledge, but by acquisition of experience and judgement.

In conclusion, the profession must have renewed confidence in its experience and judgement, and make it transparent that this is done in the interest of getting it right for each patient. This professional induction and identity should be introduced at medical school. There is not only the need to acquire knowledge and skill, but the recognition that the use of this in day to day practice is what ensures that patients are each dealt with as individuals. Medicine is a profession, and like any profession, is based on knowledge and skill, but the need to assert one's judgement plays a big part, and it is this part of the profession that others cannot access. Hence there is the potential for contradiction between the individual clinician's judgement and the autonomy of a patient's decision often based on Dr. Google! Can this contradiction be resolved by better patient engagement and less political and legal interference? Something needs to be done, and done now to safeguard the future of medicine as a profession.

References

Duncan, W. E. (1980). Osler's bookplate. *New England Journal of Medicine, 303*(18), 1067–1067. https://doi.org/10.1056/NEJM198010303031824

Hanson, M. J., & Callahan, D. (Eds.). (1999). *The goals of medicine: The forgotten issues in health care reform.* Georgetown University Press.

The Oxford Medical College, Hospital & Research Centre. (2025). *Vision and mission.* http://theoxfordmedical.org/mission_vison.htm

III.iii COMMENTARY: Medicine as a Profession

Janet Grant and Leonard Grant

This chapter presents a precise personal meditation by two practising clinicians on medicine as a profession, and a call to action. The authors begin by setting out the goals of medicine as they understand them, and then consider what constrains, affects or damages their ability to practise. In their contemplation, they list a variety of dyads which might be seen as conflicting, but which come together within the professional role. Most of these dyads present an aspect of being or becoming a clinician as opposed to patient care. So patient care was linked in an uncomfortable, oppugnant pairing with the scientific basis of medicine, focusing on the disease, time for teaching, and the clinician's own career and interests which have been shown to distance young doctors from specialties that require long-term care of the patient (Gale & Livesley, 1974). They conclude with a call to have confidence in the experience and judgement of the profession. It is upon the last line of this short reflection that we begin our theorisation.

The Identity and Future of Medicine as a Profession

Aadil and Leena Chagla are ultimately concerned with medicine as a profession. What is the nature of a profession, what sets it apart from other areas of practice and how the identity of the practitioner develops into that of the professional, are issues that have long concerned both doctors and medical educators, as the vast literature on professional identity formation attests (Sarraf-Yazdi et al., 2021).

The authors are concerned with how to 'safeguard the future of medicine as a profession', thus we begin by asking: What is the history and present of medicine as a profession?

The nature of a profession has been discussed in the literature for more than a century. Despite professionalism being a dominant concept in the lives of physicians, educators and students, there is, as yet, no agreed framework or definition (Goddard & Brockbank, 2023). It might be different in different contexts.

Doctors have long enjoyed (and fought for) a respected position as a profession (Parry & Parry, 2019). 'Doctor' carries with it not only a sense of *skill* or *expertise* (many other people are considered either experts or skilful, for example baristas, bricklayers or musicians) but a *status*. Indeed, some have argued that holding medicine as a science, rather than a practice, is a way of ensuring its status in society (Montgomery, 2006). Throughout their chapter, this tension is expressed: the authors are concerned with influences on medicine from outside forces whether 'political and legal interference' or the easier access to medical knowledge which means that 'everyone thinks they are an expert'. Aadil and Leena Chagla argue, however, that the work of the medical profession is inherently inaccessible to outsiders who do not have their judgment, cultivated through the process of practising medicine.

Although there are many characteristics attributed to a profession, there are some which are particularly important to the argument in this chapter. Centrally, professions '...develop more complex or advanced forms of knowledge bases, non-routine practices and conceptual or 'white-collar' work' (Glückler et al., 2023). This is a complex nexus of formally acquired knowledge and skill, developed in practice, through experience, within a forming mantle of values and an ethical code. The authors of this chapter are concerned that the right balance of these elements is maintained and transmitted through education and training. How the patient is viewed is central to that undertaking.

The process of becoming a professional has been similarly analysed, for it is this professional identity which is said to guide the physician's work (Rees & Monrouxe, 2018). A strong professional identity has been shown to be beneficial to healthcare practice (Monrouxe et al., 2017), a finding which resonates with the authors' experience set out in this chapter. The development of professional identity is considered to be a vital aspect of medical training (Trevino & Poitevien, 2021).

Having said that, the sometimes difficult issue of relinquishing that identity at retirement is much under-researched (Silver & Williams, 2016).

The question of who can become a professional is fraught. Race and ethnicity are largely absent or are considered irrelevant in the literature on professional identity formation, despite this literature making significant advances in understanding how trainees internalise the norms of the profession (Wyatt et al., 2021). There can exist a tension between the personal and professional identity that is difficult or impossible to navigate, as the previous two chapters demonstrate. The issues of career development raised by the authors might epitomise this tension:

> Sometimes pursuing personal milestones in one's career can be at the cost of service delivery and patient care. As physicians, it is imperative that we put our patients first.

The Importance of Practice: Polanyi's Paradox

Medicine is a fractal of society, occupying a position in the hierarchy of the context in which it finds itself. The values of a society are transmitted through experience of others and of practice. And that is also true of a profession. We can teach courses on professionalism, and students will learn that topic and pass the assessments. But some aspects of being a clinician can only develop as a function of experience. There is a necessary trajectory of learning whereby some forms of understanding are dependent on prior study and experience, whereby prior learning becomes re-evaluated in the light of subsequent experience (Slotnick, 2001). The large body of research on this topic suggests that medical professional identity, which defines values and behaviours, develops as a function of discussion, reflection and immersion in a community of practice, soaking up the ways in which things are done

(Cruess et al., 2019). Specific skills in the doctor-patient relationship can be learned in many ways, including through simulation (Bosméan et al., 2022), and through role models (Ahmady et al., 2022; Passi et al., 2013). But one student's advice still holds true: Be what you teach (Skiles, 2005).

Learning in theory and learning from practice are complementary, with practice perhaps being the more powerful, because the theory is simply a formal, and perhaps sanitised version of practice. A student cannot have the understanding of an experienced clinician. That maturity cannot be taught, it can only be developed through experience (Grant & Marsden, 1987). And that professional practice, and what has been learned from it, are difficult to represent accurately and completely. This is the paradox that Polanyi described.

Polanyi observed that there are things that we all know how to do, but do not know how to explain: We can know more than we can tell (Polanyi, 1966). This is our 'tacit knowledge'. This means that sometimes when we try to describe these things, we turn them into formulae that fail to capture the reality. Tacit knowledge is personal, built from experience, and difficult to communicate. So we can teach students about the practice of medicine and the values and skills that underpin it, but their actual personal understanding will only be built from their experience and from what they notice about that in themselves and others. It is that which develops them as a professional.

Professions each have their own knowledge cultures (Nerland, 2012) made up of the ways in which the knowledge base is produced and codified from scientific research, and reflections on practice. The knowledge culture in a profession is individually and collectively accumulated and then distributed or shared. This building of every student's and clinician's tacit knowledge makes early and continuing clinical contact, the contextualisation of their learning, and role models observed in practice, so fundamentally important (Simmenroth et al., 2023). It is their subsequent tacit knowledge that will determine their view of the patient. Polanyi, a chemist, was highly critical of the idea of 'objectivity' as representing science. Instead, as others have argued (Grant & Grant, 2023), science (both natural and social) is based on judgement and:

> …those who lauded objectivity while ignoring or rejecting the authoritative role of personal and moral elements in knowing, had opened the door to the tyranny and violence of the twentieth century. (Gulick, 2016)

Those tacit personal and moral elements are honed through the role models, practice and experience that are sometimes, and inappropriately, called the 'hidden curriculum' (Neve & Collett, 2018), which was first identified as a form of secondary socialisation of learners within the education system (Jackson, 1990).

Using Bourdieu's theory of practice (Bourdieu, 1977), other authors have analysed the tension between medical students' collective (curriculum driven) and individual trajectories (how each one navigates their way towards the ultimate curriculum imperative) (Balmer et al., 2016). The curriculum is powerful in relation to both trajectories: 'Students come to medical school with diverse histories and life experiences', however, '.....they encounter curricula that valorize competencies – common and potentially reductive standards – for what every physician should be, should know, and should be able to do' (Balmer et al., 2016).

When that personal element of learning to practise medicine is disrupted by, as the authors suggest, 'evidence-based medicine and set protocols' or, as is written elsewhere in this book, by finding your practice itself constrained or alienating, this is a very disturbing experience. It is, perhaps, a disruption to the sense of professional self that is at the core of the Aadil and Leena Chagla's tension and concern.

The Contradictions

In this chapter, the authors gesture towards two problems which they present as separate but which we would like to synthesise and explain as a contradiction.

The authors indicate that 'sometimes pursuing personal milestones in one's career can be at the cost of service delivery and patient care'. How can this be the case? How can the development of a career ever be at odds with the core function of medical practice, as the authors themselves set out at the beginning of the chapter?

The second is the tension between the desire to be patient-centred but not to subordinate professional judgement to "Dr Google". This is, without a doubt, a challenge faced by many doctors, especially primary care physicians.

We consider both of these problems to be an expression of the position of medicine as a profession. Professionalisation is not primarily measured or understood in relation to patients, although how a doctor behaves towards patients is, of course, part of this question. Rather, the profession determines and defines itself internally, in relation to other professionals. The question of outside influence (be that legal or political) is thus experienced as a threat to identity.

A profession must also be in control of the knowledge of that profession. Where professional knowledge is social and collective, it is not surprising that the centrality of practice and experience are emphasised in this chapter. In this, proficiency is developmental, and grows out of practice and social learning. And that requires a context that demonstrates the tacit knowledge that Aadil and Leena Chagla hope that entrants to the profession will acquire.

This knowledge is safeguarded by the profession itself – so is not accessible to all – thus, in order to be trusted to wield said knowledge and continue to regulate access to it, doctors must behave in a way that justifies the trust of those outside the profession (Goddard and Brockbank, 2023)

Certainly, as Aadil and Leena Chagla suggest, the expression of this contradiction could be relieved by allowing the profession more autonomy. But without considering professionalism in relation to and in conversation with people outside medicine, we wonder if this contradiction will ever be truly resolved.

References

Ahmady, S., Kohan, N., Namazi, H., Zarei, A., Mirmoghtadaei, Z. S., & Hamidi, H. (2022). Outstanding qualities of a successful role model in medical education: Students and professors' points of view. *Annals of Medicine and Surgery, 82.* https://doi.org/10.1016/j.amsu.2022.104652

Balmer, D. F., Devlin, M. J., & Richards, B. F. (2016). Understanding the relation between medical students' collective and individual trajectories: An application of habitus. *Perspectives on Medical Education, 6*(1), 36–43. https://doi.org/10.1007/S40037-016-0321-1

Bosméan, L., Chaffanjon, P., & Bellier, A. (2022). Impact of physician–patient relationship training on medical students' interpersonal skills during simulated medical consultations: A cross-sectional study. *BMC Medical Education, 22*(1), 117. https://doi.org/10.1186/s12909-022-03171-7

Bourdieu, P. (1977). *Outline of a theory of practice.* Cambridge University Press. https://doi.org/10.1017/CBO9780511812507

Cruess, S. R., Cruess, R. L., & Steinert, Y. (2019). Supporting the development of a professional identity: General principles. *Medical Teacher, 41*(6), 641–649. https://doi.org/10.1080/0142159X.2018.1536260

Gale, J., & Livesley, B. (1974). Attitudes towards geriatrics: A report of the King's survey. *Age and Ageing, 3*(1), 49–53. https://doi.org/10.1093/ageing/3.1.49

Glückler, J., Winch, C., & Punstein, A. M. (Eds.). (2023). *Professions and proficiency. Knowledge and space* (Vol. 18). Springer International Publishing. https://doi.org/10.1007/978-3-031-24910-5

Goddard, V. C. T., & Brockbank, S. (2023). Re-opening Pandora's box: Who owns professionalism and is it time for a 21st century definition? *Medical Education, 57,* 66–75. https://doi.org/10.1111/medu.14862

Grant, J., & Grant, L. (2023). Quality and constructed knowledge: Truth, paradigms, and the state of the science. *Medical Education, 57*(1), 23–30. https://doi.org/10.1111/medu.14871

Grant, J., & Marsden, P. (1987). The structure of memorized knowledge in students and clinicians: An explanation for diagnostic expertise. *Medical Education, 21*(2), 92–98. https://doi.org/10.1111/j.1365-2923.1987.tb00672.x

Gulick, W. (2016). Relating Polanyi's tacit dimension to social epistemology: Three recent interpretations. *Social Epistemology, 30*(3), 297–325. https://doi.org/10.1080/02691728.2015.1015064

Jackson, P. W. (1990). *Life in classrooms* (2nd ed.). Teachers College Press.

Monrouxe, L. V., Bullock, A., Tseng, H.-M., & Wells, S. E. (2017). Association of professional identity, gender, team understanding, anxiety and workplace learning alignment with burnout in junior doctors: A longitudinal cohort study. *BMJ Open, 7*(12), e017942. https://doi.org/10.1136/bmjopen-2017-017942

Montgomery, K. (2006). *How doctors think: Clinical judgment and the practice of medicine.* Oxford University Press.

Nerland, M. (2012). Professions as knowledge cultures. In K. Jensen, L. C. Lahn, & M. Nerland (Eds.), *Professional learning in the knowledge society* (Vol. 6, pp. 27–48). Sense Publishers.

Neve, H., & Collett, T. (2018). Empowering students with the hidden curriculum. *The Clinical Teacher, 15*(6), 494–499. https://doi.org/10.1111/tct.12736

Parry, N., & Parry, J. (2019). *The rise of the medical profession. A study of collective social mobility.* Routledge. https://www.routledge.com/The-Rise-of-the-Medical-Profession-A-Study-of-Collective-Social-Mobility/Parry-Parry/p/book/9780367001827

Passi, V., Johnson, S., Peile, E., Wright, S., Hafferty, F., & Johnson, N. (2013). Doctor role modelling in medical education: BEME guide no. 27. *Medical Teacher, 35*(9), e1422–e1436. https://doi.org/10.3109/0142159X.2013.806982

Polanyi, M. (1966). *The tacit dimension.* Doubleday.

Rees, C. E., & Monrouxe, L. V. (2018). Who are you and who do you want to be? Key considerations in developing professional identities in medicine. *Medical Journal of Australia, 209*(5), 202–203. https://doi.org/10.5694/mja18.00118

Sarraf-Yazdi, S., Teo, Y. N., How, A. E. H., Teo, Y. H., Goh, S., Kow, C. S., Lam, W. Y., Wong, R. S. M., Ghazali, H. Z. B., Lauw, S. K., Tan, J. R. M., Lee, R. B. Q., Ong, Y. T., Chan, N. P. X., Cheong, C. W. S., Kamal, N. H. A., Lee, A. S. I., Tan, L. H. E., Chin, A. M. C., … Krishna, L. K. R. (2021). A scoping review of professional identity formation in undergraduate medical education. *Journal of General Internal Medicine, 36*(11), 3511–3521. https://doi.org/10.1007/s11606-021-07024-9.

Silver, M. P., & Williams, S. A. (2016). Reluctance to retire: A qualitative study on work identity, intergenerational conflict, and retirement in academic medicine. *The Gerontologist, gnw142.* https://doi.org/10.1093/geront/gnw142

Simmenroth, A., Harding, A., Vallersnes, O. M., Dowek, A., Carelli, F., Kiknadze, N., & Karppinen, H. (2023). Early clinical exposure in undergraduate medical education: A questionnaire survey of 30 European countries. *Medical Teacher, 45*(4), 426–432. https://doi.org/1 0.1080/0142159X.2022.2137014

Skiles, J. (2005). Teaching professionalism: A medical student's opinion. *The Clinical Teacher, 2*(2), 66–71. https://doi.org/10.1111/j.1743-498X.2005.00063.x

Slotnick, H. B. (2001). How doctors learn: Education and learning across the medical-school-to-practice trajectory. *Academic Medicine, 76*, 1013–1026.

Trevino, R., & Poitevien, P. (2021). Professional identity formation for underrepresented in medicine learners. *Current Problems in Pediatric and Adolescent Health Care, 51*(10), 101091. https://doi.org/10.1016/j.cppeds.2021.101091

Wyatt, T. R., Balmer, D., Rockich-Winston, N., Chow, C. J., Richards, J., & Zaidi, Z. (2021). 'Whispers and shadows': A critical review of the professional identity literature with respect to minority physicians. *Medical Education, 55*(2), 148–158. https://doi.org/10.1111/medu.14295

Aadil S. Chagla is Professor and Head of Neurosurgery, King Edward Memorial Hospital, and Seth G S Medical College, Mumbai, India. He has made considerable original contributions to thinking about medical education emphasising giving to future generations through the process of teaching. His TEDx talk on this is at: https://www.youtube.com/watch?v=5bXGCI5b6Wk. He is a polymath representing India and the Bombay Gymkhana in cricket, as well as being an accomplished musician and classic car rally driver. This varied background informs his thoughts about education.

Leena S. Chagla is Consultant Surgeon, St Helens and Knowsley Teaching Hospitals NHS Trust, UK. She is a postgraduate specialty trainer, and President of the Association of Breast Surgery where she has led the campaign against bullying and harassment in her discipline.

Part IV

Managing the System, the Profession, and the Business of Medical Education: The Neoliberal Project

Summary

The changes and issues we see in current medical education, many expressed in the chapters of this book, are often part of the political and economic neoliberal project of our times which embodies market principles, individualisation, and regulatory control. These ultimately are of greatest benefit to vested interests and to the international trade in doctors. The widespread current drive towards universal compliance with standards, the evidence for which is missing, while its political and economic effect is clear, is the most obvious example of neoliberal control.

Just as medical education is an instrument of power and politics, it is also a business. How these factors align with, or are in contradiction to, the purposes and expressed values of a profession is a serious question. The authors of the chapters in Part IV illustrate these tensions in very different contexts. We see that when decisions about medical education and medical service are removed from the profession itself and taken over by politicians and management consultants, the market and the economy become the dominant determinants of decisions. The effects of this are a distribution of power that might not serve either the profession or communities. Following this, we have a strong complementary argument for the profession to be the leaders and decision-makers, not only for the better training of the next generations of doctors but for the better care of patients. However, concern for an increasing instrumental use of the profession to deliver others' political and business plans, is illustrated in a study from Brazil. Even within a medical school, there are tensions between academics and those who must manage the school. So political and power struggles are seen inside medical education, between medical education and politicians, between market forces and professional purposes, between the different groups who manage the business and process of medical education, between medical education and the service, and between neoliberal control and professional autonomy. And in the middle of all this is the individual doctor who is increasingly becoming a pawn in others' plans. Although in other Parts of this book the politics and power of medical education are clearly drawn in relation to international activities, we see that politics and power also drive medical education within countries, their regions and their institutions.

IV.i STATEMENT: The Marginalisation of the Medical Profession and Its Impact on Medical Education: Lessons from Sweden

Thomas Zilling

An Annual Medical Conference held by the Portuguese Medical Association (the Ordem dos Médicos) had Future Medicine as its overarching title. I was invited to give a speech entitled: *What is the Future Role for Physicians after Task Shifting and Skills Mix? Some Examples from Sweden.*

After the symposium, the moderator gathered the speakers for some debriefing and said: 'Thomas! All questions from the audience were for you and people were so shocked about your report on the transformation of healthcare in Sweden.'

This is the story about how politicians, officials and global management consulting firms have continuously tried to marginalise the medical profession in Sweden and examples of its consequences for medical education.

1 50 Years of Socialised Medicine

Healthcare in Sweden was socialised on January 1st 1970, when a new political reform forced doctors to go from being self-employed to being civil servants paid by the regional County Councils. This political reform, adopting the UK Beveridge model for healthcare, created a dramatic change in the work of the medical profession from seeing as many patients as possible to a more civil service profession where work in the outpatients' clinic was often exchanged for less stressful tasks away from patients. The political reform in Sweden created high quality care but with less accessibility for patients. Also, the management of healthcare changed. Where the medical profession had previously, to a large degree, been responsible for

T. Zilling (✉)
Department of Surgery, Lund University, Lund, Sweden
e-mail: thomas.zilling@slf.se

delivered care, politicians and officials now gradually took over the management of care through political reforms (Ström, 2020).

2 Academic Medicine Grew Stronger

One positive result of the 1970 healthcare reform was that in the 1970s and 1980s, academic medicine grew in the universities. Salaried doctors now worked only 40 hours per week which created a shortage of doctors. Thus, the number of medical students had to increase, and new medical schools opened. The length of medical education at the time was set at five and a half years and an internship of 18 months was created. This was to provide remote parts of the country with assistant doctors. Education for specialist training was regulated by the National Board of Health and Welfare and mandatory courses were financed by the government.

3 Continuing Professional Development

Before 1970, there was financing of continuing professional development (CPD) for self-employed doctors, which had never been a problem. In 1970, the Swedish government took over the financing of CPD for salaried doctors. An average of seven days per year of participation in courses and conferences occurred. In 1981, the government transferred the responsibility for financing of CPD to the County Councils. This was not considered a problem for most doctors as the pharmaceutical and medical-technical industries were contributing by sponsoring both events and participants (Swedish Medical Association, 1996). But today, financing of CPD by the medical industry is no longer accepted and the burden of paying rests largely on the doctor.

4 Reduction in Doctors' Managerial Influence

During the 1990s, Swedish politicians were constantly looking for a strategy to reduce increasing healthcare costs and solve the problem of access to care. To show political action, laws and regulations were introduced to control healthcare differently. In 1991, a new law called the "Chief Physician Reform" was rolled out. With this reform, all medical and administrative responsibilities were given to only one physician of any hospital department or health centre. The same year, the government legislated that each patient should have the right to a physician in charge of their case, a 'patient responsible doctor'. But this reform was only on paper because no one understood how to put it into practice.

These new laws and regulations resulted in less professional autonomy, and this would get worse. The medical profession, represented by the Swedish Medical Association, wanted management of care handled by medical doctors and further to tone down the politicians' direct involvement in healthcare. However, in 1997, the Health and Medical Services Act was rewritten whereby the requirement for health-care managers to have medical training was removed. Healthcare management became a separate profession. The medical profession was accused of having neglected leadership and organisational training unlike other professions, such as nurses, who now moved their position forward. The outcome of these policy changes has only been studied to a small extent. One case study describes the complexity of management and medical professionalism and the organisational needs of Swedish doctors (Kuhlmann et al., 2016). It showed that nurses usually have a strong position in middle to lower levels of management, which may include the management of doctors.

5   Joining the European Union Changes Medical Education

In 1995, Sweden joined the European Union (EU) which created a comprehensive change in Swedish basic medical education. Thus in 1997, Swedish medical education was reformed with the aim of adapting to EU standards and following the controversial Bologna process (AMEE EMSA IMFSA, 2010; Christensen, 2004). Education was now extended from five and a half to six years to end with a doctor's licence to practise. Previously, a licence to practise was awarded after completing an internship of 18 months. According to the Bologna process, all higher education in Europe must be divided into three cycles: basic level, advanced level, and post-graduate level. Also, a new points system called ECTS (European Credit Transfer System) was introduced in which the position of PhD studies was confused in both timing and process (Baptista, 2016). The new education differed from the old by more attention to project work and less time spent on traditional training and lectures.

6   Big Is Beautiful

After 60 years of financial stability, Sweden was struck by a financial crisis from 1991–93. So, there were influences on larger university hospitals to create a basis for highly specialised care and better research. In 1997, the three hospitals in Gothenburg were all merged into one, the Sahlgrenska University Hospital. These new giant hospitals with fewer beds after the merger, decreased opportunities for practical training of medical students on the wards. Instead, the core curriculum had to increase the theoretical component. To compensate for insufficient experience on the wards, training was offered in skills labs.

7   The Merger of Karolinska and Huddinge in Stockholm

In the 2002 election, the County Council of Stockholm changed hands. The merger of the two university hospitals in Stockholm, Karolinska and Huddinge, which previously had been considered as politically impossible, was now seen as the solution to several problems. The overarching motive for the merger was economic efficiency with the hope for an immediate large and quick saving. It was expected that the merger would also enhance research excellence and improve medical education.

The economic researcher Soki Choi described the merger process in Stockholm, as the "Big Bang" in which radical change occurred through a top-down approach. One year after the merger there was 'total war' between management and staff members. Eventually, management split into two groups; some were loyal to the Director and some to their medical colleagues and clinical care groups (Choi, 2011). It was quite clear that leading politicians and officials in Stockholm were stimulated by the creation of the major University Hospital in Gothenburg. They were afraid of being left behind in the areas of clinical research and highly specialised care. Instead of learning from the Gothenburg merger, Stockholm decided to follow the same track, even though a published report showed a loss of cost control. Economic problems were still reported in Gothenburg six years after the formal merger (Brorström, 2004). For the politicians in Stockholm, ideas to make care more effective and cheaper came from the United States.

8   Stockholm Value-Based Care

In the new millennium, Swedish politicians were for several years courted by consultants from the Boston Consulting Group (BCG). A Harvard Professor of Economics, Michael Porter, advocated restructuring care and emphasised the importance of competition. The patient's needs must be put at the centre and the way forward was described by Porter as Value-Based Care (Thorpe, 2007). But Porter's reform meant a change that removed the traditional medical specialities such as internal medicine, surgery, and infectious disease. These are the basis of learning for medical students and have been the backbone of professional occupational identity, acting as carriers of knowledge, research and training.

BCG had adopted Michael Porter's ideas as a business model, claiming that future healthcare requires reorganisation, and the obsolete old clinical structure must be removed. Keywords such as 'care around patients' were used to create new 'integrated competence clusters'. The old clinical department structure, which also forms the basis for medical knowledge, was scrapped and the new organisation was built around different diagnoses in a multiprofessional setting. Porter created the new concept of 'bundled payment for performance' which is based on the equation:

$$\text{Value for patients} = \frac{\text{Health outcomes that matter to patients}}{\text{Cost of delivering these outcomes}}$$

According to Porter, competition is vital so healthcare providers should compete, and more money will be given to those who deliver the best care. However, Porter's vision did not deal with the questions: How should medical education be designed when the old specialities no longer exist? What should future medical students learn?

BCG was convincing to some, and the new concept was introduced at Sahlgrenska University Hospital in 2013 and later at the New Karolinska where the politicians were eager to follow the trend. Karolinska's Director was not impressed by the new ideas which he described as 'the emperor's new clothes'. The unhappy politicians in Stockholm decided to disband the old board of Karolinska hospital and employ a business entrepreneur as chairman of a new board. With the ambition to quickly stage value-based healthcare, the board began to act operationally which could not be accepted by the hospital Director who left his position in May 2014. A new hospital Director was recruited, together with several management consultants all with the ambition to keep the backward-looking physicians out of operational decisions. In 2016, the hospital paid 36.5 million Euros to different consulting groups and 42.7 million Euros in the following year (Gustafsson & Röstlund, 2019).

9   As a Role Model for Misperceived Political Needs

Around the turn of the millennium, an intensive debate occurred about medical research and medical education.

Many university hospitals had reached a point where healthcare and the academic world had drifted apart and developed in different directions. Healthcare, which is governed by the regions, had become increasingly market-orientated with buying and selling systems and a focus on production. This in turn, put the focus on leadership, organisation, and management of care. Like all production businesses, the 21 Swedish regions developed their own systems regarding their needs for research and development.

The medical faculties, for their part, were now developing a very preclinical orientation. Furthermore, the organisation was different within government-owned universities with collegial governance, election of managers and activity characterised by committee work and a consensus culture. But universities are also governed by other fundamental values where it is essential that research is freely selected and is assessed strictly scientifically.

So a new problem arose, as the medical faculties had to produce research, and also be responsible for good medical education, specialist training and continuing professional development. For education to work, this must rest on scientific knowledge. Lack of clinical teachers was previously not a problem. Preclinical research had been linked to the physiological and biochemical era where doctors undertook preclinical research. This created a good base of teachers with a medical background. But now, former medical researchers were replaced by mathematicians, physicists, biologists, biomedical scientists, economists and more. This had some advantages; for example, modern biomedical techniques and research approaches were incorporated into medical research. However, the strong links between pre-clinical training, for example in anatomy and physiology, and clinical practice and research were lost. Fewer doctors started their careers with basic research training, and 'clinical' research was often performed by research groups lacking patient contact. Many diseases have become successful virtual research foci in grant applications, but the focus on the affected patient is lost.

With the new curricula, many basic sciences such as anatomy, histology and pharmacology disappeared at several Swedish medical universities. With this, the university also loses the corresponding teachers as well as their research. Even though the subjects remain somewhere in the curriculum, teachers with the right competence and background become a dying breed and the opportunity for regrowth is missing.

10   Epilogue

When Swedish medical faculties reformed their core curricula according to the Bologna process, the difference between content of the curriculum varied so much that people had to ask themselves if this was the same education provided in Lund as in Stockholm. Thoughts were raised regarding a national core curriculum which was soon dismissed as the various faculties considered themselves competing for the best students by offering the best programme.

Whether the new education is better or worse compared to the previous one, no-one can say. On the other hand, training medical students aims to prepare future doctors for a professional life that, irrespective of speciality, has changed dramatically. An academic career alongside the practice of medicine does not have the same merit in an organisation that primarily focuses on production. Adaptation to the Bologna process has prevented the early recruitment of medical students for research and teaching positions.

With new management where the manager is rarely a doctor, the role of a medical doctor becomes more and more like an industrial worker and the duties of academic medicine are increasingly taken over by other professions.

After three years with value-based healthcare, Sahlgrenska University Hospital in Gothenburg stopped the process in 2016. The director had ordered an evaluation, and after reading the report, she noted that it did not support the introduction of thematic reorganisation of Sahlgrenska. There is no evidence supporting value-based healthcare and this concept does not appear to be better or worse than anything else. The director concludes; 'Sahlgrenska prefers to collaborate with universities and colleges, rather than with management consultants to develop care and research' (Orstadius, 2018).

In Stockholm on the other hand, the minister of the County Council was pleased to open the new thematically organised Karolinska Hospital in June 2016. To him, there are no setbacks. Unfortunately, what he is really offering the Region of Stockholm is the world's most expensive hospital with a reduced number of beds compared to the old hospital, and with a repayment plan for 24 years. This is in a Region with an already severe lack of hospital beds and poorly developed primary care (Ennart & Mellgren, 2017). In 2018, the Swedish agency for health technology and assessment of social services (SBU) published a systematic mapping of published research on the value-based healthcare framework on the behalf of the Swedish government. According to the results, it is not possible to draw any general conclusions regarding specific effects of value-based healthcare (Dellve et al., 2018).

It is left for the future to decide whether Stockholm will reap any value for all the millions spent on consulting companies. A major problem in Stockholm is that medical professionalism has come to be viewed as a serious obstacle to the development of rationalised managerial control. The lesson learned is that with less marginalisation of the medical profession in universities and hospitals, Swedish taxpayers would have saved a lot of money and most likely gained better trained doctors and strengthened clinical research.

References

AMEE EMSA IMFSA. (2010). The Bologna Process and its implications for medical education. *Medical Teacher, 32*(4), 302–304. https://doi.org/10.3109/01421591003653047

Baptista, S. (2016). View of doctoral education through the lenses of the Bologna Process. *International Journal of Humanities and Social Science Research, 2*, 29–36. https://www.lifescienceglobal.com/pms/index.php/ijhssr/article/view/3630/2139

Brorström, R. (2004). Den stora vändningen? *Studentlitteratur.*

Choi, S. (2011). *Competing logics in hospital mergers. The case of the Karolinska University Hospital.* Karolinska Institutet.

Christensen, L. (2004). The Bologna process and medical education. *Medical Teacher, 26*(7), 625–629. https://doi.org/10.1080/01421590400012190

Dellve, L., Hellström, A., Levay, C., & Savage, C. (2018). *Value-based healthcare. A mapping of the literature.* www.SBU.SE/285E

Ennart, H., & Mellgren, F. (2017). *Sjukt Hus. Globala Miljardsvindlerier, Från Lesotho till Nya Karolinska.* Häftad.

Gustafsson, A., & Röstlund, L. (2019). *Konsulterna: Kampen om Karolinska.* Mondial.

Kuhlmann, E., Rangnitt, Y., & von Knorring, M. (2016). Medicine and management: Looking inside the box of changing hospital governance. *BMC Health Services Research, 16*(S2), 159. https://doi.org/10.1186/s12913-016-1393-7

Orstadius, I. (2018). Så tänkte Sahlgrenskas nya sjukhusdirektör då hon stoppade införandet. Sjukhusläkaren. https://www.sjukhuslakaren.se/sa-tankte-sahlgrenskas-nya-sjukhusdirektor-da-hon-stoppade-inforandet/

Ström, M. (2020). Milstolpe I svensk sjukvårdshistoria. *Läkartidningen, 117*, 10–15.

Swedish Medical Association. (1996). *Läkares Fortbildning.*

Thorpe, K. E. (2007). Redefining health care: Creating value-based competition on results. *New England Journal of Medicine, 356*(3), 316–317. https://doi.org/10.1056/NEJMbkrev57186

IV.i COMMENTARY: Politics, Neoliberalism and Proletarianisation of the Profession

Janet Grant and Leonard Grant

Thomas Zilling's account is the story of a complex system of medicine and medical education. He depicts the ways in which their equilibrium is so easily disturbed by interventions from other systems: from politics, the market, management, ideas from another context, and educational philosophies. He presents these as not only destroying a system that worked well, but in doing so, also attacking the medical profession that upheld and largely managed that system. A fundamental contradiction is being described between the medical profession and neoliberal forces. This power struggle has been enacted over many decades and has, perhaps, come to medicine very late. In the United Kingdom, taking control of the professions, beginning with teachers, was a policy of the right-wing Thatcher government in the 1980s (Gardner-McTaggart, 2021). It had been predicted over a century earlier that this would happen: where a group does not own the means of production itself, it will then be reduced to simply selling its labour power to those who do own the means of production; in Thomas Zilling's case, the local and national governments own hospitals. So the prediction can be enacted:

> The bourgeoisie has stripped of its halo every occupation hitherto honoured and looked up to with reverent awe. It has converted the physician, the lawyer, the priest, the poet, the man of science, into its paid wage labourers. (Engels & Marx, 1848)

It is this process, and the neoliberal agenda that supported it, that Thomas Zilling is describing.

Medical Education and the Healthcare Service

This chapter shows clearly that to provide the education, training, clinical experience and supervision necessary, medical education is dependent upon the healthcare service. Although many published papers discuss the relationship between medical education and the service in terms of how medical schools and their curricula will tailor themselves to the needs of the healthcare service, almost none, with very few exceptions (Khojasteh et al., 2009), discuss the dependency of medical schools on that healthcare service, or the ways in which postgraduate training and continuing professional development depend on clinical practice. This dependence introduces an economic and political weave to decisions about the practice of medicine and the design of medical education. Such concerns have been mooted in terms of the effects of providing medical education on service provision (Lee et al., 2014), while simulations in clinical training have been used rather than actual direct clinical experience to address problems of provision of clinical experience (AlHaqwi & Taha, 2015), and postgraduate doctors in training have been brought in as Teaching Fellows to mitigate disruption to the service (Hossain et al., 2021).

The political purpose of providing a healthcare service, and the professional purpose of providing health care seem to be different. A casualty of these sometimes unaligned purposes is the education and training of the next generation of doctors, and the continuing education of current clinicians. When one aspect of the system is altered, it has both planned and unplanned consequences for all other aspects.

Given the recognition that medical education depends on the quality of the hospital or primary care learning environment (Ludmerer, 2004), it seems anomalous that changes can be made to that service, such as those described by Thomas Zilling, while not considering their effect on education and training. But these changes can be understood within a neoliberal agenda.

The Rise of Neoliberalism

Thomas Zilling shares similar concerns to those of other chapter authors. These derive from the currently dominant economic and political ideas of neoliberalism. This is an outlook which began in the 1970s, at the time that Thomas Zilling reports the instigation of changes in Sweden, which has come to characterise every aspect of professional, public and private life. The growth of neoliberalism in healthcare is similarly seen across many economies. in the UK, as in Sweden, this approach has been actively encouraged and facilitated by successive governments of all parties (Humber, 2019; Park, 2012).

Neoliberalism embodies market principles, individualisation and state regulation which ultimately are of greatest benefit to the private sector, rather than the public. As this chapter shows, it is a political project which serves particular social interests (Collins et al., 2016; Waitzkin, 2018). The evidence suggests that many neoliberal policies have tended to benefit society's wealthiest at the expense of lower- and middle-income populations, as Thomas Zilling says, increasing anxiety over things like healthcare, housing, higher education and retirement, that used to be more broadly shared public goods. Neoliberalism is associated with a decline in welfare benefits and an increase in inequalities (Bambra, 2022). In the case of medicine, it is characterised by increasing commodification of health which means that costs and managerial organisation and control enter the picture. The privatisation and attendant proletarianisation and destruction of professional independence, which Thomas Zilling seems to describe, have long been sought by neoliberal forces. The case of Sweden, as described in this chapter, and the opening up of the UK NHS to market logic and its privatisation and fragmentation, are examples of the 'success' of neoliberal health policy in Europe (Mann, 2022).

As neoliberalism dominates, education is more and more organised in relation to demands of employment, mimicking the types of managerialist models of efficiency that Thomas Zilling describes (Gaspard et al., 2012). We can see this happening to medicine too through the language of mergers and cost control that he reports. Private and international capital has made huge inroads into supposedly socialised healthcare in the UK, and there is no doubt that this is also the case in Sweden

(Ramesh, 2012). This is the corollary to the events that Thomas Zilling describes—
as these changes are wrought on the profession, someone is benefitting whether that
is government coffers or private healthcare companies.

Reducing staff numbers and making those left behind work harder is a very common technique for generating more profit or decreasing costs. This is true in healthcare generally and Thomas Zilling points to it specifically—the changes to working
hours are not altruistic but presumably a cost saving exercise. The productivity of
doctors must be forced to increase to compensate, as it would in any other industry.

Neoliberalism promotes policies and an ideology that tend to encourage a greater
focus on individualism and individual responsibility, often at the expense of collective responsibility and sources of identity, such as membership of a profession.
Thomas Zilling shows us how this has worked out in Sweden in the past 50 years.

Professional Versus Managerial and Governmental Purposes: The Contradictions

Thomas Zilling's account is set within a framework of task shifting, skills mix,
employment status and salaries, reducing costs, and the inevitable decreases in professional autonomy. The opposing perspectives are that of the profession which
focuses on patient care, and that of governments and their managers (and management consultants) which focuses on efficiency. In this, the profession will be seen as
spending money, and the governments as saving money.

With the adoption of neoliberal approaches in western countries, management
control mechanisms were introduced which have had a direct effect on medical
professionalism, including medicine's role in education and training:

> In this context, governments and policymakers searched for more effective and efficient
> healthcare services, coupled with demands regarding healthcare accountability and trans-
> parency. (Numerato et al., 2012, p. 627)

Although Thomas Zilling does not say so, these demands have been accompanied
everywhere by measures designed to:

> … govern professional practices, such as auditing, clinical guidelines, knowledge manage-
> ment systems, protocols, standards, incident reporting systems, and a variety of incentive
> tools. (Numerato et al., 2012, p. 627)

Medicine seems to have embraced these neoliberal ideas. As the medical profession
has internalised the ideas of the management discourse, so medicine has come to be
dominated by these standardised and controllable processes. This has been referred
to as the 'colonisation of professionals' (Numerato et al., 2012) which has affected
both professional autonomy and the way that doctors think about their work, merg-
ing the contradictory professional and managerial cultures, to the detriment of professional autonomy, as Thomas Zilling describes. It has been argued that doctors
themselves should take up the role of managers of the healthcare service (Loh,

2015), and some have embraced this but without any significant mitigating effect on the loss of professional autonomy of their colleagues (Powell & Davies, 2016). These 'adversarial superpowers' of the profession and the managers (McKee et al., 1999) represent different interests.

The Rise of Harmonisation, Quality Assurance and Regulatory Control

Thomas Zilling's account shows a greater agenda than that experienced in Sweden alone. He discusses the much-contested Bologna Process (Cervantes & Rambaud, 2020; Kushnir, 2020; Štech, 2011), which was an invention of the European Union launched in the late 1990s, to bring into line all university education across the European space. This policy can be seen as the ultimate neoliberal project (Wihlborg, 2019) which requires compliance with one view of the structure of higher education. It is not a structure which sits well with medical education (Cumming, 2010) but is one which Sweden tried to implement.

The Bologna Process encourages the commodification and marketisation of higher education and its products (Garben, 2011). Along with its efforts towards harmonisation, competitiveness, freedom of movement, and exchange in higher education across the European community, came the need for new systems of regulation and accountability:

> The emerging European higher education system is indicative of a new architecture of regulation that shapes the nature and form of the public university in the direction of market citizenship. (Jayasuriya, 2010, p. 19)

In other words, regulation of education and its products is for economic purposes, supporting the neoliberal project. Qualifications frameworks and standards were required, supported by the promotion of European co-operation in quality assurance, which might be seen as a precursor to the even more all-encompassing and controlling trend towards the global standards and quality assurance systems that have since emerged (Rashid, 2023).

This approach to control in education was not entirely new, although its use for the market was a neoliberal development of an existing managerial and political trend. For example, at a national level, schoolteachers in the UK had already been subject to increasing control since 1984 when the governing Conservative Party abolished the Schools Council which was an independent charity advising on educational matters such as assessment, and established in its place the government-led and much more interventional Council for the Accreditation of Teacher Education (The National Archives, n.d.), which exercised control over teacher development.

With this, accreditation began its long and continuing journey as a controller of professional activity, which we now see in medical education at national and global levels, despite lack of evidence of effect, from which we might conclude that this is more about control than quality (Bedoll et al., 2021; Rashid, 2023; Rashid et al.,

2023). In medical education, the neoliberal interventions of standardisation and regulation have become synonymous with 'education' (Park, 2012), both on national and global scales (Rashid, 2021, 2022). And the concept of control brings us back to the idea of the proletarianisation of the profession.

Proletarianisation and Control of the Profession

The traditional view of a profession is that its members are self-regulating, working within some system of collegial control. But this former status quo has been eroded, and accompanied, it seems, by the deprofessionalisation and the proletarianisation that Thomas Zilling's account demonstrates (Freidson, 1984). Proletarianisation of the profession has been observed for many decades and is described as:

> ...the process by which an occupational category is divested of control over certain prerogatives relating to the location, content and essentiality of its task activities and is thereby subordinated to the broader requirements of production under advanced capitalism. (McKinlay & Arches, 1985, p. 161)

For the profession, this is accompanied by a high degree of bureaucratisation and reorganisation of services, as Thomas Zilling also indicates, and as we see in flourishing regulatory régimes, and systems of accountability and control including such processes as credentialing (Navarro, 1988).

It has been argued that physicians are not actually becoming a part of the proletariat in the sense of simply being able only to sell their labour power, even though they are losing autonomy and being organised in different ways. There are simply changes in the power that medicine retains to provide the service that each doctor would wish to provide, it is argued, and in the power relationships in society:

> ...medicine has a function – curing and caring – that is needed in any society. But how that needed function occurs depends on the power relationships in that society as reproduced in the knowledge, practice, and organization of medicine. (Navarro, 1988)

And that does not necessarily change the class position of doctors, even though it might affect their power and autonomy. So we might not fully accept the idea of proletarianisation.

Contemporaneous with the rise of neoliberalism came a growing critique of the values and power of the professions which were depicted either as self-serving, or upholding bourgeois interests rather than serving the public, lacking an altruistic focus, or creating a market for their own services (Saks, 2009). Regardless of the veracity of any of these depictions, the result has been increasing regulation of the profession, and decreasing power to organise their own work, as Thomas Zilling describes. Benefit to the public and protection of patients, is the rationale commonly put forward to support such controls:

> For all health professional groups including the still dominant medical profession, the leadership challenges in health care centrally include how their members can be persuaded to consistently serve the public good in practice where this may involve them putting the public interest before their own professional self-interests. (Saks, 2009)

Whether or not the controls put in place achieve that end, is questioned in Thomas Zilling's account which highlights more neoliberal concerns with the market and the economy rather than with patient care and the role of the profession in offering that.

References

AlHaqwi, A. I., & Taha, W. S. (2015). Promoting excellence in teaching and learning in clinical education. *Journal of Taibah University Medical Sciences, 10*(1), 97–101. https://doi.org/10.1016/j.jtumed.2015.02.005

Bambra, C. (2022). Levelling up: Global examples of reducing health inequalities. *Scandinavian Journal of Public Health, 50*(7), 908–913. https://doi.org/10.1177/14034948211022428

Bedoll, D., van Zanten, M., & McKinley, D. (2021). Global trends in medical education accreditation. *Human Resources for Health, 19*(1), 70. https://doi.org/10.1186/s12960-021-00588-x

Cervantes, P. A. M., & Rambaud, S. C. (2020). How politicized is the Bologna process? Giving way to constructive criticism. In *14th international technology, education and development conference* (pp. 9143–9148). https://doi.org/10.21125/inted.2020.2511

Collins, C., McCartney, G., & Garnham, L. (2016). Neoliberalism and health inequalities. In K. E. Smith, S. Hill, & C. Bambra (Eds.), *Health inequalities: Critical perspectives (First)*. Oxford University Press.

Cumming, A. (2010). The Bologna process, medical education and integrated learning. *Medical Teacher, 32*(4), 316–318. https://doi.org/10.3109/01421590903447716

Engels, F., & Marx, K. (1848). *The communist manifesto*. Workers' Educational Association.

Freidson, E. (1984). The changing nature of professional control. *Annual Review of Sociology, 10*(1), 1–20. https://doi.org/10.1146/annurev.so.10.080184.000245

Garben, S. (2011). *EU higher education law. The Bologna process and harmonization by stealth*. Kluwer Law International.

Gardner-McTaggart, A. (2021, May 4). *We are professionals: The proletarianisation of teachers*. SecEd. https://www.sec-ed.co.uk/content/blogs/we-are-professionals-the-proletarianisation-of-teachers.

Gaspard, J.-L., Schostak, J., & Schostak, J. (2012). Suffering and the work of emancipation through education. *Power and Education, 4*(3), 289–302. https://doi.org/10.2304/power.2012.4.3.289

Hossain, S., Shah, S., Scott, J., Dunn, A., Hartland, A. W., Hudson, S., & Johnson, J.-A. (2021). Reinventing undergraduate clinical placements with a switch to delivery by clinical teaching fellows. *Advances in Medical Education and Practice, 1429–1438*. https://doi.org/10.2147/AMEP.S336912

Humber, L. (2019). *Vital signs: The deadly costs of health inequality*. Pluto Press.

Jayasuriya, K. (2010). Learning by the market: Regulatory regionalism, Bologna, and accountability communities. *Globalisation, Societies and Education, 8*(1), 7–22. https://doi.org/10.1080/14767720903574009

Khojasteh, A., Momtazmanesh, N., Entezari, A., & Einollahi, B. (2009). Integration of medical education and healthcare service. *Iranian Journal of Public Health, 38*(Supplement 1), 29–31. https://www.academia.edu/2715638/Integration_of_medical_education_and_healthcare_service

Kushnir, I. (2020). The voice of inclusion in the midst of neoliberalist noise in the Bologna Process. *European Educational Research Journal, 19*(6), 485–505. https://doi.org/10.1177/1474904120941694

Lee, S. W. W., Clement, N., Tang, N., & Atiomo, W. (2014). The current provision of community-based teaching in UK medical schools: An online survey and systematic review. *BMJ Open, 4*(12), e005696. https://doi.org/10.1136/bmjopen-2014-005696

Loh, E. (2015). Doctors as health managers: An oxymoron, or a good idea? *Journal of Work-Applied Management, 7*(1), 52–60. https://doi.org/10.1108/JWAM-10-2015-005

Ludmerer, K. M. (2004). The clinical experience in medical education: Past, present, future. *Missouri Medicine, 101*(5), 487–490.
Mann, N. (2022). NHS privatisation is real. *BMJ, o2668.* https://doi.org/10.1136/bmj.o2668
McKee, L., Marnoch, G., & Dinnie, N. (1999). Medical managers: Puppetmasters or puppets? Sources of power and influence in clinical directorates. In A. L. Mark & S. Dopson (Eds.), *Organisational behaviour in health care: The research agenda* (pp. 89–116). Macmillan.
McKinlay, J. B., & Arches, J. (1985). Towards the proletarianization of physicians. *International Journal of Health Services, 15*(2), 161–195. https://doi.org/10.2190/JBMN-C0W6-9WFQ-Q5A6
Navarro, V. (1988). Professional dominance or proletarianization?: Neither. *The Milbank Quarterly, 66,* 57. https://doi.org/10.2307/3349915
Numerato, D., Salvatore, D., & Fattore, G. (2012). The impact of management on medical professionalism: A review. *Sociology of Health & Illness, 34*(4), 626–644. https://doi.org/10.1111/j.1467-9566.2011.01393.x
Park, S. (2012). The industrialisation of medical education? Exploring neoliberal influences within Tomorrow's Doctors policy 2009. In M. Lall (Ed.), *Policy, discourse and rhetoric: How new labour challenged social justice and democracy* (Educational Futures Rethinking Theory and Practice) (p. 52). SensePublishers Imprint.
Powell, A., & Davies, H. (2016). *Doctors and Managers: A narrative literature review.* www.nuffieldtrust.org.uk/publications/doctors-managers
Ramesh, R. (2012, December 18). Private healthcare: The lessons from Sweden. *The Guardian.* https://www.theguardian.com/society/2012/dec/18/private-healthcare-lessons-from-sweden
Rashid, M. A. (2021). *Global approaches to medical school regulation: A critical discourse analysis.* University College London. https://discovery.ucl.ac.uk/id/eprint/10135228/
Rashid, M. A. (2022). Hyperglobalist, sceptical, and transformationalist perspectives on globalization in medical education. *Medical Teacher, 44*(9), 1023–1031. https://doi.org/10.1080/0142159X.2022.2058384
Rashid, M. A. (2023). Altruism or nationalism? Exploring global discourses of medical school regulation. *Medical Education, 57*(1), 31–39. https://doi.org/10.1111/medu.14804
Rashid, M. A., Naidu, T., Wondimagegn, D., & Whitehead, C. (2023). Reconsidering a global agency for medical education: Back to the drawing board? *Teaching and Learning in Medicine,* 1–8. https://doi.org/10.1080/10401334.2023.2259363
Saks, M. (2009). Leadership challenges: Professional power and dominance in health care. In V. Bishop (Ed.), *Leadership for nursing and allied health care professions* (pp. 52–74). Open University Press.
Štech, S. (2011). The Bologna Process as a new public management tool in higher education. *Journal of Pedagogy/Pedagogický Casopis, 2*(2), 263–282. https://doi.org/10.2478/v10159-011-0013-1
The National Archives. (n.d.). *Council for the accreditation of teacher education.* Retrieved 10 December 2023, from https://discovery.nationalarchives.gov.uk/details/c/F268305
Waitzkin, H. (2018). *Healthcare under the Knife: Moving beyond capitalism for our health.* Monthly Review Press.
Wihlborg, M. (2019). Critical viewpoints on the Bologna Process in Europe: Can we do otherwise? *European Educational Research Journal, 18*(2), 135–157. https://doi.org/10.1177/1474904118824229

Thomas Zilling M.D., Ph.D. is a general surgeon specialised in oesophageal and gastric surgery. In 1991, he defended his thesis entitled 'Total gastrectomy in the treatment of gastric cancer'. The following year, he undertook postdoctoral work at the National Cancer Centre Hospital in Tokyo. He is Associate Professor in the Department of Surgery at Lund University, Sweden.

Currently he holds the position as President of the Swedish Medical Association in Southern Sweden. For many years he was Vice President for the European Association of Senior Hospital Physicians with a special interest in CPD, and initiator of the 2015 Consensus Statement of European Medical Organisations on CPD.

IV.ii STATEMENT: Medical Leadership and Management: Why Should We Bother?

Namita Kumar

Doctors love data and evidence. They like detail, they like proof, unless it was their idea. The value of medical leadership and management is in no doubt and yet those that lead and manage are still accused of 'going over to the dark side.' Is leadership and management really a haven for lazy doctors, who are not good enough to cut it clinically?

1 How Did Healthcare Management Become a 'Thing' in the UK?

From the 1960s to the late 1980s, in practical terms, hospitals were managed by the clinicians, both doctors and nurses. Therefore, compared to traditional management structures, these organisations were managed from the bottom-up. It was the clinical staff who were effectively in charge. As such, they had power to block organisational strategy and processes, if they disagreed with 'management'. There was a famous quote at the time that if Florence Nightingale was visiting an NHS hospital, she would not know who was in charge!

In 1983, a study, led by a British businessman, of the management of the UK National Health Service (NHS), was published (Griffiths Report, 1983). The enquiry had been requested by the Labour Secretary of State for Health, Sir Kenneth Robinson, to give advice on the effective use and management of staff and related resources in the NHS. It recommended that there should be:

N. Kumar (✉)
Conference of Postgraduate Medical Deans, London, UK

NHS England, London, UK
e-mail: namitakumar@doctors.org.uk

169

...a general manager at every level of the NHS from the Department of Health downward to the individual unit or hospital, who would be charged with overall managerial responsibility for the services provided and for giving the leadership required to 'stimulate initiative, urgency, and vitality' in the process of seeking ever greater efficiency (Day & Klein, 1983).

A full-time NHS Management Board would report to the supervisory board which should be multi-professional. Functions such as personnel, finance, procurement, property, scientific and technology management and service planning were to be considered at national level, while regional and district health authorities as vehicles of geographical management were suggested, with patient and public involvement.

There were obvious parallels with the private sector drawn, such as the apparent concern with levels of service, quality of the product, meeting budgets, cost improvement, productivity, motivating and rewarding staff, research and development, and the long term viability of the undertaking: all things that Parliament wanted from the NHS some 40 years ago. In the private sector, the results in all these areas would normally be carefully monitored against pre-determined standards and objectives. The NHS was being accused of stagnation and these recommendations were to help with that concern.

There were sharply opposing views about the report (Day & Klein, 1983). However, its general tenets prevailed and the key themes of overarching management responsibility, medical professional leadership, multiprofessional and public involvement, and corporate functions being accountable for their decisions, were elements of good practice we all recognise in the NHS now. The monitoring of performance against standards, whether clinical or managerial, are recognised as the basic elements of any clinical quality improvement process. But despite the implementation of general management, concerns about the NHS have remained (Hyde & Regan, 2023).

But how dark is a good management process?

2   Management and Medicine

In 2014, the Health Service Journal reviewed the impact of The Griffiths Report with the following headline: 'The Griffiths report was an attempt to entwine doctors in the management of the service' (Lewis, 2014).

So contrary to many views at the time, which were interpreted as trying to reduce the influence of doctors, it could be argued that professionalising management was needed to drive the NHS forward, and doctors were clearly stated as being part of the solution.

Since then, because of market forces, increasing competition and corporate governance pressures, hospitals have increasingly become managed by non-clinicians trained in management. This model in hospitals has been criticised for removing the dynamic and flexible nature of the traditional professional-run hospital, and being too 'top-down' in its approach. The multiprofessional clinical leadership recommended by Griffiths also appears to be lost.

This has led to loss of autonomy and decision making for doctors, resulting in some, but not all, of the frustration and loss of morale observed. Nonetheless, the concept of working professionally, in multi-disciplinary teams, is also vital, even though this may also lead to some loss of autonomy. Many of us can see the unintended consequences of decisions made elsewhere by those not near the patient, nor having ever been so. If we as physicians could have made better decisions with the resources available, surely we should not only say so but make considerable efforts to do so.

We also have a diverse medical profession while NHS boards are not, in general, representative of the communities they serve and the staff they employ. It is the job of the NHS Board to ensure that the public enjoys the full benefits of NHS services and to ensure that the organisation is focused on delivering those benefits (Coutts, 2019).

Doctors need to be at the table to help ensure these things happen. Is it not therefore logical that if we had the skills to manage in a 'professional' way, we would potentially improve patient care and quality outcomes? We could implement change more widely and have a bigger, more positive impact on health.

3 Evidence of Better Outcomes When Doctors Are Managers

The Commonwealth Fund is a private foundation that aims to promote a high performing health care system that achieves better access, improved quality, and greater efficiency, by supporting independent research on healthcare issues. One of its recommendations is to 'Engage clinicians in change and train and support clinical leaders' (Commonwealth Fund and London School of Economics and Political Science, 2017).

Studies have shown that clinical leadership is seen as key to delivering successful change. But clinicians leading change need support from local managers to ensure that local administrative systems and budgetary arrangements do not stifle change. Clinicians may also benefit from formal leadership training and opportunities to meet with peers on a regular basis. Models of medical and clinical leadership vary across sites, although management triumvirates (medical, nursing and administrative leaders) exist on paper in most sites, but the partnership of medical leaders and general managers is perceived to be more important. Doctors with high levels of engagement perform better on available measures of organisational performance than others. Looking at NHS hospital trust performance statistics, patient outcomes, mortality rates and national patient survey data, it was found that the percentage of clinicians on governing boards was low compared with international rates, but that higher representation appeared to be associated with better performance, higher patient satisfaction and lower morbidity rates (West et al., 2015).

It is reported that having a senior who is an expert in the core business of the organisation is associated with 'high levels of employee job satisfaction and low intentions of quitting (Stoller et al., 2016). Similarly, physician-leaders may know how to raise the job satisfaction of other clinicians, thereby contributing to enhanced organisational performance.

Doctors have to be managers as well as leaders in order to be effective and the most successful leaders are good managers too (Limb, 2016).

4 Reviews of Leadership and Management in the UK National Health Service (NHS)

There has been a succession of reviews of leadership and management that state that medical leadership should be a priority for the UK NHS.

In 2008, Professor John Tooke stated:

> The doctor's frequent role as head of the healthcare team and commander of considerable clinical resource requires that greater attention is paid to management and leadership skills regardless of specialism. An acknowledgement of the leadership role of medicine is increasingly evident. Role acknowledgement and aspiration to enhanced roles be they in subspecialty practice, management and leadership, education or research, are likely to facilitate greater clinical engagement (Tooke, 2008).

This has since been reinforced by other senior medical leaders.

It was recently stated that:

> The NHS is itself far from an homogenous unified organisation but rather a federated ecosystem where complex tribal and status dynamics continue to exist.
> We encourage the medical profession to examine honestly their role in setting cultures, given their unique influence in the workplace dynamic.
> We found that management tends not to be perceived – formally or informally – as a professional activity. Management lacks the status enjoyed by the established professions in health and social care (Messenger, 2022).

The Messenger Review found that the interaction between the clinical community and the rest of the workforce is a key element in setting the right culture and behaviours. The authority and influence that doctors have both in society and within the NHS, means that the medical profession does have a unique responsibility for leading behavioural change where necessary, and supporting a positive culture within their sector where all staff flourish.

5 My Conclusions

The workforce crisis in the NHS, that has required the publication of the Long-Term Workforce Plan (NHS England, 2023) is due to many contributing factors and not least that doctors, like many of those who work in healthcare, are feeling undervalued with a deep sense of the wrong decisions being made by the wrong people. How did this happen, when as a profession we still so clearly strive to do our best for patients, and are one of the groups most consistently trusted by the public (Ipsos, 2022)?

The GMC states that doctors must participate in service improvement. They must:

> Demonstrate ability to build team capacity and positive working relationships and undertake various team roles including leadership and the ability to accept leadership by others.
>
> Demonstrate awareness of the role of doctors as managers, including seeking ways to continually improve the use and prioritisation of resources. (General Medical Council, 2018)

The GMC further made leadership skills more explicit in its General Professional Capabilities Framework (General Medical Council, 2017).

Doctors tend to influence doctors, and indeed this would be further evidenced by some of the strategies used by pharmaceutical companies in using key opinion leaders to promote products. If we do need system-wide change to improve quality, innovation and retention of the workforce, how do we best influence doctors? The answer therefore is that this is usually best done through professional influence.

Being a manager and sometimes a leader, be that in delivery of clinical service as Medical Directors, education and training as Postgraduate Deans, or within our professional organisations and bodies, allows those of us with the skills and inclination to make a huge impact on patient care and quality that is system-wide. It can allow us to take the profession forwards. It is not, however, for every doctor. As we gravitate to specialisation knowing our strengths and weaknesses, we should include management and leadership outside the clinical environment.

For those of us who can do this, the profession must be supportive, as we can then collectively deliver the care we aspire to. We cannot be bystanders in poor management systems and poor decision making, that ultimately lead to poor quality of care for our patients.

We also have a responsibility for those members of our profession who come after us.

For that very reason we must all understand leadership and management, and this can only be done by education and, of course, professional influence.

References

Commonwealth Fund and London School of Economics and Political Science. (2017). *Designing a high-performing health care system for patients with complex needs: Ten recommendations for policymakers.* Commonwealth Fund and London School of Economics and Political Science. https://www.commonwealthfund.org/publications/fund-reports/2017/sep/designing-high-performing-health-care-system-patients-complex

Coutts, J. (2019, May 15). *Why talk about boards?* NHS Providers News and Blogs. https://nhsproviders.org/news-blogs/blogs/why-talk-about-boards

Day, P., & Klein, R. (1983). Two views on the Griffiths report the mobilisation of consent versus the management of conflict: Decoding the Griffiths report. *British Medical Journal, 287*, 1813–1816.

General Medical Council. (2017). *Generic professional capabilities framework.* https://www. gmc-uk.org/-/media/documents/generic-professional-capabilities-framework%2D%2D2109_ pdf-70417127.pdf#page=20

General Medical Council. (2018). *Outcomes for graduates.* https://www.gmc-uk.org/education/standards-guidance-and-curricula/standards-and-outcomes/outcomes-for-graduates/outcomes-for-graduates

Griffiths Report. (1983, October). https://sochealth.co.uk/national-health-service/griffiths-report-october-1983/

Hyde, R., & Regan, N. O. (2023). *A picture of health? Examining the state of leadership and management in healthcare.* https://www.managers.org.uk/wp-content/uploads/2023/07/a-picture-of-health-report.pdf

Ipsos. (2022). *Doctors and scientists are seen as the world's most trustworthy professions.* https:// www.ipsos.com/en-uk/doctors-and-scientists-are-seen-worlds-most-trustworthy-professions

Lewis, R. (2014, July 21). Thirty years on, the Griffiths report makes interesting reading. *Health Service Journal.* https://www.hsj.co.uk/interactive/thirty-years-on-the-griffiths-report-makes-interesting-reading/5072885.article#

Limb, M. (2016). Doctors must see themselves as managers as well as leaders. *BMJ*, cf_limbhard-decisions. https://doi.org/10.1136/bmj.i1112

Messenger, G. (2022). *Leadership for a collaborative and inclusive future.* https://www.gov.uk/government/publications/health-and-social-care-review-leadership-for-a-collaborative-and-inclusive-future/leadership-for-a-collaborative-and-inclusive-future

NHS England. (2023). *NHS long term workforce plan.* https://www.england.nhs.uk/wp-content/uploads/2023/06/nhs-long-term-workforce-plan-v1.2.pdf

Stoller, J. K., Goodall, A., & Baker, A. (2016, December 27). Why the best hospitals are managed by doctors. *Harvard Business Review.* https://hbr.org/2016/12/why-the-best-hospitals-are-managed-by-doctors

Tooke, J. (2008). *Aspiring to excellence.* MMC Inquiry.

West, M., Armit, K., Loewenthal, L., Eckert, R., West, T., & Lee, A. (2015). *Leadership and leadership development in health care: The evidence base.* https://assets.kingsfund.org.uk/f/256914/x/6577e5c839/leadership_in_health_care_report_february_2015.pdf

IV.ii COMMENTARY: The Politics of Medical Management: Empowering or Controlling?

Janet Grant and Leonard Grant

In our commentary on a later chapter written by Anne Keane, a university administrator, we note that 'university management is a contested space' (Conway, 2012) where both administrators and academics claim it to be their own. We analyse this problem in terms of social identity theory and group membership, and having analysed the contradictions, conclude that the division between these two groups can only be broken down when the institution comes together with a common purpose.

In this chapter, some of these issues are addressed by Namita Kumar who argues strongly that doctors must be the leaders and managers of hospitals, bearing in mind a responsibility to ensure that all groups within the workforce flourish within a positive culture. In this, she places doctors in a particular position of power, working in partnership with colleagues. Her interest in this derives from being a Postgraduate Dean of Medicine, with responsibility for doctors in training who rely on those hospitals for that training.

The management of hospitals, and the role of clinicians in that, has become a key topic:

> Hospitals have evolved from being professional bureaucracies to being managed professional business(es) with clinical directorates in place that are medically led (Powell & Davies, 2015).

Doctor or Manager?

The issue of the role, status and identity of doctors within the NHS is complex, and can be understood from a number of perspectives. In her chapter, Namita Kumar takes a contemporary view, from her own extensive experience. This can be illuminated if we first consider the historical context.

When the NHS was founded in 1948, it inherited hospitals which were operating on a charitable or endowment model (Brown, 2009; Riva & Cesana, 2013). The challenge was in how to transition from something based on the logic of almsgiving for the poor to a provision of medical services based on the needs of the people not the beneficence of wealthy donors. We might ask whether this has happened in any meaningful way; the NHS is continually understood on these terms (use it sensibly, don't ask for too much, don't waste resources, be grateful...). Rather than being transformed into an institution run by and for its staff and users, hospitals have moved directly from charity to sites of profit generation for private enterprise without much in between (We Own It, 2024). This framing then contextualises the 'management journey' which has been a very basic struggle over what and who the hospital is for and how funding for that is distributed. In recent times, the argument has commonly been framed as one of improving leadership and management to make the organisation more efficient and cost-effective (Ham et al., 2016). Notably, the patient is entirely absent from most of these discussions. Through all of this, as we have noted in other chapters, including that of Thomas Zilling from Sweden, the struggle of the medical profession to remain a profession has been the project of medicine, as it has been for centuries (Parry & Parry, 2018).

Hospitals, then, have been through a management journey whereby they developed from being centres of advice and healing 'managed by the clinicians, the elite professionals who had the power and influence to control the organisation', to 'managed professional businesses' subject to corporate governance and managed by non-clinicians. This model was 'criticised for removing the dynamic and flexible nature of the traditional professional-run hospital by being too top-down in its approach' which often failed to impose changes on doctors. At that point, power was restored to the professions by the development of clinical directorates at middle-management level, managed by multiprofessional clinical management teams. But these can only work if approved by senior managers at organisation level who might or might not be doctors (Loh, 2015).

As Namita Kumar points out, there are benefits in having clinicians as managers, and these are well documented (ibid.). But there are also limitations in trying to balance two identities, clinician and manager, with the danger of the identity crisis which we have seen in Part III of this book (Marnoch et al., 2000). This complex change of identity, or embracing a simultaneous and different identity (clinician and manager) is no longer uncommon. But it is still practically and emotionally difficult, involving:

> …a mutually constitutive process whereby professionals strive to make sense of and work on their perceptions of their professional identity, and negotiate a meaningful balance between that identity and their (changing) work (Vähäsantanen, 2022).

They might also have to consider their accountable relationship to their own higher manager, as well as their professional relationship to those whom they manage. They must make the organisation work, and help people to work in the organisation. As in any business, there are employees who provide the service and employees who manage the process and the people. Effectively, they are all employees of the same organisation, although with slightly different relationships to the means and process of producing its outputs.

Power and Politics in Health Service Management

Namita Kumar makes the case for physician leadership and management in the healthcare service, based on their understanding of the near-patient experience of provision of that service. She has no doubt that healthcare management must be led by doctors, since they are also, *de facto*, the leaders of clinical teams and have ultimate responsibility for clinical care. Every hospital in the UK now has a clinical career structure in management (Jarvis, 2024) and a Medical Director who is part of the senior management team. These may be rather different from the immediate line-managers who have been shown to make a difference to productivity (Shaw, 2019). Those line-managers might simply be seniors and supervisors of more junior doctors. Namita Kumar's medical managers and leaders are located a little further away from the people who provide the service. At that level in UK hospitals, there are also, however, Directors of Nursing (Indeed Editorial Team, 2022), and Directors of Medical Education (Medical Education Leaders UK, 2020). We can see immediately, that there are issues of power and politics in this apparently straightforward managerial arrangement whereby doctors are identified as the natural leaders.

All organisations are political structures:

> This means that organizations operate by distributing authority and setting a stage for the exercise of power (Zaleznik, 1970).

Namita Kumar argues that doctors are in the best position to manage hospitals, and in her case to manage the medical education that occurs within them, because they understand their functioning from a more informed perspective than career managers. The NHS is estimated to have approximately 39,000 managers making up about 3.7% of the workforce. Of those, 26.2% are nurses or health visitors and 10.5% are doctors while about 30% are other clinical staff (Nosheen, 2024). So about one third of managers in the healthcare service have no clinical experience.

The NHS has fewer managers than comparable international healthcare systems. It has been argued that more are required, not to represent those who deliver the front-line service as this chapter recommends, but contrarily:

> More managers are crucial to freeing up the time of doctors, nurses, and other professionals to do the caring (Limb, 2023).

But this is problematical if the powerbase of a manager derives from:

1. The quantity of formal authority vested in his position relative to other positions.
2. The authority vested in his expertise and reputation for competence (Zaleznik, 1970).

This might suggest that clinicians are indeed a good fit for higher management. The case could be argued either way:

> Organizational life within a political frame is a series of contradictions. It is an exercise in rationality, but its energy comes from the ideas in the minds of power figures... (Zaleznik, 1970)

Those ideas might derive from the requirements of the organisation, or of politicians, or of the profession, or the local community or patients, or the individual. These do not necessarily align, and the mechanisms of power and politics might rank-order them.

Doctors in Management: A Clash of Cultures?

The relationship between doctors and managers (whether clinical or not) in the healthcare service has not always been easy. Only 20 years after general management was introduced into the NHS, there were many areas of tension and disagreement around clinicians' involvement in management, the quality of managerial staff and clinicians' trust in them, and the balance between clinical and financial priorities (Powell & Davies, 2016).

Management has not always been an attractive proposition for doctors. Lagging far behind France, Germany, the US and Sweden, in 2014, only 10% of UK doctors expressed any interest in a management career route, recognising that:

> With many trusts now in breach of (government-set) waiting time and financial targets, the job of chief executive is increasingly likely to end in failure (Vize, 2015).

Doctors also worried that they may be disciplined by their professional regulator for events in their hospital that were outside of their control, and that they may lose their clinical skills. The introduction of leadership training for postgraduate doctors seemed to be turning that tide (Vize, 2015, p. 18). Nonetheless, there were worries that management and medical cultures might not align:

> They also fear that short term or political imperatives may place them in a conflicted position. Will they be required to compromise their values? Are safety and quality really the top priorities in the world of senior management? They are trained to analyse and then act on the basis of evidence, and operating empirically can lead to feelings of vulnerability, particularly within a culture where blame is common (ibid.).

Studies of the personal characteristics of excellent physicians show that what is thought desirable differs depending on who is making that judgement. Physicians themselves mention leadership skills (Khawar et al., 2022). However, personal characteristics are different from the defining qualities of the group of which an individual is a member, or the role which the doctor has adopted.

A Job or a Profession?

The question of the identity of doctors who move into other fields, whether that might be medical education or management, is a recurring theme in this book. This chapter adds another dimension to that tension.

We see here a tension or contradiction, also indicated in Anne Keane's chapter, between those who feel that they do the work, and those whose role is to manage or administer that. In any business or organisation, there will be those who are employed to deliver the service ('do the work') and those who are employed to manage and administer that. But whether manager or doctor, they have in common that they are employees. There is a considerable debate about whether medicine is 'just a job' (Sokol, 2017) with the doctor selling their labour power, defined in an employment contract, as any other worker does, as was predicted (Engels & Marx, 1848). Sokol (2017) believes that 'Even with morale at a low ebb, I doubt that many doctors would agree that theirs was 'just a job.'"

Some time ago, medicine did regard itself as an autonomous profession, even when most were direct employees of the NHS, but with rights, as now, to also practise privately:

> During the 1960s and 1970s, one theme recurred in British and American writing in medical sociology and health policy: that medical power was an entrenched feature of modern systems of health care. In sociological terms, medicine, with law, was the paradigmatic profession, a publicly mandated and state-backed monopolistic supplier of a valued service, exercising autonomy in the workplace and collegiate control over recruitment, training and the regulation of members' conduct (Elston, 1991).

But others feel that, in this managerial climate, medicine is no longer that profession which does practise autonomously in the workplace:

> Clock-watching has become common place, with the European Working Time Directive being the most obvious example. More troublesome for many senior doctors is the issue of job planning, which is beginning to limit the additional roles and responsibilities that doctors can undertake. ... These organizations will perceive little value in doctors spreading their wings and will treat them like factory workers, clocking on and off and filling in timesheets. Doctors in these organizations will begin to wonder whether medicine is any longer a profession (Abbasi, 2009).

We have noted in other chapters (see, for example, the commentary on Thomas Zilling's chapter) that the class position, and so the employment status and degree of autonomy of doctors, has for long placed them in a class position that they might not easily accept. We might quote again that:

> The bourgeoisie has stripped of its halo every occupation hitherto honoured and looked up to with reverent awe. It has converted the physician, the lawyer, the priest, the poet, the man of science, into its paid wage labourers (Engels & Marx, 1848).

Pay may well be much greater for a doctor than for others who are employed by the NHS (with the possible exception of managers), but the drifting class position remains. Being managed is part of that journey.

Leading and Managing in a Professional Organisation

The healthcare service is an organisation of knowledge workers, where both individual autonomy to make clinical decisions, and the not always welcome and not always complied with (Metcalfe et al., 2021) protocols or guidelines are contradictory parts of the work processes. Management and leadership in this professional service context has its own particular problems where:

… traditional conceptions of leadership and followership are problematic given the importance of individual autonomy to knowledge-based work…

…leadership in professional service firms is, above all, a process of interaction among professionals seeking to exercise influence at the individual, organizational, and strategic level. It is manifested explicitly through professional expertise, discretely through political interaction, and implicitly through personal embodiment (Empson & Langley, 2015).

We can see this reflected in Namita Kumar's call for medical leadership and management. Although a hierarchy is implied in her argument, professional environments are made up of more ambiguous and negotiated relationships amongst professional peers (Adler et al., 2008). So a doctor in management is simultaneously inside three hierarchies: their own professional medical hierarchy, the management hierarchy, and the hierarchy of professions (and others) within the organisation in which doctors are just one group. These three hierarchies might require different approaches to management. It is argued that managers in this position:

…need to be acutely aware of the implicit power structures and shifting networks of influence among their colleagues and have highly developed political skills in order to navigate and negotiate these networks of influence (Empson & Langley, 2015).

In the end, all are employees of an organisation with its own rules, perspectives, limitations and external controls, trying to make that work both as a site of employment and work identity, and to achieve its mission of caring for patients, whether as doctor or manager or both. The contradictions are complex.

References

Abbasi, K. (2009). Is medicine still a profession? *Journal of the Royal Society of Medicine, 102*(9), 353–353. https://doi.org/10.1258/jrsm.2009.09k051

Adler, P. S., Kwon, S.-W., & Heckscher, C. (2008). Perspective – Professional work: The emergence of collaborative community. *Organization Science, 19*(2), 359–376. https://doi.org/10.1287/orsc.1070.0293

Brown, M. (2009). Medicine, reform and the 'end' of charity in early nineteenth-century England. *The English Historical Review, 124*(511), 1353–1388. https://doi.org/10.1093/ehr/cep347

Conway, M. (2012). Using causal layered analysis to explore the relationship between academics and administrators in universities. *Journal of Futures Studies, 17*(2), 37–58.

Elston, M. A. (1991). The politics of professional power: Medicine in a changing health service. In J. Gabe, M. Calnan, & M. Bury (Eds.), *The sociology of the health service*. Routledge.

Empson, L., & Langley, A. (2015). Leadership and professionals: Multiple manifestations of influence in professional service firms. In L. Empson, D. Muzio, J. Broschak, & B. Hinings (Eds.), *The Oxford handbook of professional service firms* (pp. 163–188). Oxford University Press. https://openaccess.city.ac.uk/id/eprint/15427/

Engels, F., & Marx, K. (1848). *The Communist Manifesto*. Workers' Educational Association.

Ham, C., Berwick, D., & Dixon, J. (2016). *Improving quality in the English NHS. A strategy for action*. https://www.gloshospitals.nhs.uk/media/documents/The_Kings_Fund_-_Improving_quality_in_the_English_NHS.pdf

Indeed Editorial Team. (2022, November 22). *How to become director of nursing (with key skills)*. Indeed. https://uk.indeed.com/career-advice/finding-a-job/how-to-become-director-of-nursing

Jarvis, G. (2024). A day in the life of: A medical director l. *BMJ Careers*. https://www.bmj.com/careers/article/-a-day-in-the-life-of-a-medical-director

Khawar, A., Frederiks, F., Nasori, M., Mak, M., Visser, M., van Etten-Jamaludin, F., Diemers, A., & Van Dijk, N. (2022). What are the characteristics of excellent physicians and residents in the clinical workplace? A systematic review. *BMJ Open, 12*(9), e065333. https://doi.org/10.1136/bmjopen-2022-065333

Limb, M. (2023). England's 10 000 "missing managers" are holding back the NHS, says think tank. *BMJ*, 1313. https://doi.org/10.1136/bmj.p1313

Loh, E. (2015). Doctors as health managers: An oxymoron, or a good idea? *Journal of Work-Applied Management, 7*(1), 52–60.

Marnoch, G., McKee, L., & Dinnie, N. (2000). Between organisations and institutions: Legitimacy and medical managers. *Public Administration, 78*(1), 967–987.

Medical Education Leaders UK. (2020, June). *Job description – Director of Medical Education*. https://kss.hee.nhs.uk/wp-content/uploads/sites/15/2023/02/DME-role-description.pdf

Metcalfe, D., Pitkeathley, C., & Herring, J. (2021). 'Advice, not orders'? The evolving legal status of clinical guidelines. *Journal of Medical Ethics, 47*(12), e78–e78. https://doi.org/10.1136/medethics-2020-106592

Nosheen, S. (2024, February 16). *Are there too many NHS managers?* NHS Confederation. https://www.nhsconfed.org/articles/are-there-too-many-nhs-managers

Parry, N., & Parry, J. (2018). *The rise of the medical profession*. Routledge. https://doi.org/10.4324/9780429400926

Powell, A., & Davies, H. (2015). Doctors and managers: A narrative literature review. *Journal of Work-Applied Management, 7*(1), 52–60. https://www.nuffieldtrust.org.uk/publications/doctors-managers

Powell, A., & Davies, H. (2016). *Doctors and managers: A narrative literature review*. www.nuffieldtrust.org.uk/publications/doctors-managers

Riva, M. A., & Cesana, G. (2013). The charity and the care: The origin and the evolution of hospitals. *European Journal of Internal Medicine, 24*(1), 1–4. https://doi.org/10.1016/j.ejim.2012.11.002

Shaw, K. L. (2019). *Bosses matter: The effects of managers on workers' performance*. https://wol.iza.org/articles/bosses-matter-the-effects-of-managers-on-workers-performance/long

Sokol, D. (2017). Is being a doctor "just a job"? *BMJ*, j5257. https://doi.org/10.1136/bmj.j5257

Vähäsantanen, K. (2022). Professional identity in changing workplaces: Why it matters, when it becomes emotionally imbued, and how to support its agentic negotiations. In C. Harteis, D. Gijbels, & E. Kyndt (Eds.), *Research approaches on workplace learning: Insights from a growing field* (Vol. 31, pp. 29–46). Springer International Publishing.

Vize, R. (2015). Why doctors don't dare to go into management. *British Medical Journal, 350*(h922), 16–18.

We Own It. (2024, June 17). *Analysis: The NHS has lost £10 million a week to private profits since 2012*. https://weownit.org.uk/blog/analysis-nhs-has-lost-10-million-week-private-profits-2012

Zaleznik, A. (1970). Power and politics in organizational life. *Harvard Business Review, 48*(3), 47–61.

Namita Kumar, in 2003, while a doctor in training (now a specialist in Rheumatology and General Medicine) was appointed to the new UK regulatory body: the Postgraduate Medical and Education Training Board. She has held increasingly senior roles in managing postgraduate medical education as a Foundation School Director, a Postgraduate Dean, and, nationally, as Co-Chair of the English Postgraduate Deans. She is an Honorary Clinical Professor in four universities. She has been a Council member of the UK Academy of Medical Educators, and the Royal College of Physicians, and a trustee for the National Confidential Enquiry into Patient Outcome and Death. In 2023, Namita became National Dean for Postgraduate Medical and Dental Education Risk and Business Oversight.

IV.iii STATEMENT: Medical Education in Brazil: Context and Challenges

Valdes Roberto Bollela

1 Brazilian Medical Education and the Health Care System

Brazil is the fifth largest nation in the world, with 210 million people. The Brazilian population is diverse, and access to health care varies significantly from region to region. The most developed and wealthiest areas are in the South, with less developed and large areas in the North (Amazon Forest) and Northeast (semi-desert) regions.

Despite being one of the largest economies in the world, Brazil has extreme levels of inequity. Worse still, inequality threatens to reverse the country's progress in ending poverty.

In 1988, the Brazilian Constitution defined health as a universal right and a state duty. The country built the National Unified Health System (Sistema Único de Saúde—SUS) to reach this goal. SUS is the workplace for most Brazilian healthcare workers and, at the same time, is the principal educational setting for clinical training and development for medical undergraduate students and postgraduate trainees.

The country now has 2.6 doctors per 1000 inhabitants, which is quite close to the US (2.64) and Canada (2.77), and below the *OECD's* average (3.73). However, the distribution of doctors over the country needs to be rebalanced. The populated areas may reach 6.2, compared to less populated regions with 1.1 doctors per 1000 inhabitants, while large remote areas may be without a single doctor (Brazilian Federal Council of Medicine, 2023).

Since 1808, after the creation of the first medical school in Brazil, graduated doctors are automatically allowed to get a medical licence and start practising.

V. R. Bollela (✉)
University of São Paulo, Ribeirão Preto School of Medicine (FMRP-USP),
Ribeirão Preto, Brazil
e-mail: vbollela@fmrp.usp.br

© The Author(s), under exclusive license to Springer Nature
Switzerland AG 2026
J. Grant, L. Grant (eds.), *The Contradictions of Medical Education*,
https://doi.org/10.1007/978-3-031-90394-6_13

183

2   Medical Education from the Inside: Public, Private and Traditional

As this chapter is written in 2024, Brazil counts 390 medical schools. Today (June 2025), while we are doing the final review of the chapter the number of medical schools is 448, and counting. If nothing changes, in less than 12 years, Brazil will have more than one million doctors, which is twice as many as in 2024.

After 2002, the number of schools tripled (from 113 to 390), and the number of graduates more than quadrupled (10,000 to 42,000). At the beginning of the century, 50% of graduates came from public medical schools. After two decades, 76% of graduate doctors come from private medical schools in a market estimated to be worth 20 billion US dollars.

Brazilian medical schools can further be divided into public (free of charge), confessional (faith-based) non-profit, and private (for-profit) schools. Until the end of the twentieth century, public and confessional medical schools were predominant and were related to traditional research universities. After that, the number of private schools increased, and in the last 10 years, more than 90% of the new places in medical schools come from private institutions.

These schools can be divided into three main groups based on their characteristics. The public and private more traditional schools created before 2002 (Group 1); the new public medical schools started in 2002 with REUNI, the programme to support restructuring and expansion of universities in Brazil (Group 2), and private institutions, that started after 2002 (Group 3).

2.1   Group 1: Traditional Medical Schools

This group comprises state, federal, and confessional universities. The Flexnerian model strongly influenced these medical schools. They all have an associated high complexity university hospital, strong basic science departments and labs, and followed a discipline-based curriculum. This curriculum usually provided few experiences within the community, and the clinical years were centred on the hospital.

By the end of the last century, many of these schools started to review their curricula, moving towards community-based primary health care experience in the initial years, increasing the clerkship (clinical) period from one to two years, with the presence of simulation as an emerging teaching and learning strategy (Bollela et al., 2015).

2.2 Group 2: REUNI, the Restructuring and Expansion Programme of Federal Universities

In 2007, the Brazilian government decided to increase places for medical students in public education. The REUNI programme aimed to support the development of higher education in underserved areas, assuming its critical role in social and economic development. The programme increased the number of places in public universities for poorer people. It created a quota programme for low-income students (from African descent and indigenous populations), and housing and financial support to help students enter, stay and finish their studies. This action increased diversity and inclusion in the public medical schools. African-descent students increased from 1483 in 2010 to 9326 in 2019. In 2020, one-third of new medical students came from less affluent populations, and in 2024, it reached the initial proposed goal of 50%. Many REUNI medical schools were created in less developed regions, far from the wealthy economic centres, and chose to develop an integrated and community-based curriculum from scratch. These schools have no university hospitals and must build partnerships with the local health system to implement their programmes.

2.3 Group 3. Private Medical Schools

In the past two decades, for-profit private institutions have increased and now offer 75% of medical education places. Many of these schools belong to the portfolio of international corporations, spread over the country.

Following the Ministry of Education requirements, many new schools were created in underserved areas. The increased number of medical schools met challenges including poor infrastructure, shortage of doctors, lack of trained faculty members, and low articulation between the school and the local healthcare system.

The result is a wide variety of experiences, and it is hard to infer the quality of these new medical programmes because most of these schools have less than a decade of existence.

3 Regulation of Medical Education in Brazil

The Ministry of Education is responsible for regulating medical education in Brazil. It created the National System of Evaluation of Higher Education (SINAES) in 2004 and is responsible for the accreditation process of new and existing medical schools. In 2019, the World Federation of Medical Education recognised a new entity as an accreditation body in Brazil. SAEME, the Accreditation System of Medical Schools, was created by experts in medical education in partnership and supported by the Federal Council of Medicine (CFM). There is no articulation between the two systems.

In the past 10 years, during a massive political crisis in Brazil, the Ministry of Education suspended the creation of new medical schools (April 2018). However, the private sector pushed for an alternative way, and 75 medical schools were created by judicial decision during the moratorium period. Another 400 requests are waiting for the Brazilian Supreme Court decision. In September 2023, the Brazilian government launched a new programme to deal with this situation, and some medical schools were allowed to open, mainly in underserved areas.

As for the comparative quality of graduates, there are no external exams to assess the ability and readiness for autonomous and qualified practice of graduate doctors in Brazil. No matter how good or bad the learning experience is, at the end of undergraduate studies everyone will be allowed to practise medicine.

This complex situation brings many contradictions, imbalances, and challenges to Brazilian medical education. After a four-fold increase in medical graduates; the country has not changed the presence of doctors in underserved areas.

Regulation and quality assurance of medical education in Brazil did not follow the significant increase and diversity of medical schools. This situation may threaten patient safety and the sustainability of the National Health System (SUS) itself. There is an increasing tension between the fewer residency positions and the vast number of medical graduates.

The places offered in residency programmes must be aligned with health care needs, and they are not. Thousands of young doctors have started their careers in primary health care in family medicine teams without adequate training and supervision. They are not interested in staying there but only to make money until they can get a residency position in another specialty, elsewhere.

The readiness of faculty members to work as medical educators in Brazil is also a bottleneck. Despite the requirements of the Brazilian Guidelines for Medical Education (2014), adequate and effective faculty development is still an impossible dream for many trainers and faculty members.

4   How Can We Deal with This Highly Complex Situation?

Eventually, a significant movement was started involving the Ministry of Education, the Ministry of Health, the Brazilian Association of Medical Education (ABEM) representing Medical Schools, the National Council of Medical Residency (which regulates and financially supports residency programmes), the Federal Council of Medicine, the Brazilian Medical Association and their Specialty Societies' representatives. The aim was to face the problem and propose articulated and agreed solutions.

Much of this discussion was supported by a diagnostic study called Medical Demography, started in 2020 and coordinated by Prof. Mauro Sheffer from the University of São Paulo Medical School in partnership with the Ministry of Health, the Pan-American Health Organisation (PAHO), and WHO. In 2023, the Brazilian Medical Association joined the initiative to expand the data analysis. As a result of this co-operation, there are articulated actions.

Since September 2023, the Ministry of Education has imposed regulatory measures to restrict medical school opening based on clear indicators and parameters, avoiding non-technical and erratic decisions by the Supreme Court.

The National Council for Medical Residency, together with the Ministry of Health, published new regulations in April 2024 reviewing its main priorities and roles, which include:

• expansion, qualification, and structuring of residency programmes in strategic specialties for the public health system in priority locations
• improvement of the technical and pedagogical quality of medical residency programmes
• creation and expansion of the number of clinical residency programmes.

In 2024, 47% of all physicians in Brazil have no residency training. Areas such as anaesthetics, orthopaedics, psychiatry, and family medicine still have an enormous gap, considering the demand of the public health system. The government (Federal or State) funds more than 90% of all residency programmes and has now decided to review the priorities, increasing alignment between residency programmes and policies and the National Health System.

The Brazilian Association of Medical Education has been designing and implementing a progressive (beginning, middle and final) national exam with a focus on cognitive skills to gather information about medical graduates' ability for autonomous practice. The main goal is to provide medical schools with more information so that they can review and rethink their medical education towards better clinical practice and patient safety.

In March 2024, all stakeholders led by the Ministry of Education started discussion and review of the Brazilian Guidelines for Medical Education, which were first proposed in 2001 and reviewed in 2014.

Finally, in partnership with the Brazilian Association of Medical Education, the Ministry of Health, Ministry of Education and Pan American Health Organization (PAHO) launched in November 2023 a two-year project to reorganise and improve medical schools' evaluation and accreditation processes: *Medical Training Project for Brazil—A Committed Look at Social Responsibility in the 21st Century*. The project is a unique opportunity to design and implement adequate quality control for Brazilian medical education in a challenging scenario.

Hardly any of the literature, innovations, and evidence-based practice in medical education come from developing countries with diverse contexts. Medical education literature and research are predominantly European and North American and many experiences in the Global North do not apply to the Global South's reality and needs. So Brazil is trying to find its own way with one of the world's highest numbers of medical schools, but at the same time, with a consistent and strong experience of training students at all levels of the public health system.

5 Conclusion

The Brazilian model of medical education aims to deliver a physician ready to work in the national health system. This situation puts enormous pressure on the quality assurance process of medical education, which urgently needs to be addressed in Brazil. The country is establishing priorities for residency programmes based on health care needs; moving forward requires strong faculty development and collaboration initiatives among Brazilian medical educators and institutions.

All this changing movement can create a concrete opportunity for improvements and innovative practices within Brazilian medical education, which has now been articulated by the government, regulation bodies, the health care system, the Brazilian Association of Medical Education, society, and academia.

References

Bollela, V. R., Germani, A. C. C. G., Henry de Holanda Campos, H., & Amaral, E. (2015). *Community-based education for the health professions: Learning from the Brazilian experience*. International Cataloguing In-Publication Data (CIP). Brazilian Book Chamber. https://drive.google.com/file/d/1Qw14jynxYlkNXdvIbRpcQpWM5GfgWrPx/view?pli=1

Brazilian Federal Council of Medicine. (2023). *Observatório: Medical demography in Brazil*. https://demografia.cfm.org.br/dashboard/

IV.iii COMMENTARY: The Politics and Business of Medical Education, and the Lives of Doctors

Janet Grant and Leonard Grant

This chapter tells the story of the political use and control of medical education, and the business that medical education has become, against a background of professional concerns and interventions, and the decisions that doctors may make about where to settle. All these factors impinge on equity and inequity in effective access to health care. Valdes Roberto Bollela describes the range of often competing bodies that have different interests in medical education, for politics, for profit, for social development, and for the profession. He ends with the hope that these competing and differently driven bodies will now co-operate. But perhaps their differences are too great.

The Control of Medical Education

The struggle between government, profession and regulator to control medical education and the expansion of medical schools is not limited to Brazil. Medicine everywhere has too many political, professional and economic corollaries to avoid such striving for power, as has also been described, for example, in relation to England where authors have reflected:

> Medical education is important because it links the university to vital societal concerns and interests and directly to government and the state.... Will government and state work to sustain the independence of the university, partly in order to better ensure the fulfilment of their own policy goals, or will they side with the powerful societal interests because that seems to be the politically easiest path to take? Indeed there is much at stake. (Salter et al., 2016, p. 30)

Different and competing interests (professional, political and business) have given rise to different types of medical school in Brazil, as elsewhere: traditional schools, state REUNI medical schools in underserved areas, and private for-profit schools. Establishing the equal quality of such schools which are so unequal in their origins and purposes, is a challenge. A regulatory system that has two uncoordinated bodies adds to the unsatisfactory landscape: the original regulator is part of the Ministry of Education, and a new rival player in the field gained status by applying for and receiving recognition from the World Federation for Medical Education. Neither agency seems to be having the effect that might be required.

Healthcare for All and the Distribution of Doctors

The social and political rhetoric of universal healthcare for all is exposed in this chapter, for its inadequacy and perhaps emptiness. Democratic, capitalist, class-based societies, are not organised to ensure equal quality in social conditions, and that includes health and healthcare.

The author sets out the economic and social context in which medical services should be provided, and for which medicine should be learned. And he shows that access to healthcare is still uneven, despite increasing numbers of medical graduates. This same picture of maldistribution of doctors, and unequal access to health care, can be painted in most countries.

The pattern of provision of healthcare providers has been repeatedly shown to advantage higher socio-economic areas (Davis et al., 2018). This universal 'inverse care law' whereby the greater the need, the less the availability, is challenged only by 'exceptional people' (Hastings & Rao, 2001). Doctors do not choose to live and work in deprived regions, even where healthcare infrastructure is provided. Selecting students from those areas shows only weak indication that they tend to go back to work there (Dowell et al., 2015). Medicine is, in fact, a way out. Decline in commitment to working in rural areas has been shown with progress through training (McGrail et al., 2021). The aspect of Julian Tudor Hart's 'inverse care law' that is usually left out is that uneven distribution is most pronounced when medical care is exposed to market forces (Tudor Hart, 1971).

Medical Education: An Instrument of Social Mobility

Papers that address the issue of where doctors choose to live and work, rarely seem to acknowledge that education is an instrument of social mobility enabling the movement of people, including medical graduates, from poorer to richer environments (Mian, 2023). And where working in medicine does not seem attractive at all, or working in another country as a doctor seems more attractive, we cannot assume that there is a match between graduate location and numbers, or the distribution of medical schools and uptake of job vacancies, which may put further pressure on the supply of doctors to rural and deprived areas (Ferreira et al., 2023).

Although the distribution of specialised healthcare services throughout all communities may help to locate doctors in rural areas (Appleby, 2022), this is likely to be the case only where there is no social or monetary disadvantage in that. To work in a rural area requires familiarity with such a context, a sense of place where people feel connected to the natural environment, community involvement, and the self-actualisation that these things bring. But to stay in less advantageous political, social or financial environments also requires resilience (Hancock et al., 2009). Decisions about career and life are personal, even for a doctor. It would indeed take exceptional people to reject the opportunity of a more comfortable life for themselves and for their families. In Indonesia, as in other countries:

…current regulatory policies and financial incentives have not been effective in addressing the maldistribution of specialist doctors in a context of a growing private sector and predominance of doctors' income from private sources (Meliala et al., 2013).

The Limited Power of Medical Schools to Improve Health Care

The issue of health care for all cannot be solved by medical schools or medical education. It is a political, economic and social development problem. That being so, it has been argued that:

> Beyond medical education and the health service, the challenge is…to focus on broader policies that address the whole of society in remote and rural areas…
> Unless rural and remote communities are supported to flourish, encouraging doctors and their families to move or stay will remain more a matter of personal serendipity than systematic action (Maclaren et al., 2022, p. 250).

While the rhetoric of medical education usually addresses service and professional values, it would be folly to ignore the more powerful economic drivers of the field. Increases in the global health workforce have failed to address the inequities seen in WHO African and Eastern Mediterranean regions, for example (Boniol et al., 2022). Despite this, we should acknowledge that the presence of a medical school in any region can enhance its 'health, social, economic and research activity' (Hashem et al., 2022) simply through the educational and experiential activities of its staff and students. But this effect will be minor in relation to changes needed in healthcare provision which can only be addressed by fundamental political action. Such action would need to challenge the business of medical education.

The Business of Medical Education, Money and the Law

Valdes Roberto Bollela provides further evidence in his chapter of this economic (and financial) dimension of medical education, showing that it has become a business in Brazil, worth about 20 billion US dollars. Yet despite sporadic publications that look at the business and economics of medical education (Walsh, 2010), there is no systematic recognition within medical education itself that medical education has become a business making money from both education and regulation.

Medical education, unlike education in other professions, has frequently been written about in terms of its monetary value and in terms of 'the health care market' (FasterCapital, 2024; Hsieh & Tang, 2019), or even as the 'medical education industry' (Transparency Market Research, 2024), and the 'corporatization' of medical education (Lujan & DiCarlo, 2023). Legal education has been following suit in its analyses of the costs and value of a law degree (Simkovic & McIntyre, 2014), and the context of privatisation (Balan, 2023) and globalisation (Balan, 2017).

But medical education leads the field in developing into a business, with global markets and many ways of making money through, for example, the medical education consultancies that global north medical schools have established, selling curricula through such consultancies, or offering types of largely unproven international or cross-border accreditations or stamp of apparent quality for a fee, by bodies such as ACGME International (https://www.acgme-i.org), or accreditation agencies such as the Association for Evaluation and Accreditation of Medical Education Programmes (TEPDAD/Turkey) (https://tepdad.org.tr/en/accreditation-services-for-outside-of-turkey/), and non-statutory global organisations such as the World Federation for Medical Education (https://wfme.org/recognition/). This is big business.

Medical education now also has a flourishing job market and career opportunities. It is not surprising therefore, that the legislature has been involved in decisions about medical school expansion in more than one country, either to increase medical school places, as in Brazil, or to not increase them, as in Korea where a protectionist profession has argued that an increase in medical school places would lead to a 'deterioration of education and the collapse of the country's well-regarded medical system' (Park, 2024). Despite this, the number of medical school places in Korea has been incereased from 3000 to 5000. with some of the predicted chaos (Mosheim, 2025).

One solution to the problem of increasing the production of doctors, especially of doctors who will migrate from poorer to richer locations, is the somewhat uncertain outsourcing of medical education, as we see in the Caribbean (Eckhert, 2010) where island-based medical schools are for-profit, take primarily international students, do not serve their local population, and export their graduates (Morgan, 2015). This phenomenon is yet another aspect of the commodification of medical education (Hafferty et al., 2020).

Costs, Profits and Privatisation in Medical Education

In other countries, such as India, we have seen the exploitation of medical education for profit, and its gradual facilitation by changes in legislation and practice, and by the invention of public-private partnerships; in other words, the privatisation of public assets, as has been seen in the UK National Health Service (Mann, 2022). It is recognised that this will not cause more medical graduates to work in deprived areas:

All this is only about producing more doctors and not about the quality of doctors suited to our needs (Nagarajan, 2019).

In addition,

…if we want to keep health care costs down and still have access to well-qualified physicians, we also need to keep the cost of creating those physicians down…. (Asch et al., 2013, p. 1975)

The profit motive is unlikely to keep costs to the 'consumer' (the student) down. Where income is siphoned off to owners and shareholders, it is not being spent on the quality of education, nor on the communities who support that education by providing clinical experience. The first duty of a profit-making organisation is 'to deliver value to shareholders' (Walshe, 2015); reconciling this with claimed purposes of quality and social accountability may be a challenge too far.

The Rhetoric and the Reality of the Medical Education Business: A Contradiction

The business of medical education is enveloped in contradictory lines of rhetoric, deriving from politics, professional values, social imperatives and, perhaps most importantly, economics. The 'worldwide boom in private medical education', sometimes assisted by the legislature rather than the government (Knight, 2021) attests to this conclusion (Shehnaz, 2010).

Valdes Roberto Bollela illustrates that the economic imperative, in the form of new for-profit medical schools, is not necessarily accompanied by acceptable standards of education, despite medicine being the only profession to have developed a flourishing educational regulation, research and development wing of its own, which has also joined the business side of the endeavour. In this, the political imperative to increase healthcare access for voters, is perhaps in contradiction with the reality of what is required to produce medical graduates for the society that needs them (O'Dowd, 2024). At that point, where finance is needed, for-profit and private medical schools may be very useful to politicians. Although there is an argument for examining the cost of any medical school activity (Beck Dallaghan et al., 2022), that is quite different from undertaking activities within medical education for the purpose of generating income.

The Limited Effect of Medical Schools on Health Inequality

Although many claims have been made, especially in relation to arguments around social accountability, that medical schools can affect the health status of communities (Murray et al., 2012), in the end, they cannot do this in a sustainable way without political intervention. A medical school can, of course, improve the services from which their students learn, and they can offer direct help in terms of, for example, diagnostic camps and health advice. And it may be that some graduates will opt to practise where they trained, so siting schools in areas of deprivation may have some benefit. But against the social, political and economic forces, the privilege and underprivilege, that mould the lives of ordinary people, medical schools, just the like any other part of the educational system, will be limited in their effect. The provision of healthcare services is a political, not educational, issue. This should not be a cause of despair, but a trigger to realism. The task of a medical school is to produce a graduate who has learned within their own context (unless medical graduates are being produced for export) and is equipped with the skills and knowledge of medicine. If those graduates, and their teachers, choose to move into the realms of politics, economics or social reform, that is a separate strand of work which will be informed by their medical training and experience. But medical schools, even when sited in deprived areas, and even when their quality assurance is improved, and national examinations attest to that quality, cannot change society. Medical education can only address its own problems.

References

Appleby, J. (2022). Planning the healthcare workforce: How many GPs do we need? *BMJ*, o123. https://doi.org/10.1136/bmj.o123

Asch, D. A., Nicholson, S., & Vujicic, M. (2013). Are we in a medical education bubble market? *New England Journal of Medicine, 369*(21), 1973–1975. https://doi.org/10.1056/NEJMp1310778

Balan, A. (2017). Meeting the challenges of globalisation in legal education. *The Law Teacher, 51*(3), 274–286. https://doi.org/10.1080/03069400.2016.1186415

Balan, A. (2023). Neoliberalism, privatisation and marketisation: The implications for legal education in England and Wales. *Cogent Education, 10*(2). https://doi.org/10.1080/2331186X.2023.2284548

Beck Dallaghan, G. L., Lomis, K., Crow, S., & Coplit, L. (2022). Bridging educational innovation and financial offices: Using the Business Model Canvas modified for medical educators to communicate need. *Journal of Communication in Healthcare, 15*(2), 131–136. https://doi.org/10.1080/17538068.2021.1993691

Boniol, M., Kunjumen, T., Nair, T. S., Siyam, A., Campbell, J., & Diallo, K. (2022). The global health workforce stock and distribution in 2020 and 2030: A threat to equity and 'universal' health coverage? *BMJ Global Health, 7*(6), e009316. https://doi.org/10.1136/bmjgh-2022-009316

Davis, M. A., Anthopolos, R., Tootoo, J., Titler, M., Bynum, J. P. W., & Shipman, S. A. (2018). Supply of healthcare providers in relation to county socioeconomic and health status. *Journal of General Internal Medicine, 33*(4), 412–414. https://doi.org/10.1007/s11606-017-4287-4

Dowell, J., Norbury, M., Steven, K., & Guthrie, B. (2015). Widening access to medicine may improve general practitioner recruitment in deprived and rural communities: Survey of GP origins and current place of work. *BMC Medical Education, 15*(1), 165. https://doi.org/10.1186/s12909-015-0445-8

Eckhert, N. L. (2010). Perspective: Private schools of the Caribbean: Outsourcing medical education. *Academic Medicine, 85*(4), 622–630. https://doi.org/10.1097/ACM.0b013e3181d2aee1

FasterCapital. (2024, April 21). *Medical education: The business of lifelong learning: Monetizing medical education platforms.* https://fastercapital.com/content/Medical-education%2D%2DThe-Business-of-Lifelong-Learning%2D%2DMonetizing-Medical-Education-Platforms.html

Ferreira, T., Collins, A. M., Feng, O., Samworth, R. J., & Horvath, R. (2023). Career intentions of medical students in the UK: A national, cross-sectional study (AIMS study). *BMJ Open, 13*(9), e075598. https://doi.org/10.1136/bmjopen-2023-075598

Hafferty, F. W., O'Brien, B. C., & Tilburt, J. C. (2020). Beyond high-stakes testing: Learner trust, educational commodification, and the loss of medical school professionalism. *Academic Medicine, 95*(6), 833–837. https://doi.org/10.1097/ACM.0000000000003193

Hancock, C., Steinbach, A., Nesbitt, T. S., Adler, S. R., & Auerswald, C. L. (2009). Why doctors choose small towns: A developmental model of rural physician recruitment and retention. *Social Science & Medicine, 69*(9), 1368–1376. https://doi.org/10.1016/j.socscimed.2009.08.002

Hashem, F., Marchand, C., Peckham, S., & Peckham, A. (2022). What are the impacts of setting up new medical schools? A narrative review. *BMC Medical Education, 22*(1), 759. https://doi.org/10.1186/s12909-022-03835-4

Hastings, A., & Rao, M. (2001). Doctoring in deprived areas. *British Medical Journal, 323*, 409–410.

Hsieh, C.-R., & Tang, C. (2019). The multi-tiered medical education system and its influence on the health care market – China's Flexner report. *Human Resources for Health, 17*(1), 50. https://doi.org/10.1186/s12960-019-0382-4

Knight, V. (2021). For-profit medical school proposed in Montana sparks concerns. *Shots: Health News from NPR.* https://www.npr.org/sections/health-shots/2021/06/07/1002477044/once-banned-for-profit-medical-schools-are-on-the-rise-again-in-the-u-s

Lujan, H. L., & DiCarlo, S. E. (2023). We used to get money to teach students, now we teach students to get money: Medical education has become a market with credentials not knowledge the commodity! *Advances in Physiology Education, 47*(3), 521–526. https://doi.org/10.1152/advan.00065.2023

Maclaren, A. S., Locock, L., & Skea, Z. C. (2022). Valuing place in doctors' decisions to work in remote and rural locations the place of remote and rural medicine. *Future Healthcare Journal, 9*, 248–251. https://doi.org/10.7861/fhj.2022-0089

Mann, N. (2022). NHS privatisation is real. *BMJ*, o2668. https://doi.org/10.1136/bmj.o2668

McGrail, M., O'Sullivan, B., Gurney, T., Eley, D., & Kondalsamy-Chennakesavan, S. (2021). Exploring doctors' emerging commitment to rural and general practice roles over their early career. *International Journal of Environmental Research and Public Health, 18*(22), 11835. https://doi.org/10.3390/ijerph182211835

Meliala, A., Hort, K., & Trisnantoro, L. (2013). Addressing the unequal geographic distribution of specialist doctors in Indonesia: The role of the private sector and effectiveness of current regulations. *Social Science & Medicine, 82*, 30–34. https://doi.org/10.1016/j.socscimed.2013.01.029

Mian, L. (2023). The role of education in promoting social mobility. *Sociology and Criminology, 11*(2), 281–282.

Morgan, J. (2015). *Caribbean offshore medical schools and the international mobility of medical education.* Simon Fraser University.

Mosheim, T. (2025). Race to medicine "wrecking Korean universities" as dropouts soar. *Times Higher Education Supplement.* https://www.timeshighereducation.com/news/race-medicine-wrecking-korean-universities-dropouts-soar

Murray, R. B., Larkins, S., Russell, H., Ewen, S., & Prideaux, D. (2012). Medical schools as agents of change: Socially accountable medical education. *Medical Journal of Australia, 196*(10), 653–653. https://doi.org/10.5694/mja11.11473

Nagarajan, R. (2019, June 3). How medical education became a business, one policy change at a time I. *Times of India.* https://timesofindia.indiatimes.com/india/how-medical-education-became-a-business-one-policy-change-at-a-time/articleshow/69709297.cms

O'Dowd, A. (2024). Pledge to boost medical training places rings hollow, say leaders. *BMJ*, q502. https://doi.org/10.1136/bmj.q502

Park, J. (2024, May 16). Court refuses injunction on medical school expansion. *The Korea Herald.* https://www.koreaherald.com/view.php?ud=20240516050735

Salter, B., Filippakou, O., & Tapper, T. (2016). Expanding the English medical schools: The politics of knowledge control. *London Review of Education, 14*(1). https://doi.org/10.18546/LRE.14.1.04

Shehnaz, S. I. (2010). Editorial. Privatisation of medical education. Viewpoints with a global perspective. *Sultan Qaboos University Medical Journal, 10*(1), 6–11.

Simkovic, M., & McIntyre, F. (2014). The economic value of a law degree. *The Journal of Legal Studies, 43*(2), 249–289. https://doi.org/10.1086/677921

Transparency Market Research. (2024, January 12). *Medical education market to be worth USD 48.7 billion 2031, growing at 4.6% CAGR.* https://www.globenewswire.com/en/search/tag/medical%2520education%2520market

Tudor Hart, J. (1971). The inverse care law. *The Lancet, 297*(7696), 405–412. https://doi.org/10.1016/S0140-6736(71)92410-X

Walsh, K. (2010). *Cost effectiveness in medical education* (K. Walsh, Ed.). Radcliffe Publishing Ltd.

Walshe, K. (2015). Editorial. Medical schools for profit? *Annals of Medical and Health Sciences Research, 5*(3), 155–156. https://www.amhsr.org

Valdes Roberto Bollela, in 2025, is a 57 year old white man, spouse and father of a boy and a girl, who loves music, cooking and gardening. He also has been a Founder, core faculty, Fellow and Global Faculty of the US-based Foundation for the Advancement of Medical Education and Research (FAIMER) Institute in Brazil. He is Infectious Diseases Professor at the University of São Paulo, Ribeirão Preto School of Medicine (FMRP-USP) in Brazil, consultant for health professions education in Brazil and Latin America, and Academic Dean and Co-ordinator of the FMRP-USP Faculty Development Centre.

IV.iv STATEMENT: Walls and Bridges: The Professional Relationship Between Academics and Administrators

Anne Keane

1 Is There a Problem?

This reflection is predicated on the existence of unproductive divisions between some academic and administrative staff which are linked to group identity rather than personal antagonism. This is not to suggest that medical schools are gladiatorial arenas of academic and administrative conflict. There are many examples where academic and administrative staff are mutually respectful and work in tandem to achieve goals.

However, I believe that friction is significant enough to merit investigation. There are data and anecdotal evidence to show that there is an issue, although much of what follows is based on my own observations and experience. This has included a variety of senior administrative roles in medical education in universities, a medical regulatory body, and the NHS. I have, however, strenuously avoided taking sides! I have identified some common perceptions (or misperceptions), some possible reasons for divisions, and some suggestions to address them.

2 Who Are We Talking About?

'Academics', in my definition here, comprise university teachers, researchers, and clinicians with formal teaching responsibilities on undergraduate medical programmes. Academics with limited administrative responsibilities are not included.

'Administrators' comprise university staff in general or those with specialist administrative roles. The former includes course, programme, department, school,

A. Keane (✉)
Edinburgh, Scotland
e-mail: anne.m.keane@outlook.com

© The Author(s), under exclusive license to Springer Nature Switzerland AG 2026
J. Grant, L. Grant (eds.), *The Contradictions of Medical Education*,
https://doi.org/10.1007/978-3-031-90394-6_14

197

faculty, and college (for example, college of health sciences) administrators. The latter includes specialist staff in student affairs, human resources, information technology, quality assurance and external relations. It includes administrators 'locally' line-managed (in course, programme, department, school, faculty, or college structures), and administrators line-managed in central administration (for example, by the registrar's office).

3   What's the (Alleged) Problem?

Some of the main grievances that I have experienced or heard about are as follows:

3.1   Some Administrators Believe That Some Academics

- Treat administrators as second-class citizens, servants who generally remain below stairs (Greatrix, 2017).
- Want to pursue their own agenda.
- Are not interested in issues that are not directly relevant to their academic work.
- Attribute unpopular decisions to administrative animosity.
- Make interacting with them like herding cats, a view interpreted by Greatrix (who does not share it) as meaning that academics can be a bit dim and wilful (Greatrix, 2020).

3.2   Some Academics Believe That Some Administrators

- Do not know their place anymore: those who once stayed in the background are now a noisy part of the daily life of academics (Taylor, 2015).
- Are not taking care of administration so that academics can focus on academic work.
- Are not significantly contributing to universities' major missions of teaching and research.
- Are motivated by the ambition to aggrandise their own roles, maximising the power and prestige of whatever post they hold, capturing or inventing new functions (Ginsberg, 2011), thereby undermining academics' autonomy and status.
- Have/are staging an administrative coup (Greatrix, 2017), although this is not the view of Greatrix himself.

A significant difference emerges. Administrators acknowledge that academics are doing valuable work. Some academics argue that at least some administration is unnecessary and even harmful and should be stopped. Some administrators want some academics to do some things in a different way. Some academics do not want some administrators to do some things *at all*. This contrast is worth noting.

It is not possible in this context to delve into these potential sources of antagonism to confirm or refute them. The assumption is that perception can be as potent as reality.

4   Why Does It Matter?

Interaction characterised by discord rather than harmony, even among a minority of staff some of the time, is detrimental to the individuals concerned and to the university. Mutual understanding and trust create a more pleasant working environment. It can also have significant practical benefits. These include recruiting and retaining quality staff; encouraging enthusiasm and productivity; harnessing a wide variety of talents in the common interest; strengthening collaborative working; and reducing unnecessary supervision and micromanagement.

5   Potential Reasons for the Tension?

The following are hypothetical explanations for the observed beliefs and behaviours.

5.1   It is Natural

In evolutionary psychology, the urge to obtain status in organisational settings is human nature, reflecting an ancient human instinct for hierarchy: you can take the person out of the Stone Age, not the Stone Age out of the person (Nicholson, 1998).

5.2   It is Cultural

Organisational culture may be overt (for example, embedded in reporting arrangements and job descriptions) and/or covert, rooted in tacit understandings. There are also sub-cultures. Perhaps academic staff and administrators are simply in different cultures or sub-cultures?

Perhaps this scenario is apparent in academics treating their support for administrators as unusual, if not a guilty secret: "I'm just going to come out and say something that many academics would find shameful…I love my administrators" (Knight, 2017); and "It's hard to believe that a faculty member is writing this, but I do feel that most administrators do serve a useful purpose" (Kelchen, 2018).

The two cultures or sub-cultures are not necessarily antagonistic, but it indicates that there is a divide which needs to be recognised and bridged.

5.3   University Structures and Governance

University structures are generally neither flat nor flexible. Governance frameworks may be centuries old with only minor modifications in the interim. Even more modern universities may to some extent mirror these traditions and organisation. Intricate organograms and detailed remits and conduct of business regulations for the various layers of decision-making illustrate the complexity. Administrative staff may have a low, or invisible, presence in these structures.

5.4   Physical Distance

Universities may corral administrators into a central administrative building. When electronic media have become so central to the lives of practically all university staff, it may seem old-fashioned to attach any significance to physical location. But a building of administrators somewhat removed from the venues where academics are based and where teaching and research takes place, may reflect and/or encourage disconnection and factionalism.

5.5   Outnumbered

A common theme is that academics are being outnumbered by administrators. A perception is that this has changed the balance of power, with unease about the alleged declining influence and independence of academic staff. 'Nothing creates a good headline like raising the spectre of a university overrun by administrators' (Fowler, 2015).

5.6   Increased Demands

Perhaps there are more administrators because there is more administration? Student numbers and external accountability, auditing and reporting have certainly increased. There is more emphasis on the university as a business and on income generation. Internally, strategy, business planning, risk management and staff appraisal have an increasing profile.

Administrators are available to undertake much of these responsibilities, but in many cases an additional burden will also inevitably fall on academic staff. This can lead academics to question the usefulness of the growing number of administrators.

5.7   The Career Dean (or Head of School or College)

Traditionally, academics regarded deanship as something of a distraction, an interval in an academic career that would soon resume. Sometimes internal candidates were genuinely reluctant to serve as dean, and sometimes the reluctance was performative, as in Mister or Madam Speaker being dragged to the UK House of Commons' Chair. The search for deans now frequently involves recruitment consultants and international head hunting. These deans may sometimes undertake a small amount of academic or clinical work, but they are primarily managers, may have been managers for some time, and may spend the rest of their career as managers. The dean may therefore not be a familiar member of the team, a peer performing a different role for a limited time. They may be an unknown quantity with no prior links to the university. At least initially, they do not have any emotional attachment or close personal relationship to academic colleagues. They may have been chosen in preference to internal applicants.

Deans are likely to be directly affected by national and organisational strategic and business priorities, and the consequent burdens. They may be relieved that administrators can lift some of this load from their shoulders. Senior administrators may therefore have the dean's ear and may be seen by the dean or by themselves as the dean's second in command (I hesitate to use the term 'enforcer'). This can alter the dynamic between academics and senior administrative staff.

6   Is Medicine Different?

The uniqueness of medical education should not be overstated; some of the issues identified occur in other disciplines too. But undergraduate medical education has some distinct factors that may add additional complexity to the academic—administrator interface.

6.1   Medical Education

• Involves liaison with the health service both for the organisation and for management of student clinical placements.

- Is, to a significant extent, provided off-campus by teachers with clinical responsibilities.
- Is subject to additional regulation—by the General Medical Council in the UK, for example—as well as by general university quality assurance agencies.

Administrators may therefore be involved in work over and above that required to support other university disciplines. It is moot whether academic colleagues, or indeed university senior managers, recognise this additional dimension.

6.2   Clinical Academics (in My Context)

- Have another professional life as a doctor which may give them their primary identity.
- Have a strong vocation, sometimes from an early age, to be a doctor.
- Are invariably academic highflyers with postgraduate training.
- Are often from relatively affluent backgrounds.
- Disproportionately have attended private schools.

Clinical academics' clinical obligations may not be evident and understood by campus-based administrators. Many administrators also have impressive academic qualifications. Some have an affluent background and may be privately educated, but I would hypothesise that it is less common than in the medical profession. There may therefore be a greater gulf in these respects between academics and administrators than there is in many other disciplines.

6.3   Medicine Is

- A high-status profession.
- A trusted profession.
- A profession with purposes that, in broad terms, are widely understood.

This is not generally the case with administration.

So, in addition to a generic administrative and academic divide, there may be these specific issues to be considered in medical education.

7   What Can Be Done?

Many of the factors identified as potential sources of friction—including the growth in the number of administrators and the increase in oversight—may be long-term and irreversible. The following suggestions recognise that. They are also not predicated on an existing poor relationship between academics and administrators. They may be relevant even where relationships are good.

7.1   Universities Can Do the Following

Investigate

Consider whether there is an issue. Without being alarmist and suggesting there is a major problem, evaluate working relationships. Do this carefully: staff are busy and do not necessarily have the time or inclination to fill in a long questionnaire. This is particularly true if the results of previous surveys have disappeared into the university equivalent of the Bermuda Triangle. If you find out that there is an issue, do something about it.

Consider Governance

Evaluate if there is a need to make improvements to administrative representation on key committees and take any remedial action.

Send the Message that the Views of All Staff Are Important

If a review or a significant change is being considered, make sure you consult with administrators as well as with students and academic staff. Some administrators may have decades of experience, and all administrators may have useful perspectives.

Give Credit Where It Is Due

It would be unthinkable for a contributing author not to be named in a published paper: but even an herculean achievement by an administrator may remain unsung. Sometimes the significance of administration is only recognised on those rare occasions when something goes wrong. A simple public 'thank you' sends the message that all staff are valued, and acts as an incentive the next time the administrator is asked to pull out all the stops.

Academics should, of course, also be thanked, although they may receive more obvious validation through the immediate responses of a satisfied class, publication and citation of research, or positive student feedback.

Use Sensible Job Titles

Avoid obscure titles that obfuscate rather than explain what the postholder does. Confident and competent administrators—the ones you should be hiring—do not need the shield of a grandiose title. They would prefer not to have to explain their role to everyone they meet. Try to provide clear job titles that give the uninitiated a sense of the role.

The term 'non-academic' should be immediately retired. Defining someone by what they are not is rarely a good idea. The use of 'secretary' for what is really a senior management role should be carefully considered. It has a different meaning in the wider world, including in the NHS with which the 'secretary' may liaise.

7.2   Academics and Administrators Can...

Communicate

Avoid letting preconceptions based on stereotypes influence your views and interaction. Proceed on a case-by-case basis. If there is an issue, raise it courteously and try to find a solution. Eye rolling, sighing, and muttering 'typical administrator/academic' are not effective alternatives.

Liaise

Try to find a common cause. Even bureaucrats do not welcome unnecessary bureaucracy (although their definition of 'unnecessary' may differ from that of academics). Administrators and academics may feel that some of the bureaucratic demands made on them divert them away from more productive and enjoyable work. Work together to manage it in both your interests. But the temptation to form a subtle academic—administrator axis of resistance against the highest echelons of the university is probably best avoided. Probably.

Collaborate in Projects

A primary focus for more integrated working is likely to be in project work. It may already have resulted in more fluid institutional structures and cultures, with a softening of internal and external boundaries (Whitchurch, 2006). It can give academics and administrators more insight into the contribution all their colleagues can make, and cross academic vs. administrative demarcation lines.

Accept

There will always be tensions at times. Minimise them and live with it.

7.3   And Then, Academics Can…

Understand External Demands

Try not to blame administrators for work arising from university or government decisions. The administrators cannot help it. They can do their best to reduce the pain. But they will be blamed if the work is not completed on time and to the required standard. That is why they remind, badger or plead with you. The alternative is to do all the work yourself.

Have an Open Mind

Be careful about characterising some administrative roles as unnecessary. It is not always easy to have knowledge and insight into what others do, particularly if it is not in your area of expertise. It may be that the administrator has several discrete elements to their role and that the critic is only aware of some of those. If an academic is really convinced that there is no added value from a particular administrative role, they can raise it with the dean or the relevant manager in central administration. Never describe administrators as doing insignificant, unpleasant or irrelevant jobs (Spicer, 2017).

Avoid Any Hint of Condescension

There is no need to call administrators 'lovely and well-meaning' which can be seen as patronising (Greatrix, 2017) or declare "I love my administrators" (Knight, 2017). Remarks intended to be supportive may be interpreted otherwise. Your respect and cooperation are enough.

7.4   And Finally, Administrators Can…

Avoid Being Defensive

You do not have to continually justify your existence. The university created the post and put you in it. Be confident. Do not retain years of emails to cover your back or any other part of your anatomy. Defensiveness can foster a cringe factor or, conversely, officiousness. Avoid both.

Do Not Be Precious About Practical Tasks

While a senior administrator may not do it themselves, it is essential that it is done. Academics handing over a responsibility to an administrator can prevent, in my experience, a foreseeable IT glitch totally undermining an allegedly great presentation to a VIP, or chauffeuring important people around the campus in a somewhat dilapidated old minibus when sleek new models were available.

Explain

If you are asking an academic for assistance or information, explain the outcomes and benefits if they are not immediately obvious. This may not alleviate the irritation but at least it provides a rationale.

Make Some Allowances

If an academic is late for a meeting, it may be, in my observed experience, that they have just diagnosed a child with a life-threatening cancer and need to talk to the parents; or have had to section a patient having a psychotic episode. If they are regularly and predictably late however, a pointed "Thank you for joining us, I'll recap on what you've missed" may be understood. An administrator occasionally being late is unlikely to involve a life-threatening event but may be unavoidable. The occasional slipped deadline by academics or administrators is perhaps tolerable depending on the nature and significance of the task, and the degree of involvement in it of the vice chancellor! Regular unexplained absence from long-scheduled meetings, consistent unpunctuality and habitual missed targets need to be sorted out.

Be Credible

Build up personal and professional credibility. It can transcend your job title and any negativity about administration from some academic staff.

8   Conclusion

Despite the growth in projects, traditional administrative functions are likely to retain a central university role in the foreseeable future. However, it should be noted that the impact of the online, blended and distributed learning and administration model, rapidly accelerated by the pandemic, is difficult to predict.

Perhaps a change in perspective would be productive. Perhaps the major reason for tension is that some academics—and some administrators—identify the sole purpose of universities as teaching and research. That will inevitably marginalise administrators, even where it is recognised that what they do needs to be done and that they do it well. Teaching and research *are* at the core of every university. But teaching and research are activities, not outcomes. They are means, not ends. The business of universities is, amongst others, producing competent satisfied graduates ready for the next stage of their careers; and contributing to the sum of human knowledge and to improving people's lives. Both academics and administrators make a significant contribution to the achievement of those goals.

References

Fowler, K. (2015, September 3). There is no contest between academic and administrative staff. *Times Higher Education (THE)*. https://www.timeshighereducation.com/blog/there-no-contest-between-academic-and-administrative-staff

Ginsberg, B. (2011, August 28). Administrators ate my tuition. *Washington Monthly*. https://washingtonmonthly.com/2011/08/28/administrators-ate-my-tuition/

Greatrix, P. (2017, August 23). *University administrators – 'Lovely and well-meaning' but still below stairs*. Wonkhe. https://wonkhe.com/blogs/university-administrators-lovely-and-well-meaning-but-still-below-stairs/

Greatrix, P. (2020, June 3). *The university leadership challenge – From herding cats to lining up lions*. Wonkhe. https://wonkhe.com/blogs/the-university-leadership-challenge-from-herding-cats-to-lining-up-lions/

Kelchen, R. (2018, May 10). *Is administrative bloat really a big problem?* Blog. https://robert-kelchen.com/2018/05/10/is-administrative-bloat-a-problem/

Knight, C. (2017, July 28). I love my administrators! And there should be no 'conflict' with academics. *Times Higher Education*. https://www.timeshighereducation.com/blog/i-love-my-administrators-and-there-should-be-no-conflict-academics

Nicholson, N. (1998). How hardwired is human behavior? *Harvard Business Review, 76*(4), 134–147.

Spicer, A. (2017, August 21). Universities are broke. So let's cut the pointless admin and get back to teaching | André Spicer | The Guardian. *The Guardian*. https://www.theguardian.com/commentisfree/2017/aug/21/universities-broke-cut-pointless-admin-teaching?CMP=twt_gu

Taylor, L. (2015, May 28). Laurie Taylor on academics v administrators. *Times Higher Education*. https://www.timeshighereducation.com/content/laurie-taylor-on-academics-v-administrators

Whitchurch, C. (2006). Who do they think they are? The changing identities of professional administrators and managers in UK higher education. *Journal of Higher Education Policy and Management, 28*(2), 159–171. https://doi.org/10.1080/13600800600751002

IV.iv COMMENTARY: Social Identity and Group Membership in Universities

Janet Grant and Leonard Grant

Medical schools are academic organisations, either in their own right, or as part of a wider university. They have an academic mission of both conducting research and teaching, at a minimum. They are each interested in health and healthcare, as well as in being at the forefront of medical education institutions (Grbic et al., 2013). In addition to those traditional values and intentions, more recent intentions have emerged concerning prevention, diversity, focus on primary care, distribution of graduates and, importantly, cost control covering cost consciousness and cost-effectiveness in clinical practice (Valsangkar et al., 2014). But these discussions hardly ever extend to the running of the institution that will provide the education and training to meet these aspirations.

Where Does Administration Fit In?

Leadership and management are increasingly in the medical school curriculum—and in postgraduate curricula too. The importance of teamwork for effective patient management is widely recognised and promoted (Lerner et al., 2009). But the idea does not always generalise beyond patient care to the education and training infrastructure that facilitates it. That might not be surprising since relationships between healthcare professionals around actual patient care will be different from relationships between healthcare professionals or academics and administrators. The UK General Medical Council guidance on leadership and management advocates respect for colleagues (General Medical Council, 2012) but those colleagues are exclusively other healthcare professionals. Managers and administrators are rendered invisible.

The World Federation for Medical Education global standards do address governance and administration (World Federation for Medical Education, 2020), and the need for students and academic staff to participate in these, with Standard 8.3 setting out that:

> The school has appropriate and sufficient administrative support to achieve its goals in teaching, learning, and research.

However, the nature of the actual working relationship between academics and administrators is not addressed. It seems that the concept of colleagues and teams does not currently extend to the administration of the medical school. More pertinently, interpreting these issues in terms of teamwork might not be helpful. We could say that academics and administrators do not constitute a team, where:

…teams must dynamically share information and resources among members and coordinate their activities in order to fulfil a certain task—in other words, teams need to engage in *teamwork* (Schmutz et al., 2019).

And even if administrators and clinical staff were such a team, their effectiveness would be limited by the team characteristics (professional composition, team familiarity, team size), task type (routine vs non-routine tasks), and the type of performance measures used (process vs outcome performance) (Schmutz et al., 2019).

To advocate better teamworking may be a weak instrument in this context. It has been noted that since separate administrative work emerged inside universities, academics and administrators have tended to co-exist, that co-existence being characterised by tension and a 'divide' (Conway, 2012). Diminishing that divide may require a collective understanding of values, beliefs and purposes of the institution, the external influences on its operation, and the totality of work that needs to be done to enable the institution to achieve its goals (Conway, 2012).

As Conway notes (Conway, 2012):

> University management is a contested space. Administrators believe it is theirs…. On the other hand, academics still have a vested interest in ensuring the space reflects academic values underpinning their work.

The divide is sometimes blurred. In relation to medical school management, the Dean is often seen as the highest manager, and is usually a clinical academic. So that person might be identified as a senior part of the general academic team. In this narrative, they are primarily managers with an academic (and probably clinical) background, who have chosen this as their career route.

There are clearly contradictions in this situation where the academics and administrators do, in fact, arise from the same situation of intending to educate medical students and conduct research. And although there might not be mutual appreciation, in fact, neither group can exist without those other staff and functions. This tension between functional co-existence and mutual recognition is the root of the contradiction.

Social Identity Theory, Hierarchy and Group Membership

Anne Keane identifies 'unproductive divisions between some academic and administrative staff which are linked to group identity rather than personal antagonism'. Social identity is defined as a person's sense of who they are based on their group membership (Tajfel & Turner, 1986). In Anne Keane's experience, these groups are 'academics' and 'administrators'. Given the largely uncriticised importance attributed to development of professional identity in medicine (Park & Hong, 2022; Shahabi et al., 2020), it seems helpful to understand how individuals see themselves in the social context of a group or team and how this perception goes on to influence their behaviour where those group identities might not be entirely relevant.

Although we cannot explain why or how some of those group differences in identity and power are prioritised and valued over one another, in circumstances where there are group identities, there may well also be implicit or explicit hierarchies, based on knowledge, power, social status, ideas of self-worth and role. Anne Keane writes about administrators being seen as 'second-class citizens' who 'do not know their place anymore'. Depending on the rationale for group identity and hierarchy, these differences might or might not map on to the effective functioning of a medical school. Where one group, the academics or clinicians, might have a higher status in society than administrators, a flatter structure might actually apply within the medical school, but not be recognised, where neither can function without the other.

So there may be contradictions between the relative effective hierarchy of these groups in different contexts.

Anne Keane points out that these issues of groups in the organisational culture may have a detrimental effect on individuals. They may also have a detrimental effect on the organisation itself. Where such hierarchies exist, there is evidence of an erosion of positive views lower in the hierarchy about specific organisational practices, with consequent effects for implementation (Gibson et al., 2019). Anne Keane raises issues about identification and positioning of one's own group in relation to others as a significant factor for management, even though group membership can be fluid: Is the Dean an administrator or an academic? Is the administrator with a PhD (like Anne Keane) an academic in disguise? How does the clinical academic's parallel identity as a clinician affect relationships? Does a clinician's social status also count inside the institution? Anne Keane draws attention to the class and educational backgrounds of administrators, as opposed to that of academics, the latter more often coming from a situation of greater social and educational privilege, while the former also often have 'impressive academic qualifications'. In 2016, only 4% of UK clinicians came from a working-class background (Social Mobility Commission, 2016).

Behaviour is further complicated by the perceptions of group boundaries. In some societies, there are quite rigid boundaries and the groups can have no realistic aspiration of altering them. In other societies, the boundaries are less rigid and the possibility of altering the social order still exists and can influence behaviour. Examination of the medical school's organisational chart might be an interesting analytical exercise in relation to these issues. How permeable are the boundaries?

The relevance of this to the functioning of the institution is that an individual's behaviour and contribution cannot be predicted solely from their personal characteristics, as management theory might sometimes suggest (Judge et al., 2008). It is also important to understand their social context and the set of beliefs that are associated with their social role and status, and their group.

The Nature of University Administration

So far, we might be identifying contradictions between the university system, groups and hierarchy, and the professional group and its attributed hierarchy in other circumstances. It has been suggested that administration is an 'organisationally constituted formal category' whereas leadership is a 'personally constructed political category' (Ribbins, 2006). If that is so, perhaps the Dean is in the administrator group. Having said that, group boundaries are fluid, and attributed group membership might change from situation to situation. To examine this further, we need to consider the nature of university administration.

Ronald Barnett's seminal work on the idea of academic administration (Barnett, 1993), points out that academic administration is not simply a technical process, but is work that is central to the relationship between the academic administrator and the academic community. That relationship requires a 'structured discourse' between administrators and academics. The question to answer is whether they speak the same language, and whether each can become embedded in the conversations of the other. In that, Barnett draws on the work of the German philosopher and social theorist Jürgen Habermas, and depicts academics as truth-seeking, sincere in their utterances and offering understandable propositions. Importantly, the resulting conversations are critical and ongoing. This is reflected in the research-based model of managing change in a medical context that emphasises the importance of talking repeatedly and iteratively with those who will implement and be the subject of change in medical education (Gale & Grant, 1997). Talking and argument are part of the academic style. This might be in contradiction with the administrator's need to get decisions made and tasks completed, although Barnett characterises the practice of academic administration as integrated with academic practice that is founded on a conversation.

Anne Keane highlights the many ways in which each group characterises the other. The accuracy of those perceptions is an unresolved and possibly destructive issue, while their effect on relationships and action are 'as potent as reality'. The many reasons she gives for these unchallenged perceptions suggest that the organisational structure and channels of communication within institutions might require redevelopment. This might not change the hierarchy or the roles, but it might enable negotiation.

With the advent of increasing numbers of for-profit medical schools (Walshe, 2015), this relationship might be in danger of morphing from an academic one, to a business one, where administrators are managers and academics are simply employees. Hierarchies may well then change to a more industrial model.

The Contradictions

Within Anne Keane's narrative, a variety of contradictions have emerged:

Teaching and learning about management and team-working for clinical practice	and	Failure to apply this to the institution, and academic roles within it, in which that education occurs

Identity and purpose of the group of administrators	and	Identity and purpose of the group of academics

Administrators' perceived and experienced position in the hierarchy	and	Position academics attribute to administrators in the hierarchy

Perceived (lower) class and educational background of administrators	and	Academics' (especially clinicians') more privileged class and educational backgrounds.

Focused working methods of administrators	and	Discursive methods of academics

These contradictions arise from:

- Social factors (class, education)
- Roles and purposes
- Group identity
- Hierarchical position
- Knowledge and its application.

The narrative suggests ways of resolving these contradictions through investigation, communication, appreciation, appropriate attribution, collaboration, understanding, tolerance and respect. Some of these can happen at an individual level, others only at an institutional level. We have no idea whether the one without the other might constitute a new contradiction. We might agree that:

> Resolving the professional contest over this space will require not only a visible settlement about the division of labour …. It will also require new individual and collective world-views to be constructed and realised in practice to ensure that managing academic work is undertaken in ways that do not perpetuate the 'divide' into the future (Conway, 2012).

To summarise this analysis, we can say that the administration of a medical school and the academic function of a medical school are dependent upon each other. One does not and cannot exist without the other. Without administrative functions there would be no students, no materials, no booked lectures rooms, no employed staff, no cleaning, no catering, no records, no oversight. Without academic functions there would be no teaching, no research. Without either one, the purpose of the medical school would be impossible to fulfil. Therefore, we can see that the function of the medical school gives rise to these two groups—the academics and the administrators. The existence of academics and administrators is continually created and recreated through the function of the medical school. This is a key point underpinning our analysis.

Despite the origins of the two positions being within the same relation (the medical school), we also know that those two groups are not afforded the same degree of social privilege, priority or importance, and the tasks of one are seen as of lesser social and functional importance than the tasks of the other. Doctors have long enjoyed (and fought for) their status as a profession. With that comes a boundary on what knowledge is considered professional knowledge and what practices are considered professional practice. And we see this playing out in Anne Keane's narrative, with the academics wanting to maintain their position (reported as: administrators don't know their place anymore, they aren't doing their job, they are actively being obstructive) and the administrators seeking recognition and wielding whatever power they can access (reported as: administrators want academics to be interested in matters outside their academic work, academics not following procedures, expanding their roles into the academic sphere).

A resolution for this is needed. This will require a better understanding of the assumptions and concerns of both administrators and academics. Are academics thinking of a time (real or imagined) when administrators just provided a service without making any decisions or requests of their own? The relationship between academics and administrators in the university system is changing (Mok & Nelson, 2013) as a function of marketisation, limited resources, decreasing relative academic involvement in institutional decision-making, pressures for innovation and revenue-generating or market positioning initiatives, academic research being judged by funding gained and publications accepted. It has been argued that:

> In recent years, many have noted the proletarianization of the professoriate, with academic workers increasingly subordinated to institutional executives, who, in turn, respond to cost-cutting forces in business and government that control the means of scholarly production (Mok & Nelson, 2013).

Examples of industrial action taken by university academics (*UCU—University Staff Renew Strike Mandate with Historic Ballot Result*, n.d.) might support this point of view, and suggest that the tensions reported by Anne Keane might have a complex explanation.

There is also, perhaps, in the society in which this narrative is situated, a move against authority. Authority may be seen as something negative, overbearing, inappropriate. If we take the administrators as roughly equivalent to managers in industry, and the academics as roughly equivalent to the workforce, we might learn from industrial research:

> Although managers viewed the new production concepts as constituting a coherent and well-integrated system, their initiatives soon manifested important unanticipated consequences, with palpable tensions and contradictions emerging within the new regime that sharply limited its ability to elicit worker commitment and consent.
>
> Although it may be tempting to view these tensions and contradictions as anomalous events, or as simply the product of poor execution by these firms, an alternative reading sees them as a common property of workplaces undergoing the transition from one system of authority to another (Vallas, 2006).

It seems impossible to have organisation without authority. In the running of a medical school, the co-operation of many individuals is necessary, and this co-operation must be practised with great precision. Authority is necessary—the problem here being that authority is not agreed.

The resolution of the contradiction must come with the division between academic and administrator being broken down—as Anne Keane is gesturing towards in her suggestions—where all parts of the medical school come together in acknowledged common purpose.

References

Barnett, R. (1993). The idea of academic administration. *Journal of Philosophy of Education, 27*(2), 179–192. https://doi.org/10.1111/j.1467-9752.1993.tb00654.x

Conway, M. (2012). Using causal layered analysis to explore the relationship between academics and administrators in universities. *Journal of Futures Studies, 17*(2), 37–58.

Gale, R., & Grant, J. (1997). AMEE Medical Education Guide No. 10: Managing change in a medical context: Guidelines for action. *Medical Teacher, 19*(4), 239–249.

General Medical Council. (2012). *Leadership and management for all doctors.* http://www.gmc-uk.org/guidance

Gibson, C. B., Birkinshaw, J., McDaniel Sumpter, D., & Ambos, T. (2019). The hierarchical erosion effect: A new perspective on perceptual differences and business performance. *Journal of Management Studies, 56*(8), 1713–1747. https://doi.org/10.1111/joms.12443

Grbic, D., Hafferty, F. W., & Hafferty, P. K. (2013). Medical school mission statements as reflections of institutional identity and educational purpose: A network text analysis. *Academic Medicine, 88*(6), 852–860. https://doi.org/10.1097/ACM.0b013e31828f603d

Judge, T. A., Klinger, R., Simon, L. S., & Yang, I. W. F. (2008). The contributions of personality to organizational behavior and psychology: Findings, criticisms, and future research directions. *Social and Personality Psychology Compass, 2*(5), 1982–2000. https://doi.org/10.1111/j.1751-9004.2008.00136.x

Lerner, S., Magrane, D., & Friedman, E. (2009). Teaching teamwork in medical education. In. *Mount Sinai Journal of Medicine, 76*(4), 318–329. https://doi.org/10.1002/msj.20129

Mok, K. H., & Nelson, A. R. (2013). Introduction: The changing roles of academics and administrators in times of uncertainty. *Asia Pacific Education Review, 14*(1), 1–9. https://doi.org/10.1007/S12564-013-9248-Y

Park, G. M., & Hong, A. J. (2022). "Not yet a doctor": Medical student learning experiences and development of professional identity. *BMC Medical Education, 22*(1). https://doi.org/10.1186/s12909-022-03209-w

Ribbins, P. M. (2006). History and the study of administration and leadership in education: Introduction to a special issue. *Journal of Educational Administration and History, 38*(2), 113–124. https://doi.org/10.1080/00220620600554942

Schmutz, J. B., Meier, L. L., & Manser, T. (2019). How effective is teamwork really? The relationship between teamwork and performance in healthcare teams: A systematic review and meta-analysis. *BMJ Open, 9*, 28280. https://doi.org/10.1136/bmjopen-2018-028280

Shahabi, M., Mohammadi, N., Koohpayehzadeh, J., & Arabshahi, S. K. S. (2020). The attainment of physician's professional identity through meaningful practice: A qualitative study. *Medical Journal of the Islamic Republic of Iran, 34*(1), 16. https://doi.org/10.34171/MJIRI.34.16

Social Mobility Commission. (2016). *State of the nation 2016: Social mobility in Great Britain.* https://assets.publishing.service.gov.uk/government/uploads/system/uploads/attachment_data/file/569410/Social_Mobility_Commission_2016_REPORT_WEB__1__.pdf

Tajfel, H., & Turner, J. C. (1986). The social identity theory of intergroup behaviour. In S. Worchel & W. G. Austin (Eds.), *Psychology of intergroup relations* (pp. 7–24). Nelson-Hall.

UCU – University staff renew strike mandate with historic ballot result. (n.d.). Retrieved April 13, 2023, from https://www.ucu.org.uk/article/12866/University-staff-renew-strike-mandate-with-historic-ballot-result

Vallas, S. P. (2006). Empowerment redux: Structure, agency, and the remaking of managerial authority. *American Journal of Sociology, 111*(6), 1677–1717. https://doi.org/10.1086/499909

Valsangkar, B., Chen, C., Wohltjen, H., & Mullan, F. (2014). Do medical school mission statements align with the nation's health care needs? *Academic Medicine, 89*(6), 892–895. https://doi.org/10.1097/ACM.0000000000000241

Walshe, K. (2015). Editorial. Medical schools for profit? *Annals of Medical and Health Sciences Research, 5*(3), 155–156. https://www.amhsr.org

World Federation for Medical Education. (2020). *Basic medical education. WFME global standards for quality improvement. The 2020 revision.* https://www.wfme.org/

Anne Keane is a PhD social historian by background with significant experience of high-level management and administration in universities and in medical institutions. She is a regulator in national and international medical education, and in college and university education in general. She has developed quality assurance policy and systems in more than one country.

Part V
Medical Education and the Workplace

Summary

Medical education provides a vocational pathway. That being so, it is closely related to the workplace for which its graduates are primarily being prepared. As such, this relationship can be problematical. In this Part of the book, our authors, from the UK and India, explore the relationship between medical training and the workplace in which it occurs in surgery and in medicine. The tensions and contradictions between practice, training and assessment are explored. Is the doctor in training a doctor, or a learner, or even an educator also teaching those who are more junior? Does training reflect real practice? Does assessment show that a graduate is ready for independent practice? Or should we recognise that learning in the workplace cannot follow an entirely predetermined pathway, and assessment cannot entirely reflect actual practice, but can measure prerequisites for practice? Although there is a career pathway that suddenly changes a learner into an independent practitioner, the actual pathway is much different from its rationalisation. There is a central tension between the learning system and the service system, for both learner and supervisor, where, in neoliberal terms, education is a tangible, regulated product, rather than simply the 'real work of learning' by participation in real clinical practice.

V.i STATEMENT: When Does a Surgical Trainee Become Competent to Perform Surgery?

Anindya Niyogi

1 Surgical Competency and Surgical Training

Surgical competency combines technical and non-technical skills such as decision-making, communication, and leadership. Technical skills and manual dexterity are essential for a surgeon. However, excellent knowledge and experience must complement superior technical proficiency. But is there a benchmark for surgical competency?

At the time of writing, it has been more than five years since I completed training. I still ask my senior colleagues to help me during complex cases in theatres. Help is readily available in organisations such as the National Health Service. I wonder how similar situations are managed in private sectors where colleagues are competitors.

How did I learn to perform surgery? Surgical training is like an apprenticeship. I learned surgical techniques from my seniors. As a trainee, I rotated through various centres and worked with several consultants in each centre. I picked up the technical tricks I liked from my trainers and developed my technique. My technique continues to evolve with experience. There are textbooks on operative surgery; however, the techniques in practice do vary from the textbook demonstrations.

There are no standard techniques in surgery. For example, the appendicectomy approach can be a lower midline laparotomy, right lower quadrant Lanz incision, single incision or multiple port laparoscopy; the appendix base can be sealed with staplers, plastic clips or sutures. According to my current trainees, all paediatric

---

Please note: In the UK, the term 'trainee' has been replaced by 'resident'. However, we have retained the terminology as it was when this chapter was written.

A. Niyogi (✉)
King's College Hospital, London, UK
e-mail: anindya.niyogi@kcl.ac.uk

surgeons in my hospital have different techniques for circumcision, which is a standard paediatric procedure. Fortunately, the outcomes are similar as the surgeons adopt the method that works best for them. For example, for laparoscopic cholecystectomy, performance has been shown to improve throughout the first 200 operations, resulting in a 40% reduction in operative time and an ability to deal more effectively with complex cases (Voitk et al., 2001). This amount of experience is achievable in common procedures such as cholecystectomy. However, for uncommon procedures, when is the experience enough?

2   The Evolution of Surgery

Although technology in surgery has evolved significantly, surgical principles have remained the same over the decades. For example, in cholecystectomy, the cystic artery and the cystic duct are ligated and divided, and the gallbladder is removed. Various approaches can achieve this. The open surgical technique has been replaced by laparoscopy. Single-incision laparoscopy, natural orifice transluminal endoscopic surgery, and robotic surgery approaches are also used. New techniques involve new technology. All technological developments are currently in the field of minimally invasive surgery. Irrespective of the surgical approach, the surgical goal remains the same as traditional open surgery. Introducing a new technique is always associated with a learning curve and initial higher complication rates. Due to this learning curve, it is typical for senior surgeons to refrain from taking up new approaches. For example, when surgeons were asked about undergoing a cholecystectomy on themselves, most chose either conventional or mini-laparoscopy as their preferred access technique (Lima et al., 2020). Therefore, newer methods still need to be popular, even among trainees.

3   The Process of Surgical Training: Trainee to Trainer

Surgical training in my speciality is backloaded; the early years of training concentrate on simple procedures while hands-on exposure to complex procedures only happens in the final years. It is common for trainees to struggle to be signed off for all complex procedures in time, resulting in extension of the training period. The transition from a trainee (now called 'resident' in the UK) to a trainer is quite dramatic. As soon as I started as a consultant, I was expected to sign off trainees. I was signed off based on the individual perceptions of my trainers, which needed to be standardised. It took a lot of work to set a benchmark. Is being as good as me good enough?

The most challenging question is what competency standards must a trainee attain to safely treat patients without supervision? According to the 2021 paediatric surgical curriculum (McCarthy et al., 2021) in the UK, training aims 'to produce, at certification, competent doctors, able to deliver excellent outcomes for patients as consultant surgeons'. However, 'excellent outcomes' is not explicitly defined.

4 Assessment of Surgical Competencies

That takes us to the assessment of surgical competencies. Procedure-Based Assessments (PBA) are currently a mandatory tool for assessing technical competencies among surgical trainees in the United Kingdom for formative and summative purposes. PBA is procedure specific. It constitutes a checklist of scores in different domains followed by a global score (Level 0–4). Trainees are expected to improve their global scores during training. Achieving Level 4 implies reaching the standard to perform the procedure independently. Relatively common operations are called the 'index operations' for each speciality. All trainees must be competent in performing those procedures by the end of the training (Shalhoub et al., 2015).

Trainees are not assessed during all procedures they perform. They can prospectively select cases for assessment. There may be a tendency for trainees to choose cases that are more likely to be easy. The trainee can also withdraw from the assessment if their performance is insufficient. Therefore, poor performances and challenging patients can be easily excluded from the training portfolio. Thus, in the current UK system, the training portfolio may look better than the actual competency as complex cases and complications can be selectively removed from the portfolio.

There are two options to prevent selection bias: to perform PBA for all procedures during training, or randomly select patients for assessment. It is not logistically possible to undertake PBAs for all operations a trainee performs throughout the training programme. Random selection of patients may not select all index cases required in the curriculum. Therefore, the only practical way of preventing this bias is to perform PBA for all procedures during the final year of training. Only the global competency levels can be recorded instead of the detailed assessment for practicality. This way, a more transparent idea of the trainee's general performance can be obtained.

5 Assessment, Competence and Performance

The surgical certification guidance specifies the requirement of Level 4 in index procedures. However, it does not differentiate between levels 4a and 4b. Level 4a is achieved when the procedure is performed fluently without guidance or intervention. Level 4b is obtained when, in addition to attaining level 4a, the trainee could anticipate, avoid, and/or deal with the procedure's common problems and complications. Though achieving Level 4b appears more desirable, it is impossible to make Level 4b mandatory as problems and complications are variable and may not be encountered during the assessment. This problem may be solved by introducing mandatory Level 4b PBA during high-fidelity simulations of common complications and challenges in each procedure. However, this kind of simulation is not included in the UK surgical curriculum. As the literature on validating PBA in the simulated environment is lacking, further research is needed.

Surgical practice is not limited to index cases. Though some surgical skills are transferable, considerable evidence suggests that competence in one procedure does not guarantee expertise in another. The assessments are, therefore, procedure specific. Competencies in relatively rare non-index procedures are not mandatory for certification. Therefore, new consultants are likely to have deficiencies in some areas. This is not a significant issue in institutions like the National Health Service (NHS). It is a common practice to perform a complicated procedure with an experienced senior colleague. However, in other contexts where the care is provided by a single surgeon, the shortcomings in training may compromise patient safety.

6 Judging Competence, Setting Standards

When I sign a trainee off, how do I decide that the performance is at Level 4? How do I ensure that if another trainer assesses the same procedure, there will be no inter-rater variability? Absolute standard-setting is necessary to establish cut-offs for summative assessments (Pugh et al., 2015). Different procedures will have different cut-offs. Usually, the benchmarking is performed in simulated settings where the experts perform the procedure, and the trainees are assessed against that standard. The surgical techniques of experts can vary significantly. However, certain domains will remain reasonably consistent such as incision, time to complete the procedure, blood loss, the quantity of suture materials used, and complications. Standard setting should be based on consistent domains.

The process of standard-setting each procedure, which can be reliably used across the country, is challenging. The experts must be defined, regional variations must be considered, and all stakeholders should agree upon the standard steps of each index procedure. Each procedure must be performed by various blinded experts and observed by blinded experienced assessors to set the sign-off benchmark. Though there are several transferable and overlapping skills in different surgical procedures, it is known that achieving competency in one procedure does not automatically guarantee competency for another similar procedure (Marriott et al., 2011). Therefore, standard setting should be repeated separately for each complete procedure.

There is currently no standard-setting of PBAs. Therefore, based on the current evidence, we cannot confidently claim that if a trainee is assessed to be competent during a PBA, their performance was close to an expert. However, even without standardisation, inter-rater variability has been low, as the scores by blinded assessors on video recordings of performances were very similar (Beard, 2005).

There have been recommendations to include some essential intraoperative outcome parameters, such as operating time, blood loss and complications in the assessment (Beard, 2005). However, the current UK assessment tools do not have those outcome measures included. As a result, some questions remain unanswered: Was the incision made by the trainee similar to an expert? Was the procedure completed in an accepted time frame? Was the blood loss appropriate? Was the complication rate acceptable? All these aspects are essential as better technical performance has been shown to improve patient outcomes.

Introducing the Multiple Consultant Report (MCR) in the 2021 curriculum for all surgical specialities aims to reduce inter-rater variability in assessments (Bussey, 2021a, 2021b). The biannual combined report from all consultant clinical supervisors is aimed at providing a formative review of the overall progression of a trainee, based on their professional judgement, their trust in the trainee to perform 'according to supervision levels, determining the degree of oversight they need to perform safely and effectively' and consensus among seniors who supervise the trainee (Bussey, 2021b). However, PBA remains the tool for assessing technical competency.

7 Non-Technical Skills Assessment

The Non-Technical Skills for Surgeons (NOTSS) checklist is an accepted framework for assessing non-technical operating theatre skills (Yule et al., 2008). The NOTSS categories are situation awareness, decision making, communication and teamwork, and leadership. These could be non-technical skills for any discipline. Though non-technical skills complement technical skills to develop procedural competence, assessing non-technical skills is not mandatory in surgical training assessment. Adding elements of NOTTS to PBA would make the tool more comprehensive.

Surgical training and assessments are evolving. The current training system produces competent surgeons: capability-related referrals to the General Medical Council (GMC) among new consultant surgeons are extremely rare. However, standard-setting and including NOTSS and outcome parameters would make the current summative assessment of surgical competency more robust.

References

Beard, J. D. (2005). Setting standards for the assessment of operative competence. *European Journal of Vascular and Endovascular Surgery, 30*(2), 215–218. https://doi.org/10.1016/j.ejvs.2005.01.032
Bussey, M. (2021a). Judgement, capabilities and practice: How surgical supervisors make judgements about trainee readiness to practise. *The Bulletin of the Royal College of Surgeons of England, 103*(2), 94–99. https://doi.org/10.1308/RCSBULL.2021.41

Bussey, M. (2021b). Judgement, trust, consensus and the new multiple consultant report. *The Bulletin of the Royal College of Surgeons of England, 103*(7), 330–332. https://doi.org/10.1308/rcsbull.2021.124

Lima, D. L., Lima, R. N. C. L., dos Santos, D. C., Shadduck, P. P., Carvalho, G. L., & Malcher, F. (2020). Which cholecystectomy technique would surgeons prefer on themselves? *Surgical Laparoscopy, Endoscopy & Percutaneous Techniques, 30*(6), 495–499. https://doi.org/10.1097/SLE.0000000000000833

Marriott, J., Purdie, H., Crossley, J., & Beard, J. D. (2011). Evaluation of procedure-based assessment for assessing trainees' skills in the operating theatre. *British Journal of Surgery, 98*(3), 450–457. https://doi.org/10.1002/bjs.7342

McCarthy, L., Rajimwhale, A., Robb, A., & Brownlee, E. (2021). *Paediatric surgery curriculum*. https://www.iscp.ac.uk

Pugh, D. M., Wood, T. J., & Boulet, J. R. (2015). Assessing procedural competence. *Simulation in Healthcare: The Journal of the Society for Simulation in Healthcare, 10*(5), 288–294. https://doi.org/10.1097/SIH.0000000000000101

Shalhoub, J., Santos, C., Bussey, M., Eardley, I., & Allum, W. (2015). A descriptive analysis of the use of workplace-based assessments in UK surgical training. *Journal of Surgical Education, 72*(5), 786–794. https://doi.org/10.1016/j.jsurg.2015.03.019

Voitk, A. J., Tsao, S. G. S., & Ignatius, S. (2001). The tail of the learning curve for laparoscopic cholecystectomy. *The American Journal of Surgery, 182*(3), 250–253. https://doi.org/10.1016/S0002-9610(01)00699-7

Yule, S., Flin, R., Maran, N., Rowley, D., Youngson, G., & Paterson-Brown, S. (2008). Surgeons' non-technical skills in the operating room: Reliability testing of the NOTSS behavior rating system. *World Journal of Surgery, 32*(4), 548–556. https://doi.org/10.1007/s00268-007-9320-z

V.i COMMENTARY: Assessment Versus Real Performance

Janet Grant and Leonard Grant

Assessment is a never-ending quest for predictive certainty in an uncertain world. Anindya Niyogi sets out a wide range of contradictory issues in his practice as a surgeon and a trainer that might challenge the certainty that assessment strives to offer. It is in the resolution of these that the field will develop. We will look at each issue as set out, and in terms of developing the relationship between assessment, training, competence and performance. But our analytical approach leads us to ask: What is the principal contradiction here, and how does that relate to all its aspects, as described in this narrative? How does that principal contradiction enable all the other issues to exist (Mao, 1967)?

To support our analysis of the principal contradiction, we set out below all the issues identified in Anindya Niyogi's narrative and their associated problems. This analysis alone suggests a series of contradictions.

Parallel Universes of Practice, Training and Assessment?

Issue	Problem
Surgical competency consists of both technical and non-technical skills, accompanied by experience	The experience required suggests that there is no benchmark for actual surgical competency
Surgical training is an apprenticeship whereby trainees learn different approaches from different trainers. There are no standard techniques	Implicit in this is that trainees will also develop their own preferred surgical techniques. So, what should be assessed, and how does that relate to the individual surgeon's developing practice?
Surgical practice itself develops and changes. Trainers might or might not adopt new practices. Trainees need to learn them	How does a curriculum address this shifting landscape of practice, adoption, training and learning?
The learning trajectory is not smooth. Acquiring basic skills takes time and experience. Learning complex procedures is then packed into too little time	How do plans for training and assessment take into account this uneven trajectory?
The transition from trainee to trainer is abrupt. A new trainer is not far from being a trainee, yet has to judge other trainees	How can an inexperienced trainer set a benchmark to judge trainees? Given that both are still learning, how much of each is enough to enable a new trainer to assess a trainee?
The definition of a certificated clinician is that they should be able to deliver excellent outcomes for patients	There is no definition or metric for delivery of excellent outcomes. So, confirming attainment of stated competencies is the untested surrogate for that

(continued)

(continued)

Issue	Problem
Case selection bias threatens the validity of procedure-based assessments	Given that training occurs as part of providing the surgical service, it is impossible to assess all procedures conducted during training, nor to assess them all in the final year of training. Random selection of procedures to assess would leave many competencies untested. Global competencies could be assessed but would miss specific aspects of practice
Competence in high-level problem-solving skills in practice cannot be assessed since the occurrence of problems in practice is unpredictable	Although assessment of index cases might be possible, the lack of generalisability of such skills means that the new, 'fully trained' clinician, is likely to have some unassessed deficiencies which might compromise the intended 'excellent outcomes for patients'
Setting passing standards for all components of practice-based assessment is challenging, given variability in trainee and trainer practice and experience, and the opportunities offered by the service	These challenges have deterred standard setting for procedure-based assessments, although inter-rater reliability seems to be low. Some more measurable and specific intraoperative parameters and assessments of non-operative skills might add to the predictive power of the technical skills assessments if there is evidence that they improve patient outcomes

Despite all these issues, the author points out that capability-related referrals to the General Medical Council for new consultant surgeons are low. So we are left wondering whether, at least in the United Kingdom, the current training and assessment régime is sufficient, along with whatever is done to support new consultants. So what would continuing to develop better technical characteristics and predictive power of each assessment add to practice, as opposed to improving the technical analysis of the assessments themselves? The accepted criteria for effective assessments still include reliability, validity, feasibility, cost-effectiveness, acceptance, educational impact, equivalence, and catalytic effect (Norcini et al., 2011; Van Der Vleuten, 1996) Different aspects of parallel tests and test régimes have been widely discussed in the literature (Hutchison & Benton, 2009; Ketterlin-Geller et al., 2022), as has the predicative validity of formative tests for summative assessments (Meagher et al., 2009). However, the idea of testing and the practice that tests try to predict, as parallel universes which are not necessarily amenable to measurement and control, remains to be examined conceptually. Instead, the assumption seems to be simply that if we test better, the predictive validity for actual practice will be better. That might not be so.

Improving Assessments to Measure and Predict Complex Performance

Anindya Niyogi's narrative speaks to the problems associated with attempting to professionalise (and therefore standardise, regulate, and assess) a professional practice. It has been recognised for a very long time that, as he points out, clinical expertise is accompanied by variation between experts in their thinking and their practice (Apramian et al., 2015, 2016; Grant & Marsden, 1987; Henry, 2010; Stulberg et al., 2020). Expert practice is individual. This has implications for both the content and the process of postgraduate training and the extent to which either can be fully controlled. That, in turn, has implications for how best to structure the relationship between assessment and actual learning and practice. Although surgical training has developed through many stages, from apprenticeship to the control introduced by simulation (Khan & Begum, 2021), the individuality of learning, individualised training, individual trajectories of learning based on the context of training, and the need to learn through actual practice still remain. These all provide sources of variability in the development of the trainee. In the absence of evidence (what would that evidence be?) showing that any method of training is more effective than any other (Fritz et al., 2019), these are still challenges for the assessment system that tries to ensure that the trained surgeon is fit for independent practice, and so fit to train others.

Throughout his account, Anindya Niyogi is gesturing towards this problem. He readily acknowledges that there are multiple ways of conducting the same procedure and seeks to solve this problem by suggesting a system of assessment that is based on the common features of any surgical procedure. He also discusses the issue of never feeling 'ready' and the abrupt transitions between different stages in training and independent practice. The day after he completed his training, he was able to sign off trainees: but his status change was just that—something immaterial. So, if he were or were not competent to adjudicate on the standard of a trainee just before finishing training, he is or is not competent just after. That competence and confidence must develop over time. In an era of accountability, control, structure and measurement, how are we to know when that individual competence is present in each person, whether trainee or trainer?

The Principal Contradiction: Arbitrary Training Stages and Imperfect Assessments

The contradiction we are exploring here is that of attempting to benchmark, standardise, and assess the process of developing an individual practice.

There are delineated stages of professional development in training programmes, and to pass from one to another usually involves a series of assessments. The focus in medical education has often been on those assessments—either radically overhauling or modifying them, with the goal of making such assessments more fit for the intended purpose. That purpose is a check on whether a trainee is competent to move from one stage to another.

But perhaps the problem should be looked at the other way around. The different stages of training are, ultimately, arbitrary. Of course, they come with very material consequences, not least in Anindya Niyogi's UK health service, where financial remuneration is tied to the stage of training reached. So, we have a situation where people are moving from one arbitrary stage to another with a system of assessment for those stages in training. That system of assessment will always be imperfect for two main reasons. The first reason is that it is only really possible to assess a practice *within the totality of that practice*—any other form of assessment of a practice must be artificial to some degree but, we hope, representative and generalisable. The second reason for imperfection is that trainees will naturally develop in different ways and at different rates, have different challenges in their development, and have different training experiences and relationships. Under these conditions, an arbitrary move from one stage to another may not line up with the individual's trajectory, or even with a stated curriculum, so it will always feel in some way unsatisfactory, as the author of this narrative expresses.

Quantitative and Qualitative Change

We can consider here the theory of quantitative change leading to qualitative change, which has been applied in political and social sciences to examine the threshold at which the pressure of continuing quantitative changes within a system lead to a threshold where a qualitative change occurs to the system itself (Carneiro, 2000) The classic example always given is heating up water. Water rises in temperature (a quantitative change) until it reaches a certain point where it turns into steam (a qualitative change). Let us imagine the surgical trainee undergoing an apprenticeship, as Anindya Niyogi describes. The first changes will be quantitative; the trainee will learn things, be developing, be acquiring skills, be understanding the hospital and the work more and more. But at some point, there will be a qualitative change where the trainee will move into a new stage of development and will adopt new roles, new responsibilities or new confidence. The author describes this as 'my technique continues to evolve with experience', but at the same time, he has moved into the role of consultant surgeon and trainer rather than trainee. 'Evolve' is an important and revealing choice of words. Evolution is exactly this quantitative change leading to qualitative change that we are examining.

This experience of learning, of developing, of peer and self-reflection and of moving through qualitatively different stages is set alongside the felt need for 'benchmarks' for certainty. How do we know when a surgeon is competent? Anindya Niyogi talks about how easy it is for surgeons to 'game' the system—for example, by choosing easy cases on which to be assessed, or by removing those cases where their performance was inadequate. So, do we even know if a surgeon is competent through this system of assessment? The methods of workplace-based assessment were designed to try to get closer to actual performance, but the contradiction between assessment and performance is not so easily resolved. The trainee surgeon looks to achieve a pass mark on all the complex cases, not to thoroughly understand the cases. We are reminded again of how these benchmarks have real behavioural consequences, and so, of course, the trainee is not incentivised to spend time learning the skill—they are incentivised to pass the assessment, which is a proxy for performing that skill. Are those two things the same? Anindya Niyogi does not comment explicitly, but the whole of his essay suggests that the answer is 'No'. The contradiction to resolve here is how and whether we benchmark, checklist, standardise, systematise and attempt to measure the development of a trainee through increasingly managed forms of assessment. Or whether we ask how this actually relates to real performance, at present or in the future, of each individual trainee and how that, in turn, relates to the training and practice context in which each trainee finds themselves. This is a principal contradiction that has many specific aspects that the profession and its regulators grapple with. Thinking about the details of the assessment system, its purpose and its design, examining these in the light of this overarching qualitative contradiction, since this is much more than calculating predictive value, sampling requirements, or compliance with psychometric standards (De Champlain et al., 2016) and deciding how it might be resolved, is central to the debate, starting from real, untidy performance and its context.

References

Apramian, T., Cristancho, S., Watling, C., Ott, M., & Lingard, L. (2015). Thresholds of principle and preference: Exploring procedural variation in postgraduate surgical education. *Academic Medicine, 90*(11), S70–S76. Association of American Medical Colleges Medical Education Meeting. https://doi.org/10.1097/ACM.0000000000000909

Apramian, T., Cristancho, S., Watling, C., Ott, M., & Lingard, L. (2016). They have to adapt to learn: Surgeons' perspectives on the role of procedural variation in surgical education. *Journal of Surgical Education, 73*(2), 339–347. https://doi.org/10.1016/j.jsurg.2015.10.016

Carneiro, R. L. (2000). The transition from quantity to quality: A neglected causal mechanism in accounting for social evolution. *Proceedings of the National Academy of Sciences, 97*(23), 12926–12931. https://doi.org/10.1073/pnas.240462397

De Champlain, A. F., Gotzmann, A., & Qin, S. (2016). Assessing the reliability of performance assessment scores: Some considerations in selecting an appropriate framework. *Journal of Graduate Medical Education, 8*(4), 504–506. https://doi.org/10.4300/JGME-D-15-00751.1

Fritz, T., Stachel, N., & Braun, B. J. (2019). Evidence in surgical training – A review. *Innovative Surgical Sciences, 4*(1), 7. https://doi.org/10.1515/ISS-2018-0026

Grant, J., & Marsden, P. (1987). The structure of memorized knowledge in students and clinicians: An explanation for diagnostic expertise. *Medical Education, 21*(2), 92–98. https://doi.org/10.1111/j.1365-2923.1987.tb00672.x

Henry, S. G. (2010). Polanyi's tacit knowing and the relevance of epistemology to clinical medicine. *Journal of Evaluation in Clinical Practice, 16*(2), 292–297. https://doi.org/10.1111/j.1365-2753.2010.01387.x

Hutchison, D., & Benton, T. (2009). *Parallel universes and parallel measures: Estimating the reliability of test results.* https://languagetesting.info/features/2010/pupm.pdf

Ketterlin-Geller, L. R., Sparks, A., & McMurrer, J. (2022). Developing progress monitoring measures: Parallel test construction from the item-up. *Frontiers in Education, 7.* https://doi.org/10.3389/feduc.2022.940994

Khan, M. R., & Begum, S. (2021). Apprenticeship to simulation – The metamorphosis of surgical training. *JPMA. The Journal of the Pakistan Medical Association, 71*(Suppl 1), S72–S76.

Mao, Z. (1967). *On contradiction.* Foreign Language Press.

Meagher, F. M., Butler, M. W., Miller, S. D. W., Costello, R. W., Conroy, R. M., & McElvaney, N. G. (2009). Predictive validity of measurements of clinical competence using the Team Objective Structured Bedside Assessment (TOSBA): Assessing the clinical competence of final year medical students. *Medical Teacher, 31*(11), e545–e550. https://doi.org/10.3109/01421590903095494

Norcini, J., Anderson, B., Bollela, V., Burch, V., Costa, M. J., Duvivier, R., Galbraith, R., Hays, R., Kent, A., Perrott, V., & Roberts, T. (2011). Criteria for good assessment: Consensus statement and recommendations from the Ottawa 2010 conference. *Medical Teacher, 33*(3), 206–214. https://doi.org/10.3109/0142159X.2011.551559

Stulberg, J. J., Huang, R., Kreutzer, L., Ban, K., Champagne, B. J., Steele, S. R., Johnson, J. K., Holl, J. L., Greenberg, C. C., & Bilimoria, K. Y. (2020). Association between surgeon technical skills and patient outcomes. *JAMA Surgery, 155*(10), 960–968. https://doi.org/10.1001/JAMASURG.2020.3007

Van Der Vleuten, C. P. M. (1996). The assessment of professional competence: Developments, research and practical implications. *Advances in Health Sciences Education, 1*, 41–67.

Anindya Niyogi, the author of this reflection, is a consultant paediatric surgeon in London who also has a Master's degree in Health Professions Education. He is a widely experienced national examiner and designer of clinical assessments. He is co-founder and teacher on an international virtual education programme for paediatric surgery.

V.ii STATEMENT: Postgraduate Surgical Training and the Workplace: A Developing Mismatch

Kadambari Dharanipragada and Evangeline Mary Kiruba Samuel

This chapter presents the opinions of a surgical teacher and a postgraduate resident in surgery.

1 The Teacher's View

Postgraduate (PG) trainees (called 'residents' in India) learn on the job, as part of the healthcare team with a specific role, progressing steadily, accruing experiences that would result in them becoming independent practitioners. The three year training period can be seen as an initiation into their chosen speciality, during which a rich variety of experiences is necessary to put the trainee at the threshold of independent practice and lifelong learning. This method of training has been the norm for several decades. Yet, in our perception, many factors have adversely affected that training.

2 The Resident's View

As a schoolgirl who had dreamt of becoming a surgeon, the day the admission list into postgraduate courses was released was probably the happiest of my life. I spent many nights before starting my PG training, dreaming of how I was going to fulfil

K. Dharanipragada (✉)
Jawaharlal Institute of Postgraduate Medical Education and Research (JIPMER),
Puducherry, India
e-mail: kadambari1909@gmail.com

E. M. K. Samuel
The Institute of Child Health and Hospital for Children, Chennai, India

231

all my ambitions, and make significant strides forward for my department and my field. Even though I had worked as an intern in the same department, I had superficial knowledge, at best, about how the department functioned and the various intricacies and obstacles that a resident has to face to come out at the other side. Therefore, when I finally set foot into the department as a surgical resident, I realised that there were many lessons in store for me.

A great thing about training as a surgical resident in India, is the sheer number of cases that come your way. In the outpatients' department (OPD), wave after wave of patients flood into the room, with no two individuals having the same complaints. The steep load leads to constant repetition, which forms a habit of identifying patterns, which lies at the crux of making a fast provisional diagnosis, in distinguishing the emergency from the elective and in anticipating complications. In a teaching hospital like ours, the number of patients that a resident sees is not their choice; they must attend the OPD until every patient is settled. The maxim to 'try, try and try again until you succeed' is nowhere more apt than in surgical specialities and hence, in a country like India, with its vast magnitude of various diseases, surgical residents are blessed with a wide and extensive exposure.

2.1 Work Intensity

But the large patient load in India creates intense work pressure on the residents. Surgery, by nature, is not for the weak-hearted. Long hours on your feet, emergencies that may occur at any time or place, the very physical nature of the work that requires extreme endurance and the debilitating effects a complication has on the psyche—all these take an intense physical, mental and emotional toll on the resident. Many new trainees, including me, anticipate this, but are in no way prepared for the magnitude of the impact it would have on us.

Coupled with the workload is the traditionally unforgiving heavy-handedness of seniors and the guilt that follows when simple, avoidable mistakes occur due to oversight, carelessness or plain, simple tiredness. In my time as a surgical resident, I have seen more than half of the residents resign due to inability to cope with the pressure and competition. The justification I have heard is that it is the duty of the course to toughen up the residents to face a field as unforgiving and challenging as surgery. However, I feel it is important to strike a balance. Residents are more likely to work with enthusiasm, less likely to make silly mistakes and will be more eager to learn when they are adequately rested and fed.

To address this, we could ensure that all residents equally share the workload, keeping rotational duties within a surgical unit to attend to emergencies, and to give residents a weekend day off in sequence. Specific tasks could be assigned to specific residents who then have to report the progress personally to the senior resident in charge. A consultant or senior resident could be assigned as a mentor to each junior resident, to guide them through any difficulties that they may face and to provide advice. It is important for trainees to understand that it is not the quantity of work they do that matters but the quality. Small measures, in total, would make a large difference to the quality of life during residency which would then improve the quality of work done by surgical residents.

2.2 Supervision

A wonderful aspect of surgical training in India is the experience and qualification of the professors working in teaching hospitals who strive to inspire in trainees a desire for perfection in their work. To rise to a position of eminence in India which is overflowing with highly qualified surgeons, takes a special dedication to the mission of training young surgeons as well as outstanding credentials.

I have been motivated during my clerkship and internship by my unit's caring and committed seniors and consultants who made untiring efforts to push me to learn the basic tenets of surgical care, who impressed on me the importance of clear concepts and who painstakingly took me through every suture and knot, correcting me patiently at every step. However, not all residents in all programmes are as blessed, leading to a disparity in skills, knowledge and work ethic between graduates of different institutes or sometimes even within the same institute but within different units.

2.3 Assessment

Compounding the issue is the method of assessment of surgical graduates, with one theoretical examination at the end of a three year course that tests only traditional book-knowledge. The logbook and thesis that the course expects the residents to complete are mostly taken as formalities to be rushed through and sometimes even partially fabricated, amidst the whirlwind of ward work. This leads to a large imbalance between different residents and sometimes, glaring potholes of knowledge in certain important areas.

One way to circumvent this may be to keep regular and strict assessment checkpoints throughout residency, both practical and theoretical. For example, before changing from one unit to another, all residents should be asked to independently perform certain surgical procedures under the direct supervision of a consultant who will score them and who can tell them where they can improve. Before passing from one year to another, residents should have completed a set number of selected, essential surgeries under supervision, and would not be allowed to progress without fulfilling their quota. This would ensure that all graduates fulfil a minimum standard before being allowed to obtain their degree, and allow for a more uniform training programme across the country. Care should also be taken to ensure that trainees have skill in their hands but also learn the equal importance of perioperative management, and develop an empathetic attitude and control their hubris and so have the courage and wisdom to learn from their past mistakes.

2.4   Infrastructure and Training Opportunities

India, being a developing country, has its own difficulties with respect to infrastructure and available resources, as a result of which our country has not yet incorporated all technical advances in medical science into day-to-day practice. With respect to surgery, this pertains mostly to minimal access surgery and newer instrumentation. Minimal access surgery has been widely integrated into surgical practice in the west but as of now, there is only a small percentage of surgeons in India who are proficient in such techniques.

Looking forward, the skyline of surgery is slowly shifting away from open procedures. However, Indian surgical graduates who will enter into a world that is slowly being dominated by these techniques, have a very limited exposure to it. Very few residents would be allowed to assist in such procedures, much less perform even simple ones independently. This leaves our trainees unequipped to face the world of independent surgical practice.

To address this, minimal access surgery should be incorporated into surgical education; for example, a surgical resident would be required to perform a laparoscopic appendicectomy or cholecystectomy before graduation. This might require compulsory simulation and training programmes for residents to familiarise themselves with the skill set required to become proficient in laparoscopic surgery.

Our country's training programmes have produced a generation of great surgeons but in order to achieve our full potential, it is important to recognise the lacunae that currently exist in our medical education system and try to fill them. In many ways, the reputation of a hospital rests on the shoulders of the surgical department due to the multiple disciplines that are tied to it. Therefore, India must utilise the bright young minds that dare to take up the mantle and to not just meet, but exceed the standards set by the rest of world, in order to provide the best medical care for our patients.

3   Our Concerns

As teacher and resident, we share concerns about surgical training which are, we believe, shared by our colleagues from our own departments and other branches of postgraduate (PG) training as well.

3.1   The Selection Process

The problem begins at the time of selection into the PG programme. In India, selection is on the basis of a multiple-choice test. There are many reasons why this system is flawed:

1. Students sometimes select a speciality that is easier to enter, without having a particular interest in it. They may have attempted to secure a PG position several times and do not want to go through the test again.
2. There is pressure from their parents to choose a particular speciality.
3. The speciality in question is an 'end speciality' such as orthopaedics or ophthalmology, which does not require them to go further up the training ladder to sub-specialty training.
4. The students have no particular choice of speciality and are willing to enter any programme just to acquire a PG degree.
5. One particularly disturbing scenario for us is when a student selects surgery but is actually interested in another speciality where there are no vacancies. This usually ends with them leaving the course after a few months.

These situations are not common, but occur often enough to be troubling. In those cases, we are faced with wondering how to train students who are not interested in the speciality?

3.2 Mismatch Between Need for Training and Training Opportunities

The general framework of the PG training programme is to provide tasks of increasing complexity and increased responsibilities in patient care areas over the first three years. Junior residents are closely supervised by senior residents and the teaching faculty. In general surgery training, this would mean that they would perform increasingly complex surgical procedures both in emergency and elective patient care settings. So adequate opportunities must be provided for all the trainees to become competent at independently performing certain operative procedures by the end of three years.

With a recent national mandate to increase the number of training positions in all specialities, the number of operating opportunities for the individual trainee have decreased. In some private institutions, the number of patients seen is not proportionate to the number of postgraduate residents. Trainees therefore can complete the course with very little operative experience. This has a definite impact on their future performance. For instance, if they decide to progress to subspeciality training immediately, the lack of adequate experience in general surgical skills hampers their progress in the chosen subspeciality. If they decide to continue in general surgery as a senior resident, they lack confidence in decision making because of their inadequate experience. Moreover, to compensate for lack of surgical experience, service planners would potentially take away operative opportunities from PG trainees which would in turn affect their training adversely.

3.3   Patient Safety, Time and Resources for Training

There are also tensions between the needs of PG training and patient care. Concerns for patient safety can limit the opportunities for practising new skills on patients. Skills labs have recently been mandated by the regulatory National Medical Commission (NMC) but most institutes lack even the most basic equipment.

The academic programme for PG training consists of journal clubs, short presentations of topics of current interest and clinical case discussions, in addition to the daily ward round. The bedside is a very valuable teaching spot and trainees gain important tips on managing a variety of clinical problems and the rational use of tests. They also can observe the consultant interacting with the patient. However, it often happens that the physical demands of working as a junior doctor in a busy clinical environment leave them too tired to read their books regularly, causing them to fall behind in their studies and sometimes unable to answer questions posed by the consultant during rounds.

3.4   Research

During the PG course, as a mandatory requirement, trainees must conduct a supervised research project over one and half to two years. They attend a workshop on basic research methodology and learn the processes of presenting a research proposal to the Institute Review Board and the Ethics Committee for approval, and of conducting a small project. Sadly, the sincerity with which they conduct the study and the authenticity of the data that they collect are sometimes in question. This could happen either because the supervisor chooses a topic which the trainee does not understand or has no interest in, or the trainee is simply not interested in research and goes through with the project because it is mandatory.

Either way, the credibility of the study is in doubt and the trainee does not learn the principles of good research.

3.5   Assessment

In most centres in the country, there is just one summative assessment at the end of three years, as mandated by the regulatory body. A different, formal assessment programme employed to monitor progress of the trainee through the period of training would keep a check on the quality of the training programme while ensuring that trainees are maintaining standards of performance.

4   Conclusions

A resident enters the programme with a lot of hope and expectation. Most try to derive as much as possible from that training while coping with the shortcomings. The improvements that are required to make the training more robust are certainly feasible. Some training of teachers is required particularly in observation and feedback so that residents understand where they stand and what they need to do to improve. But for the most part, what is needed is to rely on our judgements and on our experience as teachers to do what is best for our trainees.

V.ii COMMENTARY: Service Versus Training: An Apparent or Real Contradiction?

Janet Grant and Leonard Grant

Although this chapter presents an analysis of postgraduate training in one specialty in one institute in one country, many of the points made apply almost universally. First, we will look at the generalisability of the analysis, and then we will ask why this might be the case.

Transitions and Disjunctions. Not Continuum

Although the details of postgraduate training in medicine are specific to its context, its challenges are common to many systems. And although the stages of medical education are often referred to as a 'continuum', nothing could be less accurate. The characterisation of these stages as 'a series of linked, but independent silos' (Iobst & Holmboe, 2015) is probably more appropriate. That authors refer to the 'transition' rather than the 'progress' to postgraduate training tells us that medical education is a series of discontinuities or junctions rather than a continuum (Jonker et al., 2022; van den Broek et al., 2017; Wijnen-Meijer et al., 2010). For many, the transition to postgraduate training is an issue of 'work readiness' (Monti et al., 2020; Padley et al., 2021), and therein lies the heart of a contradiction that we see examined in this chapter.

Doctor, Learner or Other?

While basic medical education takes place within a structured university environment and the learners are exclusively students, postgraduate medical education usually takes place within the work environment where the learners are actually primarily practising doctors, albeit under decreasing supervision, but doctors nonetheless, undergoing a process of professional induction in the workplace towards independent practice.

> …considerable learning takes place without the prompts of any educational process or curriculum, or indeed teachers or trainers …. The simple notion revealed is that learning is an intrinsic part of work (Boud, 2016, p. 159).

That 'situated learning' which occurs in the context of practice with colleagues in a 'community of practice' (Lave & Wenger, 1991) is an essential component of this stage of training (Mann, 2011). But it requires support to ensure the effectiveness of self-directed and independent learning typical of an apprenticeship (So, 2023).

There is a balance to achieve within the symbiosis of working and learning. At that point, as a doctor, the trainee will have an associated line of accountability, and perhaps employment. As a trainee, there is another line of accountability and perhaps registration. These two lines may well be separately managed.

And for the postgraduate doctor, they may also have different professional identities. Or they may develop identities which are neither doctor nor trainee but might be educator in their own right as Anindya Niyogi has also described in the previous chapter, depending on what the period of postgraduate training intends (de Lasson et al., 2016; Gill, 2013; Haruta et al., 2020; Sethi et al., 2018). For each parallel identity, the postgraduate doctor may well judge the experience differently. And those competing identities, accountabilities and judgements may well contribute to stress and burnout at this stage of professional development (Monrouxe et al., 2017).

How Common Are These Problems?

The issues for postgraduate training in surgery that the two authors of this chapter raise, concern selection into the specialty, the ability to offer sufficient graduated and supervised experience, clinically overworked and tired trainees (but a lot of exposure to cases), tensions between the needs of the service and the needs of training, ineffective research training, assessments that fail to monitor progress or practice, unsympathetic seniors (but also caring and committed ones), burned-out trainees (causing a large attrition rate), poor and inconsistent work planning for residents to ensure both the service and training, and inadequate infrastructure to support training and modern practice.

But first, how typical are these observations of other countries and systems?

In Australia, problems of applying for specialty training are reported (O'Sullivan et al., 2021). In Japan, organisational cultures have been identified as impeding the changes in postgraduate training needed to reflect epidemiolocal and demographic development, along with gender biases in medicine (Honda et al., 2022). In Ireland, the tensions between the education and service systems were also clear:

> *Organisation and conditions of work* and *Time to learn with senior doctors during patient care* were rated as the most difficult areas in which to make improvements (Kilty et al., 2017).

In Europe, the challenge of organising effective postgraduate training changed with changes in working conditions:

> Shift patterns in the era of the European Working Time Directive could result in the trainer and the resident not seeing each other for several days leading to unsettled restrictive educational practice as patient follow-up is lost (Sandhu, 2018).

In Africa, similar challenges have been identified in relation to clinical training opportunities, lack of relevant curricula for postgraduate training, resource constraints, inconsistent supervision and high levels of stress among postgraduate trainees (Talib et al., 2019).

In the United Kingdom, similar problems have been reported:

> Life as a trainee can be challenging, with unfamiliar working environments, inadequate inductions, continuous assessment and examinations, relocations or long commutes, and a lack of belonging. Therefore, trainees often feel undervalued, lacking control, and disillusioned with medicine (Rimmer, 2023, p. 1783).

In relation to the assessment system, this has been a challenge for workplace-based postgraduate training which is less predictable, structured and curriculum-driven than education in a medical school where cohorts of students have the same experiences with the same intended outcomes. Although tests of knowledge and skill seem essential, the transposition of undergraduate assessment models to the postgraduate phase has long been questioned, with a greater balance of formative assessment recommended as each trainee forges their own path through practice (Marshall, 1993). So a different approach is appropriate:

> …to shift the emphasis in workplace-based assessment from assessment of trainee performance to the learning of trainees. Only then will workplace-based assessment gain credibility in the eyes of trainees and supervisors (Driessen & Scheele, 2013).

Transposition of educational models from basic medical education to the postgraduate phase sets up contradictions.

The 2021 UK General Medical Council's survey of postgraduate trainees showed that the quality of training was generally good, despite lost training opportunities and problems completing workplace-based assessments. The working environment was seen as supporting that training, but heavy workloads put about 15% of trainees at risk of burnout (General Medical Council, 2021).

The Service Versus the Training System

From these examples, and many more, it is clear that the challenges, and the strengths, discussed by the authors of this chapter are common to many systems of postgraduate medical education which struggle to reconcile the conditions of the service with the process of education and training. It seems that these problems are widespread because healthcare systems are stretched and are separately managed from the education and training system:

> Health care systems internationally are under strain, facing increasing demands with limited resources…. Although patients have shorter hospital stays, inpatients are sicker and healthcare has become more complex and expensive …. Short staffing and overcrowding are often features of the environments in which doctors learn…. (Wiese et al., 2017)

System managers are trying to manage patient throughput and staffing (Barati et al., 2016; Davies, 2006), while education managers are trying to manage the education and training of postgraduate doctors. These two management systems have different structures, purposes and accountability and so are not necessarily aligned. It may be that the management of the educational thread is formal, or it may be that there is very little educational support and management (Sierocinski et al., 2022) and the recorded quantified experience of being a doctor is regarded as sufficient (Kadmon et al., 2017).

Why Does Postgraduate Training Work?

Given these problems, it is important to note Dr. Evangeline's observation that:

> Our country's training programmes have produced a generation of great surgeons.

How can all these contradictory claims be true simultaneously?

It has been argued that learning in the workplace in an apprenticeship mode, offers 'pedagogically rich activities', whereby those participating learn, rather than continuing the model of 'being taught':

> …the process of utilizing, applying, and monitoring the use of our knowledge brings about change to it (i.e. learning). Often, the learning through our engagement in everyday activities is the reinforcing, refining, and extending of what we know, can do, and value (Billett & Noble, 2020).

As Dr. Evangeline would agree:

> …at its best, engagement in authentic goal-directed work tasks comprise opportunities to engage in both routine and nonroutine problem-solving and being able to access understandings, procedures, and values through others' perspectives and rationales, all of which can have particular potency for effective learning (Billett & Noble, 2020).

The Contradictions

In our analysis, the problems and challenges identified, and the strengths of the phase of postgraduate training, derive from the contradictions and tensions of competing professional identities (doctor vs trainee; doctor vs trainer), and essentially separate management of the learning process and of the service environment. There seems to be no point at which these parallel lines are aligned in one system; their purposes, ownership, responsibility, influences, accountability and management are not unified:

> Developing a culture of education integral to service delivery requires engagement from all stakeholders and collaboration between the clinical and educational leadership frameworks (Gawne et al., 2020).

For example, even though changes in the structure of postgraduate training in the UK were politically rather than professionally or educationally driven to produce the medical workforce that was needed, the management of the context of training, the service, did not change (Grant, 2007).

Where postgraduate training takes place in the context of service, as effective postgraduate training must, such issues are an inevitable consequence of different management structures and purposes for the service and for training. And yet, the two are inextricable for the postgraduate doctor:

> …considerable learning takes place without the prompts of any educational process or curriculum, or indeed teachers or trainers …. The simple notion revealed is that learning is an intrinsic part of work… Little of the learning that takes place in conjunction with work is systematic, structured or even planned. It arises out of the exigencies of work itself and is a response to the everyday challenges the conduct of any activity throws up (Boud, 2016, p. 159).

If that is the case, then a different way of thinking about, and managing, postgraduate training is required, simply because, at this stage:

> The management of learning can only be partially influenced by the educator, and the learner necessarily has much greater responsibility for managing and organising their own learning than is the case in conventional courses (Boud, 2016, p. 169).

The medical education literature is awash with calls and interventions to develop the skills of self-directed learning (Liu & Sullivan, 2021; Lu et al., 2023; Murad et al., 2010; Ricotta et al., 2022). And yet, the management of medical education is possibly one of the most controlled and controlling of any professional training. There is an unresolved contradiction in these two lines of rhetoric. That being so, why perpetuate, for postgraduate training, an educational model that is typical of an undergraduate, institutionally planned and controlled curriculum process?

References

Barati, O., Sadeghi, A., Khammarnia, M., Siavashi, E., & Oskrochi, G. (2016). A qualitative study to identify skills and competency required for hospital managers. *Electronic Physician, 8*(6), 2458–2465. https://doi.org/10.19082/2458

Billett, S., & Noble, C. (2020). Utilizing pedagogically rich work activities to promote professional learning. *Éducation et Didactique, 14*(3), 137–150. https://doi.org/10.4000/educationdidactique.7943

Boud, D. (2016). Taking professional practice seriously: Implications for deliberate course design. In F. Trede & C. McEwen (Eds.), *Professional and practice-based learning educating the deliberate professional preparing for future practices.* Springer.

Davies, S. (2006). Health services management education: Why and what? *Journal of Health Organization and Management, 20*(4), 325–334. https://doi.org/10.1108/14777260610680122

de Lasson, L., Just, E., Stegeager, N., & Malling, B. (2016). Professional identity formation in the transition from medical school to working life: A qualitative study of group-coaching courses for junior doctors. *BMC Medical Education, 16*(1), 165. https://doi.org/10.1186/s12909-016-0684-3

Driessen, E., & Scheele, F. (2013). What is wrong with assessment in postgraduate training? Lessons from clinical practice and educational research. *Medical Teacher, 35*(7), 569–574. https://doi.org/10.3109/0142159X.2013.798403

Gawne, S., Fish, R., & Machin, L. (2020). Developing a workplace-based learning culture in the NHS: Aspirations and challenges. *Journal of Medical Education and Curricular Development, 7.* https://doi.org/10.1177/2382120520947063

General Medical Council. (2021). *Experiences and challenges in postgraduate medical education.* https://www.gmc-uk.org/-/media/documents/somep-2021-chapter-2_pdf-88509765.pdf

Gill, D. (2013). *Becoming doctors: The formation of professional identity in newly qualified doctors.* London University. https://discovery.ucl.ac.uk/id/eprint/10020735/1/__d6_ Shared$_SUPP_Library_User%20Services_Circulation_Inter-Library%20Loans_IOE%20 ETHOS_ETHOS%20digitised%20by%20ILL_GILL,%20D.pdf

Grant, J. R. (2007). Changing postgraduate medical education: A commentary from the United Kingdom. *Medical Journal of Australia, 186*(S7), S9–S13. https://doi.org/10.5694/j.1326-5377.2007.tb00958.x

Haruta, J., Ozone, S., & Hamano, J. (2020). Doctors' professional identity and socialisation from medical students to staff doctors in Japan: Narrative analysis in qualitative research from a family physician perspective. *BMJ Open, 10*(7), e035300. https://doi.org/10.1136/ bmjopen-2019-035300

Honda, M., Inoue, N., Liverani, M., & Nagai, M. (2022). Lessons learned from the history of post-graduate medical training in Japan: From disease-centred care to patient-centred care in an aging society. *Human Resources for Health, 20*(1), 54. https://doi.org/10.1186/s12960-022-00752-x

Iobst, W. F., & Holmboe, E. S. (2015). Building the continuum of competency-based medical education. *Perspectives on Medical Education, 4*(4), 165–167. https://doi.org/10.1007/ S40037-015-0191-Y

Jonker, G., Booij, E., Vernooij, J. E. M., Kalkman, C. J., ten Cate, O., & Hoff, R. G. (2022). In pursuit of a better transition to selected residencies: A quasi-experimental evaluation of a final year of medical school dedicated to the acute care domain. *BMC Medical Education, 22*(1), 807. https://doi.org/10.1186/s12909-022-03871-0

Kadmon, M., Ten Cate, O., Harendza, S., & Berberat, P. O. (2017). Postgraduate medical education-an increasingly important focus of study and innovation. *GMS Journal for Medical Education, 34*(5), 1–6. https://doi.org/10.1007/s10459-013-9444-x

Kilty, C., Wiese, A., Bergin, C., Flood, P., Fu, N., Horgan, M., Higgins, A., Maher, B., O'Kane, G., Prihodova, L., Slattery, D., Stoyanov, S., & Bennett, D. (2017). A national stakeholder consensus study of challenges and priorities for clinical learning environments in postgraduate medical education. *BMC Medical Education, 17*(1), 226. https://doi.org/10.1186/s12909-017-1065-2

Lave, J., & Wenger, E. (1991). *Situated learning: Legitimate peripheral participation.* Cambridge University Press.

Liu, T.-H., & Sullivan, A. M. (2021). A story half told: A qualitative study of medical students' self-directed learning in the clinical setting. *BMC Medical Education, 21*(1), 494. https://doi. org/10.1186/s12909-021-02913-3

Lu, S. Y., Ren, X. P., Xu, H., & Han, D. (2023). Improving self-directed learning ability of medical students using the blended teaching method: A quasi-experimental study. *BMC Medical Education, 23*(1), 616. https://doi.org/10.1186/s12909-023-04565-x

Mann, K. V. (2011). Theoretical perspectives in medical education: Past experience and future possibilities. *Medical Education, 45*(1), 60–68. https://doi.org/10.1111/j.1365-2923.2010.03757.x

Marshall, J. (1993). Assessment during postgraduate training. *Academic Medicine, 68*(Suppl. 1), S23–S26.

Monrouxe, L. V., Bullock, A., Tseng, H.-M., & Wells, S. E. (2017). Association of professional identity, gender, team understanding, anxiety and workplace learning alignment with burn-out in junior doctors: A longitudinal cohort study. *BMJ Open, 7*(12), e017942. https://doi. org/10.1136/bmjopen-2017-017942

Monti, M., Brunet, L., & Michaud, P. A. (2020). Transition to postgraduate practice: Perceptions of preparedness and experience of the daily work of junior residents. *Swiss Medical Weekly, 150*(4748), w20370. https://doi.org/10.4414/smw.2020.20370

Murad, M. H., Coto-Yglesias, F., Varkey, P., Prokop, L. J., & Murad, A. L. (2010). The effectiveness of self-directed learning in health professions education: A systematic review. *Medical Education, 44*(11), 1057–1068. https://doi.org/10.1111/j.1365-2923.2010.03750.x

O'Sullivan, B., McGrail, M., Gurney, T., & Martin, P. (2021). Barriers to getting into postgraduate specialty training for junior Australian doctors: An interview-based study. *PLoS One, 16*(10), e0258584. https://doi.org/10.1371/journal.pone.0258584

Padley, J., Boyd, S., Jones, A., & Walters, L. (2021). Transitioning from university to postgraduate medical training: A narrative review of work readiness of medical graduates. *Health Science Reports, 4*(2). https://doi.org/10.1002/hsr2.270

Ricotta, D. N., Richards, J. B., Atkins, K. M., Hayes, M. M., McOwen, K., Soffler, M. I., Tibbles, C. D., Whelan, A. J., & Schwartzstein, R. M. (2022). Self-directed learning in medical education: Training for a lifetime of discovery. *Teaching and Learning in Medicine, 34*(5), 530–540. https://doi.org/10.1080/10401334.2021.1938074

Rimmer, A. (2023). How can we make life better for doctors in postgraduate training? *BMJ, 382*, 1783–1784. https://doi.org/10.1136/bmj.p1783

Sandhu, D. (2018). Postgraduate medical education – Challenges and innovative solutions. *Medical Teacher, 40*(6), 607–609. https://doi.org/10.1080/0142159X.2018.1461997

Sethi, A., Schofield, S., McAleer, S., & Ajjawi, R. (2018). The influence of postgraduate qualifications on educational identity formation of healthcare professionals. *Advances in Health Sciences Education, 23*(3), 567–585. https://doi.org/10.1007/s10459-018-9814-5

Sierocinski, E., Mathias, L., Freyer Martins Pereira, J., & Chenot, J.-F. (2022). Postgraduate medical training in Germany: A narrative review. *GMS Journal for Medical Education, 39*(5), Doc49. https://doi.org/10.3205/zma001570

So, H. (2023). Postgraduate medical education: See one, do one, teach one…and what else? *Hong Kong Medical Journal, 29*, 104. https://doi.org/10.12809/hkmj235145

Talib, Z., Narayan, L., & Harrod, T. (2019). Postgraduate medical education in sub-Saharan Africa: A scoping review spanning 26 years and lessons learned. *Journal of Graduate Medical Education, 11*(4s), 34–46. https://doi.org/10.4300/JGME-D-19-00170

van den Broek, W. E. S., Wijnen-Meijer, M., Ten Cate, O., & van Dijk, M. (2017). Medical students' preparation for the transition to postgraduate training through final year elective rotations. *GMS Journal for Medical Education, 34*(5), Doc65. https://doi.org/10.3205/zma001142

Wiese, A., Kilty, C., Bergin, C., Flood, P., Fu, N., Horgan, M., Higgins, A., Maher, B., O'Kane, G., Prihodova, L., Slattery, D., & Bennett, D. (2017). Protocol for a realist review of workplace learning in postgraduate medical education and training. *Systematic Reviews, 6*(1), 10. https://doi.org/10.1186/s13643-017-0415-9

Wijnen-Meijer, M., ten Cate, O. T. J., van der Schaaf, M., & Borleffs, J. C. C. (2010). Vertical integration in medical school: Effect on the transition to postgraduate training. *Medical Education, 44*(3), 272–279. https://doi.org/10.1111/j.1365-2923.2009.03571.x

Kadambari Dharanipragada is a Professor in the JIPMER Department of Surgery, and a surgeon educator with more than 25 years of experience teaching undergraduates and postgraduates. She believes in a continuous process of improvement in her practice of teaching and looks for opportunities to learn how she can achieve that.

Evangeline Mary Kiruba Samuel completed her MBBS and Masters in General Surgery from the Jawaharlal Institute of Postgraduate Medical Education and Research (JIPMER), Puducherry (India) and, at the time of writing was pursuing her M.Ch. Paediatric Surgery from the Institute of Child Health and Hospital for Children, Chennai (India). She is passionate not only about surgery but about its teaching to students in order to spark their interest and inspire them to take up the field.

V.iii STATEMENT: Training During the Real Work of After-Admitting Ward Rounds

Gordon Caldwell

1 Background

In 2004, I sat in a lecture at the Royal College of Physicians of London becoming increasingly frustrated and angry at the design of the new workplace-based assessments (WBA) being promoted for doctors in the pre-specialty Foundation Programme (FP) which covers the first two years after medical school, as part of the much criticised new system of postgraduate training called Modernising Medical Careers (MMC) (Tooke, 2008). I decided to immediately develop my own formative feedback process for my team on after-admitting ward rounds. I implemented this the next morning and developed the process over the subsequent 13 years.

2 Problems with Workplace-Based Assessments

I felt there were many problems with the WBAs, which were supposed to be formative and improve trainees' expertise in the work of doctoring. There seemed to be a belief that being a doctor consisted of many small pieces of competence that, glued together, somehow made a proficient medical practitioner. There was also an assumption that there was one way to do each part of the work and that it would be easy to get a group of clinical supervisors to agree on the level of a trainee's performance and offer the same advice for improvement. Further, although the process was being marketed as formative, the assessment forms were summative on a seven-point scale.

G. Caldwell (✉)
Lorn and Islands Hospital, Oban, UK
e-mail: drgordon.caldwell@gmail.com

245

The assessments also had to be 'trainee driven'. In my experience, the WBAs were artificial and time consuming. The trainee had to ask for an assessment, whereas my belief, as the accountable clinician, was that I had to actively train my team to provide high quality safe care. An apprentice master (Caldwell, 2011) wants to see the apprentices developing and flourishing whilst ensuring the artwork is to his exacting standards.

3   Uses of Workplace-Based Assessment

I had some experience of using mini-CEX and could see the value of formative feedback to help a trainee develop expertise. I had been thinking about the way a driving instructor trains a learner driver. Instructors have to support 'learning whilst doing' on real roads whilst keeping themselves and other road users safe. I wanted to develop a process to be used during the real work of ward rounds to develop the members of the team, whilst keeping patients safe.

A theme in the books I read (Benner, 2001; Black et al., 2003) was that in a formative process, the apprentice master does not have to assess exactly where the apprentice is on some measurable scale, but has to identify recommendations for the apprentice to try out, to improve their proficiency. The official mini-CEX form gave seven levels of performance, each with a descriptor. One day I asked MMC staff to do a mini-CEX on the psychiatrist who interviewed Patch Adams in the film of that name. I asked the non-clinicians to watch the psychiatrist and offer one piece of advice the doctor could try in his next consultation. The MMC clinicians were to use the form and mused over seven-point scales and descriptors, unable to offer the psychiatrist any advice for improvement within the timescale. The non-clinicians had several simple ideas for the psychiatrist to try next time. The complexity of the MMC process and its demand for consistency, reliability and validity actively precluded opportunities to offer recommendations for improvements. Another advantage of a formative feedback process is that there is no ending to the possibility of further improvement. But in the MMC process, if the trainee reached Foundation Programme completion competency, there was no impetus to improve further. In a proper formative process, the trainee could be encouraged to perform even better and perhaps complete initial specialty exams during Foundation.

4   How I Developed the Formative Feedback Process

Developing a formative feedback process to use during the morning ward rounds after a period of acute admitting, was as far away as possible from a semi-simulated 'Examine the chest' mini-CEX as a timetabled event, separate from the world of the real practice of the art of medicine. I envisaged the reward for me being well organised ward rounds with team members developing in expertise.

I thought the process might fail because doctors could be exhausted and unable to learn at the end of a night shift. I also doubted my ability to provide feedback when work had been substandard.

I needed some documentation to serve as a framework for the feedback. I also wanted to teach higher level trainees to run ward rounds, so I needed the documentation to support good organisation of the work.

I wanted the process to emphasise the importance of teamwork. The WBAs were individualistic, but clinical practice depends on teamwork. Within three weeks I included this:

> This is a team assessment – one team member's assessment may be brought down by e.g. poor prescribing by another member of the team, or brought up if we all work effectively together to care for the patients.

As I travelled back to Worthing, I designed a form to organise the work and provide feedback on the management of the first case that a doctor presented to me on the round. I divided the areas of performance into the following domains:

Domain	Notes
Is the patient acutely ill?	Could the doctor identify a patient needing more urgent attention? (The Foundation Programme did not seem to value this as an important ability)
Organisation of notes and charts	There should be a place for everything and everything in its place. If not, time and mental effort is spent only in finding information
Case presentation and summary	Some presentations were short, logical, engaging and thorough but others could be verbose, scattered, and incomplete
Management plan	Did the plan for investigations and treatment make sense?
Plan for ongoing assessment and review	What monitoring is required and when does the patient require a review of progress?
Prescribing drugs, fluids and oxygen	Emphasis on legibility and accountability
Arranging appropriate tests	Were too many or too few tests requested? Could the doctor interpret the results?
Rapport with the patient	At the bedside, could I see that the patient trusted the doctor who had done the admitting work?

At that stage, I graded performance as 'Excellent', 'Competent' or 'Improve, please', but later I removed all such categorisation. I found it too easy to give scores and not recommendations for improvement.

The domains changed frequently over the years. For example, after a year, I had already started allowing the senior trainees to lead rounds under supervision. An important new domain was a 'Learning Ticket'. One of the junior doctors said I was not being challenging enough when I kept on telling her how good her performance was. I then started giving a learning task such as:

> Come back in a week with a tutorial on the absorption of Vitamin B12 and its role in cell metabolism.

Adding a specific learning point was a challenge to me to produce some directed learning. However, I know my knowledge is very limited so I could direct staff to read up on topics I should know:

> You quoted the CURB-65 score for management of community acquired pneumonia (CAP), what were the diagnostic criteria for CAP in the studies?

In this way, we combined organisation of the work and structure for training.

I also reasoned that the process could work better if the junior doctors or other staff were given an opportunity to provide feedback on my role as leader. On the first form the domains were:

- Professional role model
- Prioritising round appropriately
- Treating all healthcare workers with respect
- Treating patients with respect
- Made diagnoses and problems clear to the team
- Made investigation and treatment plan clear to the team
- Made plan for assessment of progress and need for review clear to the team
- Reviewed investigations and commented on the need for tests
- Reviewed prescribing and made reasons for changes clear
- Clear, effective communications with patients and relatives
- Providing positive feedback on good performance
- Ability to correct errors and provide feedback on unsatisfactory performance in a considerate manner
- Use of teaching and training opportunities.

I found the feedback from this process valuable. Early on, a medical student commented that I had not explained clearly the changes I had made in a patient's prescription. This made me explain more clearly thereafter. A senior trainee challenged me about why I had the junior doctor present the case at the bedside, rather than a preliminary discussion in a quiet private room. I changed my process on the next round and have never reverted to the old way. The senior trainees commented that having to provide feedback on my performance made them realise how much work is involved in leading ward rounds. This in turn helped them to develop their processes for leading rounds.

I believe that having a structure and being overtly keen to take feedback made it easy for observers to provide feedback. I hope that this requesting feedback was also role modelling how I would want future Consultants to behave. We are all team members and should acknowledge we are not perfect and can respond to constructive advice to try for improvement.

5   The Team Assessment and Feedback Process

I went into work early to ensure that I had a clear overview of the impending cases. My plan was to do the feedback on the first case each junior doctor presented, not only so that it was easy to remember, but also because it left the type of case as a random event, rather than the trainee cherry picking a 'good' case.

Whilst the junior doctor presented the case, I jotted notes on the form. Immediately after the case review was completed, I provided some verbal feedback. I tried to say "And" not "But":"

> Your clinical reasoning and clinical management were excellent AND to be better next time please write fewer words, more legibly and write the names of the medications in capitals.

Once the round was finished, I typed up my comments and circulated the completed form to all members of the team by email, including those junior doctors who were not at the ward round. From the first day I was pleased with the response from trainees, who appreciated that I was trying to develop their expertise (Caldwell, 2006). I found it easy to point out good practice:

> Your Problems List was comprehensive, and you had a sensible plan for each problem. This made it easy for me to grasp the case.

I found it challenging to provide advice for improvement. I was tempted to overload feedback for improvement and so tried to limit the number of points:

> Next time please clearly state date and time you started your clerking and write your name and GMC number legibly.

Once a staff member had shown they could respond to such simple basic advice then I could move onto more complex issues like Problem Lists.

6   How I Spotted Poor Performance

I thought I would be poor at acknowledging poor performance because I prefer to avoid confrontation and difficult conversations. I found that it helped to have the feedback form with descriptors, which made it easier for me to say:

> Your case presentation was well organised and made sense, however I cannot easily read your handwriting and you wrote extensive notes. Next time could you try to write fewer words and write more legibly?

There was only a handful of instances in 14 years when there was a serious weakness in performance. I did not announce such serious weaknesses in oral or public feedback and took the matter up in private with the trainee and, if necessary, with the postgraduate medical education team. In this type of event, the trainee usually needed extra support: one was caring for a dying parent, one was in the early stages of a psychosis. In only one case was there a very serious issue and the evidence I was able to provide contributed to the GMC being able to end a long running case with suspension of the doctor from the medical register.

7 One Thing Leads to Another

I saw that I could specifically develop the senior trainee's ability to be ward round leader (Levett & Caldwell, 2014). I was able to entrust leading rounds to them and provide feedback on their clinical expertise and leadership skills. I was fortunate to see several of them return to our hospital as fine Consultants.

My attention to performance on ward rounds led to an interest in quality and safety at the point of care. We developed a ward round checklist and a 'check and correct' process for improving safe prescribing (Conroy-Smith et al., 2011; Mohan & Caldwell, 2013) which improved patient safety and served as training tools. Several previous members of our team contributed to a joint publication by the Royal College of Physicians and Royal College of Nursing on recommendations for best practice on ward rounds (Kirthi et al., 2012). A report on organising care at the NHS frontline was stimulated by our work (Ham & Berwick, 2017). I learned so much because of my desire to train staff.

8 Evaluation

I kept the typed forms and a record of the staff members. I did not have any data from before the changes I implemented. After five years, I contacted staff through social media and was surprised that half of those who had experienced the process completed a questionnaire. I collected a further year's feedback from staff and interviewed 10 doctors. I was reassured my process resulted in doctors who were more confident in their expertise and who claimed that my process had advanced their development as doctors and resulted in improvements in how they did their work and in their self-confidence. Trainees preferred it to the WBAs, partly because they did not have to ask in advance for an assessment, and so the process was more real, and they could not cherry pick a case (Caldwell, 2013).

I shall finish with a verbatim comment from a junior trainee who had become a bit jaded and cynical:

> You made a comment to individualise the patient and I found that my Consultants like that. You know, no-one can remember a community acquired pneumonia, whereas they can remember, you know, "A French teacher with a dog called Bob, with pneumonia." It has had a really good effect on daily life with Consultants, and on my knowing my patients.

All that work would have been worthwhile for me for that one comment alone.

The art of medicine is a human endeavour. I have had a great reward in being an apprentice master helping to shape the work of the medical artists of the future generation.

References

Benner, P. (2001). *Novice to expert: Excellence and power in clinical nursing practice, commemorative edition*. Prentice-Hall.

Black, P., Harrison, C., Lee, C., Marshall, B., & William, D. (2003). *Assessment for learning: Putting it into practice*. Open University Press.

Caldwell, G. (2006). Real-time assessment and feedback of junior doctors. Improves clinical performance. *The Clinical Teacher, 3*(3), 185–188.

Caldwell, G. (2011). Whatever happened to apprenticeship learning? *The Clinical Teacher, 8*(4), 272–275. https://doi.org/10.1111/j.1743-498X.2011.00456.x

Caldwell, G. (2013). An evaluation of a formative assessment process used on post take ward rounds. *Acute Medicine, 12*(4), 208–213.

Conroy-Smith, E., Herring, R., & Caldwell, G. (2011). Learning safe prescribing during post-take ward rounds. *The Clinical Teacher, 8*(2), 75–78. https://doi.org/10.1111/j.1743-498X.2011.00432.x

Ham, C., & Berwick, D. (2017). *Organising care at the NHS front line. Who is responsible?* The King's Fund.

Kirthi, V., Ingham, J., Lecko, C., Amin, Y., Temple, R. M., Hughes, S., Soong, J., Currie, L., Duff, L., Lees, L., Caldwell, G., Desai, T., Herring, R., Abdi, Z., Stewart, K., Patterson, L., & Davies, J. (2012). *Ward rounds in medicine. Principles for best practice*. RCP.

Levett, T., & Caldwell, G. (2014). Leadership training for registrars on ward rounds. *The Clinical Teacher, 11*(5), 350–354. https://doi.org/10.1111/tct.12167

Mohan, N., & Caldwell, G. (2013). A considerate checklist to ensure safe daily patient review. *The Clinical Teacher, 10*(4), 209–213. https://doi.org/10.1111/tct.12023

Tooke, J. (2008). *Aspiring to excellence*. Final report of the Independent Inquiry into Modernising Medical Careers. http://www.asit.org/assets/documents/MMC_FINAL_REPORT_REVD_4jan.pdf

V.iii COMMENTARY: Neoliberalism, Globalisation, and the Real Work of Learning Medicine in Practice

Janet Grant and Leonard Grant

Gordon Caldwell's experience draws a picture of the contradiction between the apparent current direction of medical education at postgraduate level, and the actual professional, vocational development of the practitioner. Setting his analysis in the context of actual patient care highlights this tension and the distancing of current ideas of education from that practice, that 'real work'.

The account presented by Gordon Caldwell gestures towards the neoliberal turn in education. In this analysis, we first remind ourselves what neoliberalism is as an economic and social ideology and how it is relevant to the problems the author identifies in relation to workplace-based assessments.

Neoliberalism in Medical Education

The origin of neoliberalism can be traced back to the 1970s and takes as its focus policies of economic liberalisation, privatisation, free trade, deregulation, and reductions in government spending (Harvey, 2005). Although conceptually the emphasis is on the economy's operation on market principles, the reality is that neoliberalism is only made possible through state intervention including in the forms of new laws, regulations, policies towards privatisation and the resultant government interventions when vital businesses inevitably fail (Humber, 2019). Underpinning a neoliberal approach is the maintenance of order, and so requires both regulatory actions and organising actions (Foucault, 2008). Postgraduate training in the United Kingdom, and medical education globally, has both in abundance.

The effects of neoliberalism are felt widely. It is characterised by increasing inequality, insecurity, and dislocation while reducing social protections and collective identities (Humber, 2019; Smith et al., 2016). Neoliberalism is not just a political ideology but a project serving particular social interests. The benefits of neoliberalism are felt by only a small, specific, and usually privileged, section of society (Harvey, 2005).

Education has not escaped the effects of neoliberialism. With the reduction in state funding and in the increase in tuition fees, higher education in Britain has become commodified (McKeown, 2022), students are dubbed 'consumers' and academics compete with each other for job security. The business language of performance benchmarks, auditing and cost-benefit analysis find their way regularly into educational environments. We are supposed to believe that consumer choice within the market is the ultimate guarantor of democracy (Ball, 1994; Harris, 2007). But the neoliberal turn ultimately altered the relationship that students have with their institutions, promoting education as a tangible product or an investment towards future employment reward (Peters cited in Park, 2012).

Gordon Caldwell does not see education like this himself, and so finds himself in opposition to the dominant educational ideology. On the one hand, he identifies himself as an apprentice master (Caldwell, 2011). On the other hand, he is identified in his job as a consultant and trainer, and as such, he is required to implement systems that do not arise from the supervised practice that he shares with his trainees. For him, postgraduate training is about learning from real work, with its unpredictability, and about the work-based, practical relationship between apprentice and apprentice master.

Unavoidably, medicine, and healthcare generally, in Britain have been affected by neoliberal ideology. Successive governments since before 1990 have actively encouraged private enterprise within the NHS (Humber, 2019). This model is enabled by the idea that healthcare is a commodity to be bought and sold on the market. If healthcare is a commodity, so too is the doctor whose production line is clearly set out.

The Effects of Neoliberalism in Practice

Within medical education, we can see this logic play out in the form of standardisation. Standardised curricula and high-stakes testing, and the standardised approach to formative assessment that Gordon Caldwell describes, focus instruction on limited skills and knowledge, resulting in quantitative data that can be measured and compared in the product of the educational pipeline. There is a focus on outcomes, not process, which is supposed to allow performance to be compared but actually creates a system upon which future job security and benefits are conferred (Park, 2012).

Doctors' working practices have become increasingly compartmentalised, epitomised by the long-criticised fashion of competency-based medical education (Boyd et al., 2018; Grant, 1999), each item being measured against defined outcomes. The author identifies this at play in the workplace-based assessments:

> There seemed to be a belief that being a doctor consisted of many small pieces of competence that, glued together, somehow made a proficient medical practitioner.

However, as correctly identified in this piece, practical knowledge cannot be made explicit, monitorable, and measurable, despite the best efforts of the neoliberal medical education managers and regulators (Park, 2012). Famously, a lot of knowledge is tacit: 'We know more than we can tell" (Henry, 2010; Polanyi, 1966). So professional knowledge cannot be codified as something to be meaningfully measured. Rather, it is something that must be developed through practice, with the guidance of the apprentice master, as Gordon Caldwell has theorised. As such, the formative assessment system that the author developed, is rooted in practice, and is real work driven, not driven by spurious outcomes or milestones.

Medical Education, Neoliberalism, Regulation and Bureaucracy

It has been claimed that we are living in a post-bureaucratic era (McSweeney, 2006), although Gordon Caldwell's experience of the system of workplace-based assessment (WBA) which he was supposed to implement, might suggest that we are still very much in a bureaucratic era which has been condemned in the strongest of apocalyptic terms (Charlton, 2010). Bureaucracy has become a necessary part of the neoliberal project (Hibou, 2015). It was characterised by Max Weber (Weber, 1947) as having certain qualities that we see described in this chapter: rules and procedures, records, and impersonal and hierarchical processes (in opposition to the participatory approach that the author developed). But these are not described in medical education as bureaucratic processes; they often are presented as necessary for standardisation and accountability, for the audit trail, for reliability and validity (Moonen-van Loon et al., 2013). For example, in postgraduate medical education in the UK, a certain *number* of WBAs must be completed and this number amounts to the summative aspect of what is presented as a formative process which focuses on the attainment of competencies in the atomised manner that Gordon Caldwell objects to. These have pushed WBA towards the formalisation and structure (Hurst & Prescott-Clements, 2018) that seem to Gordon Caldwell to be contrary to an approach based on actual professional practice, even though his own approach also has, perforce, paperwork and records.

The Drive towards Management and Global Standardisation

Medical education is increasingly seen as a design and management problem (Armstrong et al., 2004; Khanna et al., 2021) against a background of regulatory standards, inspection, compliance and accreditation. We live in an era of regulation (Aftab et al., 2021), despite lack of evidence of its effect. Such regulation, equally without evidence of effect, has now moved, perhaps problematically, on to a global stage (Rashid, 2021; Rashid et al., 2023). Gordon Caldwell's concerns at the level of his own ward rounds and his identity as an apprentice master, are part of this all-pervading approach to the management of medical education, often under the unproven guise of improving quality, while actually underpinned by the 'epistemicidal' efforts to export the practices of the global north to the global south (Naidu, 2021), identified as the era of global standards and accreditation (Weisz & Nannestad, 2021). This extends globally the concerns raised above about the neoliberal approach to the maintenance of order requiring both regulatory actions and organising actions (Foucault, 2008).

So regulation, standardisation and managed systems have become synonymous with medical education both locally and globally; meeting such requirements seems to Gordon Caldwell antithetical to the vocational development of trainees in the context of real practice. At the global level, this presents a challenge to the needs and qualities of the local context (Rashid, 2021; Rashid et al., 2023; Rashid & Griffin, 2023). At the level of Gordon Caldwell's ward round, this plays out as a challenge to his role as apprentice master, supporting and guiding trainees in their developing art of medicine.

Education in the Profession

As medical education becomes increasingly defined by a bureaucratic, regulatory, controlling and controlled perspective typical of the neoliberal project, arguments are being put forward in other professional domains, that practice must be informed by a humanism that recognises contextual awareness, critical thinking and individual moral autonomy (Herbel, 2018). In other words, we can trust an apprentice master to develop their apprentices and to make judgements about their progress in practice.

Gordon Caldwell is, essentially, arguing for an emancipatory, professional approach to training, as explained here:

> In contrast to bureaucracies, … which force individuals into specified patterns of interaction, the social structure in the post-bureaucratic organizations is seen as founded on an "organic" communitarian system.… More specifically, it is made up from webs of affect-laden relationships among individuals, relationships based on personal loyalties that interweave and reinforce one another. Furthermore, these relationships are anchored in a commitment to a set of values, norms, and meanings, which are rooted in a shared history and identity… (Maravelias, 2003)

This is quintessentially the nature of learning in a profession, particularly at postgraduate level, where learning is situated in the context of practice and the professional community supports that learning as part of the shared work of patient care (Webster-Wright, 2009; Wenger, 1998). The effects of external over-control on the centrality of the workplace in learning in the professions is well-established (Eraut, 1994, 2004). This has been thoroughly explored by de Cossart (a surgeon) and Fish (a teacher educator), who argue that over-control and regulation are damaging to professional practice and education, turning both into:

> …purely technical practices in which we have lost sight of the creativity, sensitivity, flexibility and courage to produce personal rather than protocol-driven decisions… (Fish, 2012)

Instead, they argue for a 'moral mode' of education and practice which develops the whole person, and gains learning from practice through 'transformative reflection' (de Cossart & Fish, 2020). This is typified by Gordon Caldwell's approach to the development of his trainees through being open to feedback himself and engaging with them on what they want. This shared path to development seems to result in a satisfied, happy, and confident practitioner, perhaps starting to address the acknowledged problems of workplace culture in medicine (Shanafelt et al., 2019), by developing positive relationships rather than authoritative and perhaps alienating 'leadership' (Aggarwal & Swanwick, 2015; Strand et al., 2015). Although

Caldwell's approach is not a panacea, it is a contribution to moving away from the oppressive aspects of postgraduate medical training (Averbuch et al., 2021). Gordon Caldwell is always careful to emphasise his team. This is important in enabling his intentions to be based on agreement on what sorts of behaviours and approaches are acceptable and not acceptable. This is contrary to the top-down approach through standard setting. Instead, what Caldwell demonstrates is an ongoing continued negotiation between practitioner apprentice master, the trainee, patients, and other healthcare staff.

It has been suggested that after neoliberalism, academic organisations might be characterised by a more appropriately professional community (Cole & Heinecke, 2020). Gordon Caldwell demonstrates one small but powerful intervention that can start the journey down that liberating path for postgraduate medical education.

References

Aftab, W., Khan, M., Rego, S., Chavan, N., Rahman-Shepherd, A., Sharma, I., Wu, S., Zeinali, Z., Hasan, R., & Siddiqi, S. (2021). Variations in regulations to control standards for training and licensing of physicians: A multi-country comparison. *Human Resources for Health, 19*(1), 91. https://doi.org/10.1186/s12960-021-00629-5

Aggarwal, R., & Swanwick, T. (2015). Clinical leadership development in postgraduate medical education and training: Policy, strategy, and delivery in the UK National Health Service. *Journal of Healthcare Leadership, 7*, 109–122. https://doi.org/10.2147/JHL.S69330

Armstrong, E. G., Mackey, M., & Spear, S. J. (2004). Medical education as a process management problem. *Academic Medicine, 79*(8), 721–728. https://journals.lww.com/academicmedicine/Fulltext/2004/08000/Preparing_Graduates_for_the_First_Year_of.00002.aspx

Averbuch, T., Eliya, Y., & Van Spall, H. G. C. (2021). Systematic review of academic bullying in medical settings: Dynamics and consequences. *BMJ Open, 11*(7), e043256. https://doi.org/10.1136/bmjopen-2020-043256

Ball, S. J. (1994). *Education reform: A critical and post-structural approach.* Open University Press.

Boyd, V. A., Whitehead, C. R., Thille, P., Ginsburg, S., Brydges, R., & Kuper, A. (2018). Competency-based medical education: The discourse of infallibility. *Medical Education, 52*(1), 45–57. https://doi.org/10.1111/medu.13467

Caldwell, G. (2011). Whatever happened to apprenticeship learning? *The Clinical Teacher, 8*(4), 272–275. https://doi.org/10.1111/j.1743-498X.2011.00456.x

Charlton, B. G. (2010). The cancer of bureaucracy: How it will destroy science, medicine, education; and eventually everything else. *Medical Hypotheses, 74*(6), 961–965. https://doi.org/10.1016/j.mehy.2009.11.038

Cole, R. M., & Heinecke, W. F. (2020). Higher education after neoliberalism: Student activism as a guiding light. *Policy Futures in Education, 18*(1), 90–116. https://doi.org/10.1177/1478210318767459

de Cossart, L., & Fish, D. (2020). *Transformative reflection for practicing physicians and surgeons: Reclaiming professionalism, wisdom and moral agency.* The Choir Press/Aneumi Publications.

Eraut, M. (1994). *Developing professional knowledge and competence.* Falmer.

Eraut, M. (2004). Informal learning in the workplace. *Studies in Continuing Education, 26*(2), 247–273.

Fish, D. (2012). *Refocusing postgraduate medical education: From the technical to the moral mode of practice.* Aneumi Publications.

Foucault, M. (2008). *The birth of biopolitics: Lectures at the Collège de France, 1978–79* (G. Burchell & M. Senellart, Eds.). Palgrave Macmillan.

Grant, J. (1999). The incapacitating effects of competence: A critique. *Advances in Health Sciences Education, 4*(3), 271–277. https://doi.org/10.1023/A:1009845202352

Harris, S. (2007). *The governance of education: How neo-liberalism is transforming policy and practice.* Continuum International Publishing Group.

Harvey, D. (2005). *A brief history of neoliberalism.* Oxford University Press.

Henry, S. G. (2010). Polanyi's tacit knowing and the relevance of epistemology to clinical medicine. *Journal of Evaluation in Clinical Practice, 16*(2), 292–297. https://doi.org/10.1111/j.1365-2753.2010.01387.x

Herbel, J. (2018). Humanism and bureaucracy: The case for a liberal arts conception of public administration. *Journal of Public Affairs Education, 24*(3), 395–416. https://doi.org/10.1080/15236803.2018.1429819

Hibou, B. (2015). What is neoliberal bureaucracy? In *The bureaucratization of the world in the neoliberal era. An international and comparative perspective.* Palgrave Macmillan.

Humber, L. (2019). *Vital signs: The deadly costs of health inequality.* Pluto Press.

Hurst, Y. K., & Prescott-Clements, L. (2018). Optimising workplace-based assessment. *The Clinical Teacher, 15*(1), 7–12. https://doi.org/10.1111/tct.12730

Khanna, P., Roberts, C., & Lane, A. S. (2021). Designing health professional education curricula using systems thinking perspectives. *BMC Medical Education, 21*(1), 20. https://doi.org/10.1186/s12909-020-02442-5

Maravelias, C. (2003). Post-bureaucracy – Control through professional freedom. *Journal of Organizational Change Management, 16*(5), 547–566. https://doi.org/10.1108/09534810310494937

McKeown, M. (2022). The view from below: How the neoliberal academy is shaping contemporary political theory. *Society, 59*(2), 99–109. https://doi.org/10.1007/s12115-022-00705-z

McSweeney, B. (2006). Are we living in a post-bureaucratic epoch? *Journal of Organizational Change Management, 19*(1), 22–37. https://doi.org/10.1108/09534810610643668

Moonen-van Loon, J. M. W., Overeem, K., Donkers, H. H. L. M., van der Vleuten, C. P. M., & Driessen, E. W. (2013). Composite reliability of a workplace-based assessment toolbox for postgraduate medical education. *Advances in Health Sciences Education, 18*(5), 1087–1102. https://doi.org/10.1007/s10459-013-9450-z

Naidu, T. (2021). Southern exposure: Levelling the Northern tilt in global medical and medical humanities education. *Advances in Health Sciences Education, 26*(2), 739–752. https://doi.org/10.1007/s10459-020-09976-9

Park, S. (2012). The industrialisation of medical education? Exploring neoliberal influences within Tomorrow's Doctors policy 2009. In M. Lall (Ed.), *Policy, discourse and rhetoric: How new labour challenged social justice and democracy* (Educational futures rethinking theory and practice, 52). SensePublishers Imprint.

Polanyi, M. (1966). *The tacit dimension.* Doubleday.

Rashid, M. A. (2021). *Global approaches to medical school regulation: A critical discourse analysis.* University College London. https://discovery.ucl.ac.uk/id/eprint/10135228/

Rashid, M. A., & Griffin, A. (2023). Is west really best? The discourse of modernisation in global medical school regulation policy. *Teaching and Learning in Medicine, 1–12*, 504–515. https://doi.org/10.1080/10401334.2023.2230586

Rashid, M. A., Ali, S. M., & Dharanipragada, K. (2023). Decolonising medical education regulation: A global view. *BMJ Global Health, 8*(6), e011622. https://doi.org/10.1136/bmjgh-2022-011622

Shanafelt, T. D., Schein, E., Minor, L. B., Trockel, M., Schein, P., & Kirch, D. (2019). Healing the professional culture of medicine. *Mayo Clinic Proceedings, 94*(8), 1556–1566. https://doi.org/10.1016/j.mayocp.2019.03.026

Smith, K. E., Hill, S., & Bambra, C. (Eds.). (2016). *Health inequalities: Critical perspectives* (1st ed.). Oxford University Press.

Strand, P., Edgren, G., Borna, P., Lindgren, S., Wichmann-Hansen, G., & Stalmeijer, R. E. (2015). Conceptions of how a learning or teaching curriculum, workplace culture and agency of individuals shape medical student learning and supervisory practices in the clinical workplace. *Advances in Health Sciences Education, 20*(2), 531–557. https://doi.org/10.1007/s10459-014-9546-0

Weber, M. (1947). *The theory of social and economic organization* (T. Parsons, Ed.; Translation). Oxford University Press.

Webster-Wright, A. (2009). Reframing professional development through understanding authentic professional learning. *Review of Educational Research, 79*(2), 702–739. https://doi.org/10.3102/0034654308330970

Weisz, G., & Nannestad, B. (2021). The World Health Organization and the global standardization of medical training, a history. *Globalization and Health, 17*, 96. https://doi.org/10.1186/s12992-021-00733-0

Wenger, E. (1998). *Communities of practice: Learning, meaning, and identity.* Cambridge University Press.

Gordon Caldwell was Consultant Physician and Clinical Lead at Lorn and Islands Hospital in Oban, Scotland. He was previously Postgraduate Clinical Tutor with overall responsibility for the training of all postgraduate doctors at Worthing Hospital, England, and a member of the NHS England Emergency Care Improvement Support Team. He has written extensively about education in the workplace and represents the voice of clinicians who are dedicated to preparing the next generation of specialist doctors and improving patient care despite overwhelming bureaucracy.

Part VI
The Power and Politics of Curriculum

Summary

We define a curriculum as:

...a managerial, ideological and planning document that should:

- tell the learner exactly what to expect including entry requirements, length and organisation of the course or programme and its flexibilities, the assessment system and methods of student support
- advise the teacher what to do to deliver the content and support the learners in their task of personal and professional development
- help the institution to set appropriate assessments of student learning and implement relevant evaluations of the educational provision.
- tell society how the school is executing its responsibility to produce the next generation of doctors appropriately. (Grant, 2019)

The power and politics of curriculum are central to all medical education endeavours. The educational process is for the reproduction or development of the status quo. It is in the curriculum and its enactment, that the power and politics of medical education are most exposed. Arguments around medical education curricula can focus on many different aspects:

- Principles of design
- Content and outcomes
- Methods and sites of learning
- The role of teachers
- Beliefs about learning and learners
- Ownership and relation to the profession that the curriculum intends to reproduce
- The symbolism that the curriculum has in terms of placing the medical school on a national or global stage.

The curriculum, and the way in which it is developed and implemented, will have intended and unintended effects. But the curriculum process always suggests in all of these, the beliefs and values that underpin it. Power and politics play a central role in the struggle for control.

Thus a curriculum is never a neutral, objective document, but reflects the values, beliefs and frames of reference of those who write it. The extent to which a written curriculum is translated into teaching and learning practice depends, in turn, on the values and beliefs of both learners and teachers in their own contexts. In that relationship between the theory and the practice of curriculum is found the hidden curriculum, which perhaps tells us more about the multiple truths of teachers, learners and institutions than anything that is written.

VI.i STATEMENT: Basic Science in Medical Education: Switching It Up

Susan Jamieson

This chapter explores discourses around the basic science component of the undergraduate medical curriculum and aims to provoke thinking about new approaches. The need for new thinking arises from four problems:

- A traditional view of the necessity, content and timing of the basic science component of medical education leads to basic science overload at the beginning of the medical course. This might be seen by learners as a hurdle to be overcome before starting 'real medicine'.
- Medical education must accommodate constantly emerging themes and priorities such as leadership development, teaching skills and professional identity formation. Accommodating these certainly presents a challenge for undergraduate curriculum managers and if new themes are shoe-horned into the already crowded early, 'non-clinical' years, the time available for basic sciences is further squeezed.
- Unrealistic expectations about the nature of the basic science component fail to take account of the fact that whilst medical doctors may be predisposed towards science, their primary purpose is to be medical practitioners, and few will become scientists in their own right.
- How do we future-proof basic science learning to ensure that future clinicians will be able to identify, understand, critique and apply what is *then* relevant science, to solve clinical problems that we cannot necessarily predict?

S. Jamieson (✉)
School of Medicine, Dentistry & Nursing, University of Glasgow, Glasgow, Scotland, UK
e-mail: susan.jamieson@glasgow.ac.uk

© The Author(s), under exclusive license to Springer Nature
Switzerland AG 2026
J. Grant, L. Grant (eds.), *The Contradictions of Medical Education*,
https://doi.org/10.1007/978-3-031-90394-6_18

1 The Accepted View of Basic Science in the Medical Curriculum

Since Flexner's time, it has been generally accepted that basic science is essential to underpin medical education, so undergraduate medical students traditionally spend at least two years focusing on basic sciences. Whilst the literature incorporates arguments about the proportion of science versus the humanities, it does not seem to be contested that there is a place for basic science, in its own right. It is commonly understood that clinicians use basic science knowledge to construct mental representations in memory, sometimes called schema, which associate specific clinical features and management options with specific conditions, and thereby facilitate clinical diagnosis and management.

There is experimental and research evidence to show that medical students use basic science knowledge in their clinical reasoning (Boshuizen & Schmidt, 1990). In contrast, experienced clinicians appear to have built sophisticated schemata related to each clinical condition, which can be rapidly called into play to facilitate clinical problem-solving (Boshuizen & Schmidt, 1990; Patel & Groen, 1986). However, when experts are confronted with unfamiliar problems, for which they have no ready schema, they utilise their basic science knowledge to reason analytically about the problem (Grant & Marsden, 1987; Norman, 2005; Norman et al., 1994). Thus, whilst experts may not seem to use basic science, in fact it is important in developing their schemata and expertise, and they still use it in challenging situations. This provides a strong rationale for teaching basic science to medical students. But how best do we go about it?

2 Questioning the Status Quo

With reason, medical educators collectively subscribe to the notion that clinical science and clinical practice should be underpinned by a sound understanding of basic science. We describe medical doctors as scientists and we revere 'scientific', generally positivistic biomedical research. We largely expect basic science to be learned early in a medical career and we invest a lot of time in testing our learners' understanding and application of basic science knowledge. In 'traditional' curricula, or even in 'modern' integrated curricula, the focus of the early years is still on basic science, and it is politically and academically difficult to challenge the necessity, content and timing of the basic science component in medical education. However, we owe it to our medical learners and to their future patients to do just that by asking:

- *Should* we teach basic science in a medical curriculum and *why* should we teach it?
- *What* basic science should we teach and *how* should we teach it, *when* should we teach it, and *who* should teach it?
- Do we teach basic science that has traditionally been perceived as relevant, or do we try to prepare students for unknown situations?

The evidence that doctors use basic science to develop schemata and expertise, and to address challenging clinical situations, provides an answer to the first question: yes, we should teach basic science, because it is needed for developing clinical expertise and in clinical practice. We are then left to answer the remaining questions.

3 Which Basic Science Disciplines?

The overarching question is: What basic science should we teach? We can first think about this in terms of which basic science disciplines. There are well-rehearsed arguments about the explosion of scientific information since the late twentieth century and the coincidental reduced time in the undergraduate medical curriculum for basic science teaching. Difficult decisions follow about which basic science disciplines should be taught, and how much curriculum time each should be given. Such decisions are often political, where stakeholders have beliefs, prejudices and vested interests. For example, tradition (or lack of imagination) colours what is considered to be 'basic science'. Even now, when one asks which are the basic sciences, a well-worn answer is 'anatomy, physiology and biochemistry'. So-called 'new' basic science disciplines of, for example, behavioural science, epidemiology, statistics and health-care economics, may need to fight for their corner of the curriculum. Some sciences, such as anatomy, are probably championed because their relevance to medicine seems obvious, but even here other considerations may be at play, such as the prestige attached to medical schools with anatomy departments, where cadaveric dissection is offered to students and popularly regarded as an essential rite of passage in medicine. Decisions about basic science in the curriculum are also inextricably linked to the availability of staff with relevant expertise, although this is perhaps less the case with the expansion of online and blended learning. The academic careers of some basic scientists may also be linked with their discipline's status in the medical curriculum.

4 How Much Basic Science?

The question of 'What basic science?' can also be interpreted in terms of the amount of basic science. Views change. In 1993, the UK General Medical Council (GMC) published a generic curriculum for undergraduate medical education, *Tomorrow's Doctors,* which led to a reduction in the amount of scientific information that medical students were expected to learn (General Medical Council, 1993). Medical educators were encouraged to teach core basic science concepts. However, in subsequent editions of *Tomorrow's Doctors* (General Medical Council, 2003, 2009), there was a re-emphasis on science.

There had been indignant protests from basic scientists whose own discipline was 'squeezed' and a wave of surveys by learned bodies, trying to ascertain how much basic science was incorporated in the new undergraduate courses. In 2005, when I worked as a senior manager in an undergraduate medical school, we undertook an internal curriculum review. Seven senior scientists (including an anatomist, academics with expertise in infection and immunity and pharmacology, and a biochemist) were asked to review the basic science content of the curriculum, to suggest where more of a specific science was needed, and also to identify what basic science(s) might be cut out of the curriculum.

It is hardly surprising that three areas considered to be underrepresented were infection, molecular biology and pharmacology. In addition, whilst it was recognised that anatomy was represented, its coverage was regarded as 'basic'. Moreover, no basic science topics were identified as 'extraneous material' that could be dropped, perhaps because it was all genuinely perceived as necessary, or because of professional courtesy to fellow scientists. The review team may also have identified specific disciplines as under-represented because the curriculum was integrated and, at that time, was delivered with a high proportion of problem-based learning (PBL), so it was difficult for someone not intimately familiar with all of the PBL scenarios across Years 1 and 2 to appreciate where relevant disciplines were incorporated.

The GMC itself also commissioned an evaluation of the effects of *Tomorrow's Doctors* (Grant et al., 2007) which showed that:

Overall, there are two areas of concern that thread their way through all phases of the study:

- that the scientific basis of medicine is no longer taught and learned adequate to need
- that the teaching and learning methods now used exacerbate this problem.

And there is a third point that is important for the writing of future guidance:

- *Tomorrow's Doctors*, while allowing local interpretation, failed to provide sufficient guidance on the necessary core of medical education.

The re-emphasis on science was also driven by wider concerns, such as patient safety, when publications about prescribing errors led to renewed focus on the teaching of pharmacology.

5   What Depth of Basic Science?

We may also think about 'What basic science?' in terms of the level at which it should be understood. It may be difficult for any basic science specialist to resist the temptation to include material in their teaching that is of particular interest to them, and difficult to recognise what is truly needed by learners at a particular level. As a basic scientist myself, a cell biologist, I recognise the enthusiasm of fellow basic scientists to encourage medical learners to appreciate the relevance and excitement of their discipline! Indeed, as far back as 2001, I published a letter in *Medical*

Education, advocating the relevance of cell biology in the medical curriculum (Jamieson, 2001). Scientists may also legitimately take the position that if we are to subscribe to the notion of the 'doctor as a scientist' (General Medical Council, 2003), then it is reasonable to expect them to have a scientist's understanding of basic science disciplines; perhaps the tension comes from expecting a student at the early stages of their medical career to have an understanding as sophisticated as a senior basic scientist?

Clinicians may also be unclear about how much basic science to present to students. It was not uncommon in my experience as a curriculum manager for a specialist in, for example, dermatology to cram an hour-long lecture with details of every growth factor or structural protein or (patho-)physiological mechanism that might conceivably be relevant to skin biology or to skin conditions ranging from eczema to melanoma, contributing to the curriculum overload problem.

To summarise thus far, whilst we may accept that a basic science component is necessary in medical education, and that basic science knowledge facilitates the development and practice of clinical reasoning, we cannot seem to agree on what basic science should be taught: neither the specific disciplines, nor the amount, nor the level at which it should be understood. No wonder that undergraduate medical learners come to regard basic sciences as an endurance test!

6   Space to Teach Basic Sciences

The questions of how, when and by whom basic sciences are or should be taught may be considered in terms of finding curriculum space to teach basic sciences.

6.1   Traditional Space Squeezed

The traditional delineation of basic and clinical sciences has broken down with the trend for horizontal integration of different basic sciences in systems-based curricula; and for vertical integration of basic sciences with clinical sciences (Hassan, 2013). The intention with systems-based learning may include recognition that medical conditions typically involve more than one physiological system. For example, diabetes involves at least the cardiovascular, endocrine, gastro-intestinal and renal systems. The rationale for integration is to help the learning of basic science by giving it a clinical context. Integration of basic and clinical sciences was common in UK medical school curricula following publication of the first edition of *Tomorrow's Doctors* (General Medical Council, 1993).

The time traditionally given to the teaching of basic science has been further squeezed by the introduction of early clinical experience; simulation-based education to address concerns over patient safety, and student feedback regarding a perceived lack of clinical experience and concomitant lack of confidence in their performance in technical and non-technical skills; and assistantships or shadowing periods just prior to graduation. Integrated curricula tend—at least in a UK context—to incorporate early clinical experience. As a former curriculum manager, I can attest that the possibility of early clinical experience was attractive to prospective students and enjoyed by our Year 1 students.

In addition, there is a need to accommodate formative and summative assessments conducted at a national level (including – in the UK – the Situational Judgement Test and the Medical Licensing Assessment). There is also enthusiasm from some quarters to bring registration with the GMC forward to the point of graduation, rather than one-year post-graduation. In response to some of these pressures, curriculum managers have moved the teaching of specific knowledge and skills to an ever earlier point in the undergraduate medical curriculum, where possible.

6.2 Finding Space

How do we respond to the squeeze on curriculum space for basic science teaching, even in the early years? To some extent fuelled by necessity during the COVID pandemic, basic scientists have already responded by using blended or online models, whereby students engage with basic science material outwith class time, with the latter reserved for group tutorials and clinical experience (simulated or work-based). However, there still seems to be an expectation that students will independently learn a substantial body of basic science at an early stage.

We should also consider whether there really is a need for all medical students to learn all basic sciences, and to learn them prior to doing any clinical work. Perhaps medical educationalists need to return to that vexed question of the core basic science curriculum and think of it not as a mix of the core biochemistry curriculum, plus the core cell biology curriculum, plus the core physiology curriculum, and so on; but as a generic science curriculum comprised of unifying, or threshold, concepts. Exposure to and engagement with specific basic sciences could occur throughout the curriculum, via events such as student projects, taster days, and student-selected components (Lindsley et al., 2024). In contrast, the detailed knowledge base of basic science disciplines relevant to particular clinical specialities (e.g., neuroscience for neurologists) could be organised by leaders of clinical placements in later years of the undergraduate curriculum, and/or by the relevant postgraduate curriculum, working in collaboration with academic basic scientists. Given that the learners would by then be mainly based in the clinical workplace, greater use would need to be made of blended learning for the basic science aspect.

7 Arguments Against Changing from Early Basic Science

One argument against shifting the basic science curriculum to later in a medical career is a possible detrimental impact on development of clinical reasoning skills. It is sometimes said that the distinction between medicine and other healthcare professions is the focus on science in medicine, which leads to the hallmark ability of medical doctors to solve clinical problems. Even if we agree that medical doctors require an enhanced understanding of basic sciences relevant to their speciality, their earlier clinical exposure could emphasise non-technical skills (communication, team-working) and patient care, which are essential for all healthcare professionals. Aligned clinical reasoning curricula could initially focus on teaching intellectual concepts such as cognitive bias, and practical skills such as history-taking for collecting data to inform clinical reasoning, which would not necessarily require significant basic science knowledge. Gradually, in more senior years, on longer placements, a combined approach of blended learning and workplace learning could allow relevant basic science knowledge to be learned and applied in context. Thus detailed teaching of relevant basic science could be part of undergraduate clinical placements in a particular specialty, or during postgraduate specialty training. Motivation to learn would potentially be enhanced by appreciating the relevance of the science, and (in postgraduate years) because the individual has chosen that specialty.

8 Future Proofing the Curriculum

Turning to the question of how to future-proof the basic science curriculum: perhaps we need to emphasise aspects that are common to all basics sciences, which is not in the details peculiar to, say, anatomical knowledge or cell biology knowledge and so on, but in scientific ways of thinking that may facilitate future appreciation and learning of any basic science. Thus the core concepts of a generic science curriculum in the early undergraduate years would not be so much about detailed knowledge of how the body works; rather, the focus would be on transferable scientific concepts such as measurement, levels of evidence, critical thinking, and application of the scientific method.

9 Switching It Up

In summary, contradictions related to the basic science component of a medical curriculum may be addressed by 'switching it up'; that is, changing the way we currently do things—changing our expectations, changing our focus and changing the timing of when basic science appears in the curriculum. The basic science component would begin with an early focus on transferable concepts that underpin all basic sciences, with one-off or short-term exposure to specific basic sciences, and more detailed basic science content being aligned with clinical placement in a particular specialty, or during postgraduate specialty training.

References

Boshuizen, H. P. A., & Schmidt, H. G. (1990). *The role of biomedical knowledge in clinical reasoning by experts, intermediates and novices*. https://files.eric.ed.gov/fulltext/ED321714.pdf

General Medical Council. (1993). *Tomorrow's doctors*. Recommendations on Undergraduate Medical Education.

General Medical Council. (2003). *Tomorrow's doctors* (2nd ed.).

General Medical Council. (2009). *Tomorrow's doctors* (3rd ed.).

Grant, J. (2019). Principles of curriculum design. In T. Swanwick, K. Forrest, & B. O'Brien (Eds.), *Understanding education: Evidence, theory and practice* (pp. 71–88). Wiley Blackwell.

Grant, J., & Marsden, P. (1987). The structure of memorized knowledge in students and clinicians: An explanation for diagnostic expertise. *Medical Education, 21*(2), 92–98. https://doi.org/10.1111/j.1365-2923.1987.tb00672.x

Grant, J., Roberts, T., Maxted, M., Boursicot, K., Chambers, K., Kilminster, S., & Marshall, J. (2007). *An investigation of the explicit and implicit purposes in tomorrow's doctors and an analysis of the impact of possible environmental changes on the knowledge, skills, attitudes and behaviours required of medical graduates*. General Medical Council and CenMEDIC, London.

Hassan, S. (2013). Concepts of vertical and horizontal integration as an approach to integrated curriculum. *Education in Medicine Journal, 5*(4). https://doi.org/10.5959/eimj.v5i4.163

Lindsley, J. E., Abali, E. E., Asare, E. A., Chow, C. J., Cluff, C., Hernandez, M., Jamieson, S., Kaushal, A., & Woods, N. N. (2024). Contribution of basic science education to the professional identity development of medical learners: A critical scoping review. *Academic Medicine, 99*(11), 1191–1198. https://doi.org/10.1097/ACM.0000000000005833

Jamieson, S. (2001). Cell and molecular biology in the medical curriculum. *Medical Education, 35*(1), 85–86. https://doi.org/10.1046/j.1365-2923.2001.0862d.x

Norman, G. (2005). Research in clinical reasoning: Past history and current trends. *Medical Education, 39*(4), 418–427. https://doi.org/10.1111/j.1365-2929.2005.02127.x

Norman, G. R., Trott, A. D., Brooks, L. R., & Smith, E. K. M. (1994). Cognitive differences in clinical reasoning related to postgraduate training. *Teaching and Learning in Medicine, 6*(2), 114–120.

Patel, V. L., & Groen, G. J. (1986). Knowledge based solution strategies in medical reasoning. *Cognitive Science, 10*(1), 91–116. https://doi.org/10.1207/s15516709cog1001_4

VI.i COMMENTARY: The Politics of Curriculum: Ideology and Power

Janet Grant and Leonard Grant

Power and the Curriculum

The power struggles and decision-making processes around curriculum design have been studied for a long time, recognising that:

> The curriculum is ... a contested space, a 'jungle' (Bolman & Gallos, 2011) where power struggles between different tribes and territories play out ... which leads to topics or perspectives being included or excluded.... (Becher & Trowler, 2001; McKimm & Jones, 2018, p. 520)

Those power struggles can be at the institutional level of different groups involved in a specific curriculum design process, or at the level of sections of society for whom a curriculum might try to reproduce or challenge current power structures and social relations. These might be about social class in wider society, or about interest groups within a system to which the curriculum is an induction. In either case, the curriculum adopts and transmits its ideologies.

Any curriculum, as Susan Jamieson illustrates, is a selection of intended outcomes, content and process. Competing ideologies take different views about each of these (Apple, 2019) and the most powerful ideology is likely to have the most influence. This is important because the curriculum offers a view of how to understand the world being studied. In Susan Jamieson's case, that world contains basic scientists and clinicians. It confers preferential legitimacy on some types of knowledge and view. That being so, whoever controls the curriculum gains or retains power, whether that is academic (in this case), ideological, economic or social. Susan Jamieson's discussion of the presentation and role of basic sciences in the medical curriculum epitomises these struggles on a small scale.

Curriculum Design in Medicine

Despite many real and ever-present struggles around curriculum, medical education has tended to see curriculum design as a simple matter of sequential steps, perhaps based on some identification of 'needs' (Kern et al., 2009), or as ill-defined 'modernisation' (Achike, 2016) often accompanied by concerns, such as Susan Jamieson expresses, about how certain topics will be organised and learned, and their relative importance (Goldie et al., 2004; Jeyakumar et al., 2020; Kruschinski et al., 2011; Turney, 2007; Wylie & Thompson, 2007). Curriculum design in medicine has also been affected by beliefs and fashions about teaching and learning: both problem-based and integrated curricula are examples of designs based on well-pro-moted ideas about teaching and learning, not on evidence (Hassan, 2013; Trullàs et al., 2022). Medicine is unmatched in generating '?-based' learning methods (Challa et al., 2021). In all this, educational research provides us with little evidence to guide curriculum choices, so decisions tend to be made in a context of power. Curriculum design is a political process, the aim of which has been seen as cultural reproduction (Bourdieu & Passeron, 1977) which maintains rather than challenges the status quo, despite cosmetic changes. This problem may be the basis of the issues discussed by Susan Jamieson in this chapter, if the culture to be reproduced is that of medicine as it is. On the other hand, by distributing basic science around clinical medicine, this may challenge the power status quo.

The Contradictions

Susan Jamieson's view of the contradictions of curriculum are that medicine, col-lectively, recognises that basic science underpins medical education and is funda-mental in supporting clinical reasoning. And yet, clinical medicine is, in practice, the more valued. Accordingly, the undergraduate curriculum is front-loaded with basic science. And yet, time for learning basic science is progressively decreased, as clinical experience, medical humanities, and learning non-technical skills and pro-fessional attributes are introduced into the early years of medical school. There are debates about incorporating political awareness into the apparently infinitely expandable medical curriculum (Paterson, 2023), cultural competence (Shapiro et al., 2006) which has been superseded by the construct of cultural humility (Yu et al., 2023), and awareness of social justice (Ambrose et al., 2014; Harindranathan, 2023). New views of the scope of medical practice mean that there is a seemingly endless array of topics that might be taught. The same problem occurs at earlier stages of education where '…schools are seen as the place where children will be inoculated against all social ills, or taught all the virtues…', the red flag corollary of which is that '…people wanted more of every subject in the school curriculum, but did not want a longer school day or year.' (Levin, 2008).

However, in his analysis of the contradictions of medical education in relation to politics and social justice, Bleakley explains that:

> There is a block in medical education about what 'curriculum' can mean or be. There is an endless argument about content – what should and should not be 'in' the curriculum. This mistakes syllabus for curriculum…. (Bleakley, 2021, p. 8)

Most debates about what medical students should learn, and when and how they should learn it, are based on views about what is required to practise medicine (such as basic science or communications skills), or what is required to protect the prac-tice of medicine (such as ethics or politics), or about the order in which those things should be learned (reflected in ideas about curriculum structure and organisation) and the associated methods of learning (reflected in rhetoric around how students learn, new teaching methods and the actual practice of continuing traditional teach-ing methods).

These ideas are rarely based on arguments about the trajectory, or pathway, of learning that is required in order to reach that final and personal arrangement of knowledge and skill within the individual clinician (Grant & Marsden, 1987). That trajectory can be seen cognitively, as the way in which knowledge and skill are acquired, organised, stored, added to, retrieved, used, and altered in memory, leading to developmental progression (Huang, 2021; Piaget, 1952), as has been studied in other areas of education (Luo et al., 2020). Or it can be seen procedurally, as in ideas, for example, of situated learning, or as the arrangement of content and context. In these, the lived developmental learning experience of the student cannot be ignored (Membrive et al., 2022).

It might seem that such decisions only require evidence about the best way to learn. While this might be useful, there is no evidence to suggest that one way of learning, or one curriculum design is better than any other. Education and learning are both too complex to be described in simple solutions.

Every doctor and medical teacher will take their own view. At secondary school level, it has been pointed out that:

> …an important element of the politics around education is that everyone has gone to school, so just about everyone has a feeling of being knowledgeable and a personal response to educational issues. (Levin, 2008)

But without a rational and supported theory of knowledge (Lehrer, 2018) and of learning trajectory, and a conceptual framework for curriculum (Chater, 1975; Totté et al., 2014), experience is an uncertain basis for decision-making.

So the problem described by Susan Jamieson is a fractal of bigger issues. And those issues are cited in the power and politics which play out in both national and global contexts. It has been argued that:

> Medical education and its sanctioning structure and agency are confirmed as forceful political enterprises. (de Leeuw, 2012)

This is seen in the relationship between the theory and practice of curriculum. Susan Jamieson's proposals may well be accepted on paper, but be altered in practice, as her consultations with specialists might suggest. Such changes might succeed or fail within the context of influence (the ideological and political basis of the new plan), the context of text production (where will the resources to support the new arrangement come from?), or the context of practice (how will the new arrangements be interpreted by teachers?) (Crawford, 2000).

Contesting the Curriculum: The Politics of Cultural Capital

Fundamentally, curriculum decisions are based on vested beliefs and arguments about what should be taught (although people often prefer to think of this as what should be learned), and how it should be taught and assessed. In the absence of definitive evidence of the effectiveness of any particular curriculum design or teaching method, curriculum is a contested area at all levels and locations of education.

A medical school curriculum is a reflection of the relative institutionalised cultural capital (qualifications, status, educational credentials, values, ideas) of the groups contesting its contents and processes (Bourdieu, 1986). So basic scientists, clinicians and educational designers have a political interest in the curriculum, in terms of their own positions, beliefs, values, purposes and academic place. As more players enter the field, in the form of new topics to add to the curriculum as Susan Jamieson describes, the sources of cultural capital that can be drawn on within the constraints of time and resources, become more keenly contested. Susan Jamieson chooses to respond to this by distributing her own academic area, and cultural capital, across the curriculum. She defends this in persuasive arguments about the role of basic sciences in clinical problem solving and in clinical specialty knowledge. Although, in doing so, the identity of the basic sciences may be lost. If they are, then their institutionalised cultural capital is also lost.

Medical education is not alone is debating curriculum. It is important to everyone at all levels in all contexts because education has the function of producing the next generation, and we all take a view about what qualities that generation should display.

Arguments and opinions abound in relation to what knowledge should be taught and about how that knowledge should be taught. Even if we prefer to employ the rhetoric of 'learning' rather than 'teaching', within any formal educational system, the process is still ultimately controlled by the teacher. To that extent, for example, the culturally limited and … 'possibly superficial (and probably doomed)…' idea of 'learner centredness' (Schweisfurth, 2019) is an enforced choice of the teacher. And the choices that are made, are dependent upon the power, position and beliefs of the parties involved. Curriculum choices are therefore political.

The political analysis of curriculum design might involve consideration of the institutional structure and processes around which curriculum decisions are made, how issues arise around curriculum decisions, and the ways in which decisions are eventually made when different points of view, associated with different types of cultural capital, exist (Levin, 2008). Susan Jamieson's argument is a rehearsal for addressing each of these, made more complicated by the credible claim that:

> Expertise in a subject area – and even expertise in teaching the subject – does not necessarily equate to expertise in constructing a curriculum. (Levin, 2008)

Teachers, content and process advocates, 'authorities', 'trend-setters and followers' and practitioners may see the issues of curriculum content and process quite differently. Research and evidence may play a small role or no role at all, although the inclusion of prescribing in the UK undergraduate medical curriculum might be an exception to this rule (Magavern et al., 2023; Medical Schools Council, 2023; Rothwell et al., 2015), while '…even small incidents can turn into significant political issues if they press the right buttons for enough people' (Levin, 2008). What we are left with is decision-making based on debate and political power.

> Although curriculum is a fundamental part of the framework of schooling, curriculum decisions and choices are shaped in large measure by other considerations – ideology, personal values, issues in the public domain, and interests. … Political processes are driven by interests, and particularly by the most vocal interests. (Levin, 2008, p. 22)

Curriculum and Ideology

Ideology and politics arise from the material world. They are dialectically related to material conditions. A curriculum is a statement of ideology (Apple, 2019). It expresses the beliefs and values of its developers about the form and function of the curriculum in the world that it serves or challenges (Schiro, 2007). Understanding the ideologies of self and others, and the conceptual frameworks and values that underpin them, can help in curriculum discussions, and in the resolution of disagreements, although even those, ultimately, will be based on power. The exercise of power is facilitated by the lack of evidence to support curriculum decisions.

Where there is no evidence, we are left with argument, beliefs, ideology and power. Those might manifest themselves in contests based on fashion and belief in relation to context, culture, professional and social beliefs and values, theories and ideas of learning, as well as the pragmatics of resources (Grant, 2019). Or curriculum decisions might be made on the basis of wanting to be identified with a powerful group or movement. The uptake of problem-based learning or competency-based curricula could be seen in those terms.

Education is a socially constructed process (Grant et al., 2013), and if we are aware of that, then we will also be conscious of the reasons why we make choices in curriculum design. The current fashion for competency-based curricula cannot be explained on the basis of evidence, but can only be understood as a choice that takes its lead from others: as a matter of the power of practice and compliance.

In this morass of confusion, how are curriculum decisions made? We can only conclude that this is a political process (Grant et al., 2013), designed to hand on the culture of its referent dominant society (Kelly, 2009). So changing a curriculum is a much larger matter than simply deciding on new content and process. And the central argument, as Susan Jamieson illustrates, will always focus on:

> … the whole issue of the nature of knowledge and the question whether any body of knowledge has or can have an intrinsic, objective, absolute value or status. (Kelly, 2009)

The same issues apply to benchmarks, learning outcomes, programmes of study, beliefs about learning, and standards (Kelly, 2009). Each of these is controversial, especially so in the absence of a body of evidence or an articulated theory of curriculum that sets out the value of certain types and bodies of knowledge, how that knowledge is to be understood and used, what might constitute balance in a curriculum, and how those decisions should be made and reviewed. Susan Jamieson illustrates the politics and power of all of this.

References

Achike, F. I. (2016). The challenges of integration in an innovative modern medical curriculum. *Medical Science Educator, 26*(1), 153–158. https://doi.org/10.1007/s40670-015-0206-7

Ambrose, A. J. H., Andaya, J. M., Yamada, S., & Maskarinec, G. G. (2014). Social justice in medical education: Strengths and challenges of a student-driven social justice curriculum. *Hawai'i Journal of Medicine and Public Health, 73*(8), 244–250.

Apple, M. (2019). *Ideology and curriculum* (4th ed.). Routledge.

Becher, T., & Trowler, P. (2001). *Academic tribes and territories: Intellectual enquiry and the culture of disciplines*. McGraw-Hill Education.

Bleakley, A. (2021). *Medical education, politics and social justice. The contradiction cure*. Routledge.

Bolman, L. G., & Gallos, J. V. (2011). *Reframing academic leadership*. Jossey-Bass.

Bourdieu, P. (1986). The forms of capital. In J. Richardson (Ed.), *Handbook of theory and research for the sociology of education* (pp. 241–258). Greenwood.

Bourdieu, P., & Passeron, J.-C. (1977). *Reproduction in education society and culture*. Sage Publications.

Challa, K. T., Sayed, A., & Acharya, Y. (2021). Modern techniques of teaching and learning in medical education: A descriptive literature review. *MedEdPublish, 10*(1), 10.15694/mep.2021.000018.1.

Chater, S. S. (1975). A conceptual framework for curriculum development. *Nursing Outlook, 23*(7), 428–433.

Crawford, K. (2000). The political construction of the 'whole curriculum'. *British Educational Research Journal, 26*(5). https://doi.org/10.1080/01411920020007823

de Leeuw, E. (2012). The politics of medical curriculum accreditation. *International Journal of User-Driven Healthcare, 2*(1), 53–69. https://doi.org/10.4018/ijudh.2012010108

Goldie, J., Schwartz, L., McConnachie, A., & Morrison, J. (2004). The impact of a modern medical curriculum on students' proposed behaviour on meeting ethical dilemmas. *Medical Education, 38*(9), 942–949. https://doi.org/10.1111/j.1365-2929.2004.01915.x

Grant, J. (2019). Principles of curriculum design. In T. Swanwick, K. Forrest, & B. O'Brien (Eds.), *Understanding education: Evidence, theory and practice* (pp. 71–88). Wiley Blackwell.

Grant, J., Abdelrahmen, M. Y. H., & Zachariah, A. (2013). Curriculum design in context. In K. Walsh (Ed.), *Oxford textbook of medical education*. Oxford University Press.

Grant, J., & Marsden, P. (1987). The structure of memorized knowledge in students and clinicians: An explanation for diagnostic expertise. *Medical Education, 21*(2), 92–98. https://doi.org/10.1111/j.1365-2923.1987.tb00672.x

Harindranathan, P. (2023, May). Social justice as part of medical education. *Times Higher Education*. https://www.timeshighereducation.com/campus/social-justice-part-medical-education

Hassan, S. (2013). Concepts of vertical and horizontal integration as an approach to integrated curriculum. *Education in Medicine Journal, 5*(4). https://doi.org/10.5959/eimj.v5i4.163

Huang, Y.-C. (2021). Comparison and contrast of Piaget and Vygotsky's theories. *Advances in Social Science, Education and Humanities Research, 554*, 28–32. https://doi.org/10.2991/assehr.k.210519.007

Jeyakumar, A., Dissanayake, B., & Dissabandara, L. (2020). Dissection in the modern medical curriculum: An exploration into student perception and adaptions for the future. *Anatomical Sciences Education, 13*(3), 366–380. https://doi.org/10.1002/ase.1905

Kelly, A. V. (2009). *The curriculum. Theory and practice*. Sage Publications Limited.

Kern, D. E., Thomas, P. A., & Hughes, M. T. (2009). *Curriculum development for medical education. A six-step approach* (2nd ed.). Johns Hopkins University Press.

Kruschinski, C., Wiese, B., Eberhard, J., & Hummers-Pradier, E. (2011). Attitudes of medical students towards general practice: Effects of gender, a general practice clerkship and a modern curriculum. *GMS Zeitschrift Fur Medizinische Ausbildung, 28*(1) Doc16. https://doi.org/10.3205/zma000728

Lehrer, K. (2018). *Theory of knowledge*. Routledge.

Levin, B. (2008). Curriculum policy and the politics of what should be learned in schools. In F. M. Connelly, M. F. He, & J. Phillion (Eds.), *The SAGE handbook of curriculum and instruction* (pp. 7–24). SAGE Publications, Inc. https://doi.org/10.4135/9781412976572.n1

Luo, F., Israel, M., Liu, R., Yan, W., Gane, B., & Hampton, J. (2020). Understanding students' computational thinking through cognitive interviews. In *Proceedings of the 51st ACM technical symposium on computer science education* (pp. 919–925). https://doi.org/10.1145/3328778.3366845

Magavern, E. F., Hitchings, A., Bollington, L., Wilson, K., Hepburn, D., Westacott, R. J., Sam, A. H., Caulfield, M. J., & Maxwell, S. (2023). UK prescribing safety assessment (PSA): The development, implementation and outcomes of a national online prescribing assessment. *British Journal of Clinical Pharmacology*, Epub ahead of print. https://doi.org/10.1111/BCP.15919

McKimm, J., & Jones, P. K. (2018). Twelve tips for applying change models to curriculum design, development and delivery. *Medical Teacher, 40*(5), 520–526. https://doi.org/10.108 0/0142159X.2017.1391377

Medical Schools Council. (2023, November 9). *New doctors should pass a prescribing skills test before they qualify to improve safety for patients.* https://www.medschools.ac.uk/news/ new-doctors-should-pass-a-prescribing-skills-test-before-they-qualify-to-improve-safety-for-patients

Membrive, A., Silva, N., Rochera, M. J., & Merino, I. (2022). Advancing the conceptualization of learning trajectories: A review of learning across contexts. *Learning, Culture and Social Interaction, 37*, 100658. https://doi.org/10.1016/j.lcsi.2022.100658

Paterson, A. (2023). *Does the medical classroom need a healthy dose of politics?* London School of Economics, Essays in Education. https://blogs.lse.ac.uk/highereducation/2023/03/09/ could-the-medical-classroom-do-with-a-healthy-dose-of-politics/

Piaget, J. (1952). *The origins of intelligence in children.* International University Press.

Rothwell, C., Nazar, M., Chaytor, A., Portlock, J., Husband, A., & Nazar, H. (2015). Teaching safe prescribing to medical students: Perspectives in the UK. *Advances in Medical Education and Practice*, 279–295. https://doi.org/10.2147/AMEP.S56179

Schiro, M. S. (2007). *Curriculum theory: Conflicting visions and enduring concerns* (1st ed.). Sage Publications.

Schweisfurth, M. (2019). *Is learner-centred education 'best practice'?* https://www.unicef.org/ disabilities/files/UNICEF_Right_to_Education_Children_Disabilities_En_Web.pdf

Shapiro, J., Lie, D., Gutierrez, D., & Zhuang, G. (2006). 'That never would have occurred to me': A qualitative study of medical students' views of a cultural competence curriculum. *BMC Medical Education, 6*(1), 31. https://doi.org/10.1186/1472-6920-6-31

Totté, N., Huyghe, S., & Verhagen, A. (2014). *Building the curriculum in higher education: A conceptual framework.* https://blog.associatie.kuleuven.be/petrsu/files/2013/11/ Buildingthecurriculum_TottC3A9_Huyghe.pdf

Trullàs, J. C., Blay, C., Sarri, E., & Pujol, R. (2022). Effectiveness of problem-based learning methodology in undergraduate medical education: A scoping review. *BMC Medical Education, 22*(1), 104. https://doi.org/10.1186/s12909-022-03154-8

Turney, B. (2007). Anatomy in a modern medical curriculum. *The Annals of The Royal College of Surgeons of England, 89*(2), 104–107. https://doi.org/10.1308/003588407X168244

Wylie, A., & Thompson, S. (2007). Establishing health promotion in the modern medical curriculum: A case study. *Medical Teacher, 29*(8), 766–771. https://doi.org/10.1080/01421590701477407

Yu, H., Flores, D. D., Bonett, S., & Bauermeister, J. A. (2023). LGBTQ+cultural competency training for health professionals: A systematic review. *BMC Medical Education, 23*(1), 558. https://doi.org/10.1186/s12909-023-04373-3

Susan Jamieson is a cell biologist, educator and research supervisor. She is now Emerita Professor and was formerly Professor of Health Professions Education in the University of Glasgow's School of Medicine, Dentistry and Nursing, and Director of their Health Professions Education programme. Prior to that she was Director of Year 1 and then Deputy Head of Glasgow's Undergraduate Medical School, initially responsible for the early (bioscience) years of the curriculum and latterly specialising in educator development. Her research interests include critical thinking, socio-constructivism, basic sciences in medical education, and curriculum.

VI.ii STATEMENT: Is the Current Integrated Approach to the Medical Curriculum Obscuring What Students Need to Learn for Clinical Practice?

Rebecca Gillibrand

1 Changes in the Medical Curriculum

As medical knowledge has increased, the undergraduate curriculum has had to adapt to include an ever-expanding volume of new material. Regulation of medical education and training in the United Kingdom is through the General Medical Council, and, following the publication of *Tomorrow's Doctors: Recommendations on Undergraduate Medical Education* (General Medical Council, 1993), the curriculum has undergone marked changes in more recent years. The more traditional structure of pre-clinical and clinical years has largely been replaced by an integrated, systems approach to learning (Mattick et al., 2004) which has resulted in some subjects traditionally regarded as core elements and taught as 'blocks', with their own assessment system and exam papers, becoming increasingly marginalised. Although this integrated approach has followed a general trend in education at all levels (Drake & Reid, 2020), it is important to consider if this is appropriate in medical education and if it supports the needs both of the practising doctor and of the medical profession (Buja, 2019).

2 The Background to These Changes

Historically, medical education in the UK has developed from the three independent apprenticeship-based professions of surgeon, physician and apothecary (Clarke, 2009) which formed the basis of the traditional pre-clinical and clinical curriculum. This was reflected in healthcare provision before the advent of the First World War

R. Gillibrand (✉)
North Middlesex University Hospital, London, UK
e-mail: rebeccagillibrand@doctors.org.uk

J. Grant, L. Grant (eds.), *The Contradictions of Medical Education*, https://doi.org/10.1007/978-3-031-90394-6_19

in 1914, which consisted of a disjointed system of local physicians, pharmacists, voluntary hospitals and endowed institutions. The experiences and lessons of the two World Wars led to the establishment of the National Health Service in 1948 (Beveridge, 1942; Tangye, 1920). Aligned with this was consideration of training doctors to meet the needs of the new health service (Goodenough, 1944), and the establishment of the Conference of Deans of Provincial Medical Schools and the Conference of Deans of London Medical Schools; now the Medical Schools Council (Medical Schools Council, 2020). This background continues to shape healthcare provision and education today in the UK.

The Medical Act of 1983 set out the mandate for the formation of the General Medical Council (GMC), including its responsibilities toward medical education. It was in response to this Act that the Education Committee of the GMC published *Tomorrow's Doctors* (General Medical Council, 1993). The Education Committee recognised that evolution of the medical education system had resulted in an unco-ordinated curriculum with split pre-clinical and clinical components and loss of a defined overview of course aims. It set out several recommendations aimed at reducing the amount of factual learning required, with preference given to 'foster-ing the critical study of principles and the development of independent thought'. The Committee defined the required attainments of a newly qualified doctor as a core curriculum to be supplemented by special study modules where the student could choose to study areas of interest to them in greater depth. A key recommenda-tion was that:

> The core curriculum should be systems-based, its component parts being the combined responsibility of basic scientists and clinicians integrating their contributions to a common purpose, thus eliminating the rigid pre-clinical/clinical divide and the exclusive departmen-tally based course. (General Medical Council, 1993)

As a result of this, the integrated curriculum, in a wide variety of forms, has steadily become the accepted model for undergraduate medical education. There is still no evidence to support that.

3   The Integrated Curriculum and Its Dangers

Integration has been defined as 'a fully synchronous, trans-disciplinary delivery of information between the foundational sciences and the applied sciences throughout all years of a medical school curriculum' (Brauer & Ferguson, 2015).

It could be argued that by integrating the curriculum, however, previously stand-alone subjects may become obscured or even lost as their distinct status disappears. In his discussion of integrated learning, Loftus (2015) uses the example of problem-based learning to highlight some of the associated challenges. This scenario may be used to discuss a wide range of subjects including anatomy, physiology, pathology, pharmacology and social considerations; however, as he points out, it remains for the medical school to determine which components are regarded as core learning material.

The impact of potentially obscuring some subjects becomes increasingly important at the postgraduate training level, as newly qualified doctors select their specialty training schemes. According to a workforce census conducted by the UK Royal College of Pathologists, there are serious pressures on the current pathology workforce, with only 3% of departments having sufficient staffing, and over a quarter of pathologists being over the age of 55 and so approaching retirement (The Royal College of Pathologists, 2018). The College also recognises that the absence of specific undergraduate pathology teaching has negatively influenced recruitment.

4 The Disconnection Between Undergraduate and Postgraduate Curricula

Postgraduate training in the UK follows a well-prescribed path. New graduates must first complete two years of foundation training which is designed to help them develop the required skills and competencies to manage acutely ill patients. After successful completion, they can then apply for specialist training including in general practice (British Medical Association, 2020). Postgraduate curricula and assessments are designed by The Academy of Medical Royal Colleges, the Royal Colleges and the Faculties in accordance with GMC guidelines (General Medical Council, 2017) and approval. In order to take part in specialty training, postgraduates must enrol with the appropriate Medical Royal College or Faculty (or intercollegiate body) which allows them to record their training documentation and progress, resulting in recommendation for the certificate of completion of training or equivalent, when eligible (Council of Postgraduate Medical Education Deans, 2020).

There are 37 specialties listed under the 2021 recruitment plans of the National Health Service (Health Education England, 2023). The majority of these reflect specialties in which the undergraduates will have had direct experience such as medicine, surgery, emergency medicine and general practice. There are, however, several specialties that have become heavily integrated into the undergraduate curriculum thereby losing their distinct and visible status.

With this loss of recognition as a specific entity at undergraduate level, there is a real risk of a disconnection developing between the undergraduate curriculum and the needs of the medical profession and service. Pathology provides an example of a group of subjects (including cellular pathology, microbiology, and clinical biochemistry) that have historically formed a core part of the pre-clinical undergraduate curriculum, but which are now often taught in an integrated manner with little representation in final examinations. This position is not reflected at postgraduate level, however, and pathology remains a defined specialty within medicine with its own training schemes and professional body, The Royal College of Pathologists. *Tomorrow's Doctors* (General Medical Council, 1993), and its more recent incarnation *Outcomes for Graduates* (General Medical Council, 2018), recognise that pathology in practice is central to the diagnostic process and that it is essential that the graduate doctor can not only request appropriate tests but is also able to understand and interpret the results correctly. The cellular pathologist also forms a core member of multidisciplinary team meetings where patients are discussed with a view to planning treatment, and is recognised as such in internal and external peer review.

5   Additional Effects of Service Reorganisation

An additional problem arises in the provision of teaching and training in some fields where there is national reconfiguration and centralisation of services. Following the publication of Lord Carter's review of pathology services in 2009, there was a significant reorganisation of pathology provision nationally which has resulted in the development of pathology hubs with less or no medical representation at some hospitals, including those sites involved in medical undergraduate training (Lord Carter of Coles, 2009). This has, in turn, had an effect on teaching and education. Cellular pathology is already seeing a shift to recruiting non-medically qualified biomedical scientists to undertake additional training in order to report cases within a defined framework (Lishman & Sturdgess, 2017). As the number of academic pathologists also declines, this only serves to compound the problem (Brockmoeller et al., 2019).

There are, therefore, real challenges to be met in ensuring interesting and relevant teaching for students. If these challenges are not met, this could have an impact on student knowledge and their understanding of the core role of the pathologist in patient diagnosis and treatment, and consequently adversely affect patient care and future recruitment to the specialty.

6   The Case for Teaching in Context Rather Than Integration

Interactive teaching is provided at our institution by pathologists and is constructed around vignettes, surgical specimens and autopsies. It incorporates discussion on which samples are appropriate for diagnosis and how they are processed, as well as developing understanding of pathological terms and likely diagnoses within defined clinical scenarios. A key aim of these sessions is to give the students the opportunity to understand the relevance of pathology within the multidisciplinary team delivering patient care. It receives good student feedback and is well attended.

On asking what experience of pathology the final year students have at the start of a teaching session, the answer is invariably 'very little', However, once the clinical scenarios are presented and the discussions start, little pieces of knowledge often start to surface. This would perhaps suggest that the overview necessary to understand the subject is obscured within the integrated systems teaching that they have received. Our experience has been that by giving students the opportunity to have interactive teaching with a pathologist, they are able to consolidate their learning and to learn from an actual practitioner how the discipline works in practice. These impressions are supported by the findings of a project conducted by Rae et al. (2017)

which looked at potential benefits of including pathologists in anatomy teaching sessions. They found that having pathologists available during dissection of the bodies, and being able to discuss the cause of death with those pathologists, resulted in greater understanding of clinico-pathological correlation as well as raising student interest in pathology. The benefits of role modelling as part of the teaching and learning experience have also been highlighted in relation to how pathology teaching could be developed to improve student engagement (Maley et al., 2008).

A study looking at how to improve the experience of learning pathology for undergraduates, compared multidisciplinary strategies with traditional approaches to teaching undergraduate pathology and found that teaching modules combining lectures with clinical scenarios and virtual microscopy to supplement conventional laboratory teaching was received well (Gopalan et al., 2018). Interestingly though, integration of lectures with problem-based learning (PBL) and clinical skills sessions, although well received overall, received the lowest score on the rating of learning experiences (39% of students disagreed or were neutral). This could suggest that teaching in context rather than integration was valued more highly by the students.

This idea is further supported by Diaz-Perez et al. (2014) who compared the exam results of a student group taught by traditional methods (lectures and laboratory sessions) with a group taught using digital pathology with clinico-pathological correlation. The results for the digital pathology with clinico-pathological correlation group were better, again supporting the view that teaching in context is important.

Our experience, and that of other groups, would therefore suggest that by teaching in context we can enhance the undergraduate experience and maintain the presence of these subjects. We can relate our subjects to the clinical situation and highlight their role in diagnosis and treatment planning, rather than see them being taught in a completely integrated manner, perhaps by non-practitioners. We can then better support the needs of students in their postgraduate careers and raise the profile of our professions with the aim of promoting interest and recruitment in the future.

7 Conclusion

The establishment of the integrated curriculum within the medical undergraduate educational framework has followed changing practice in other areas of education resulting in the loss of some topics and negatively affecting the identity of others. This has raised significant challenges in providing important and relevant teaching to students which, if not met, may have an impact on student knowledge and core understanding, and may potentially affect patient care and recruitment to those medical specialties. Learning a discipline is also about learning about that discipline in practice, and by taking opportunities to teach these subjects in context we can support the integrated curriculum and provide a more effective learning experience whilst maintaining subject identity.

References

Beveridge, W. (1942). *Social Insurance and Allied Services Report*.

Brauer, D. G., & Ferguson, K. J. (2015). The integrated curriculum in medical education: AMEE Guide No. 96. *Medical Teacher, 37*(4), 312–322. https://doi.org/10.310 9/0142159X.2014.970998

British Medical Association. (2020). *Medical Training Pathway*. https://www.bma.org.uk/ advice-and-support/studying-medicine/becoming-a-doctor/medical-training-pathway

Brockmoeller, S., Young, C., Lee, J., Arends, M. J., Wilkins, B. S., Thomas, G. J., Oien, K. A., Jones, L., & Hunter, K. D. (2019). Survey of UK histopathology consultants' attitudes towards academic and molecular pathology. *Journal of Clinical Pathology, 72*(6), 399–405. https://doi. org/10.1136/jclinpath-2018-205568

Buja, L. M. (2019). Medical education today: All that glitters is not gold. *BMC Medical Education, 19*(1), 110. https://doi.org/10.1186/s12909-019-1535-9

Clarke, E. (2009). History of British medical education. *Medical Education, 1*(1), 7–15. https:// doi.org/10.1111/j.1365-2923.1966.tb02062.x

Council of Postgraduate Medical Education Deans. (2020). *A reference guide for postgraduate foundation and specialty training in the UK. The Gold Guide 8th edition*. https://www.copmed. org.uk/images/docs/gold_guide_8th_edition/Gold_Guide_8th_Edition_March_2020.pdf

Diaz-Perez, J. A., Raju, S., & Echeverri, J. H. (2014). Evaluation of a teaching strategy based on integration of clinical subjects, virtual autopsy, pathology museum, and digital microscopy for medical students. *Journal of Pathology Informatics, 5*(1), 25. https://doi. org/10.4103/2153-3539.137729

Drake, S. M., & Reid, J. L. (2020). 21st century competencies in light of the history of integrated curriculum. *Frontiers in Education, 5*. https://doi.org/10.3389/feduc.2020.00122

General Medical Council. (1993). *Tomorrow's doctors. Recommendations on undergraduate medical education*.

General Medical Council. (2017). *Excellence by design - Standards for the development and design of postgraduate medical curricula*. https://www.gmc-uk.org/education/ standards-guidance-and-curricula/standards-and-outcomes/excellence-by-design

General Medical Council. (2018). *Outcomes for graduates*. https://www.gmc-uk.org/educa- tion/standards-guidance-and-curricula/standards-and-outcomes/outcomes-for-graduates/ outcomes-for-graduates

Goodenough, W. (1944). Training of doctors: the Goodenough Committees report. *British Medical Journal, 4359*(2), 121–123.

Gopalan, V., Kasem, K., Pillai, S., Olveda, D., Ariana, A., Leung, M., & Lam, A. K. Y. (2018). Evaluation of multidisciplinary strategies and traditional approaches in teaching pathology in medical students. *Pathology International, 68*(8), 459–466. https://doi.org/10.1111/pin.12706

Health Education England. (2023). *Medical specialty recruitment*. https://medical.hee.nhs.uk/ medical-training-recruitment/medical-specialty-training

Lishman, S., & Sturdgess, I. (2017). *The role of biomedical scientists in histopathol- ogy reporting. A joint statement from the Royal College of Pathologists and the Institute of Biomedical Scientists*. https://www.ibms.org/resources/documents/joint- statement-on-the-histopathology-reporting-qualification

Loftus, S. (2015). Understanding integration in medical education. *Medical Science Educator, 25*(3), 357–360. https://doi.org/10.1007/s40670-015-0152-4

Lord Carter of Coles. (2009). *Report of the Review of NHS Pathology Services in England*. www. dh.gov.uk/publications

Maley, M. A. L., Harvey, J. R., Boer, W. B. de, Scott, N. W., & Arena, G. E. (2008). Addressing current problems in teaching pathology to medical stu- dents: Blended learning. *Medical Teacher, 30*(1), e1–e9. https://doi.org/10.1080/ 01421590701753575

Mattick, K., Dennis, I., & Bligh, J. (2004). Approaches to learning and studying in medical students: validation of a revised inventory and its relation to student characteristics and performance. *Medical Education, 38*(5), 535–543. https://doi.org/10.1111/j.1365-2929.2004.01836.x

Medical Schools Council. (2020). *Introduction to the Medical Schools Council.* https://www.medschools.ac.uk/media/2525/introduction-to-msc-002.pdf

Rae, G., Cork, J. R., Karpinski, A. C., McGoey, R., & Swartz, W. (2017). How the integration of pathology in the gross anatomy laboratory affects medical students. *Teaching and Learning in Medicine, 29*(1), 101–108. https://doi.org/10.1080/10401334.2016.1194761

Tangye, C. E. (1920). The Dawson report. *Public Health, 34*, 42–44. https://doi.org/10.1016/S0033-3506(20)80029-8

The Royal College of Pathologists. (2018). *Meeting pathology demand. Histopathology Workforce Census.* https://www.rcpath.org/uploads/assets/952a934d-2ec3-48c9-a8e6e00fcdca700f/Meeting-Pathology-Demand-Histopathology-Workforce-Census-2018.pdf

VI.ii COMMENTARY: Curriculum Integration and the Trajectory of Learning: Practice and Theory from a Postgraduate Perspective

Janet Grant and Leonard Grant

In the previous chapter we considered the threatened position of basic sciences in the curriculum, and the power struggles around curriculum design. In this chapter, a specialty is also arguing for its distinct place in the medical school curriculum. The arguments around power and decision-making are similar but not the same. In relation to basic sciences in the curriculum, the power struggles were located between different groups and sections of society. But in this chapter, Rebecca Gillibrand locates the struggle as being between ideas of curriculum structure and their unintended effects. The idea that curriculum decisions are based on vested beliefs and arguments still holds true. But here, they are beliefs about curriculum design which have consequences for her specialty.

The Integrated Curriculum: A Popular Belief

The integrated curriculum first appeared in medical education around the 1980s and has gained in popularity ever since (Brauer & Ferguson, 2015). This popular belief in medicine followed on from many years of integrated curriculum development in primary and secondary schools (Drake & Reid, 2020) which, perhaps, are rather different from medical schools in their intention.

Discussions of the integrated curriculum in medical education tend to rely on arguments rather than analysis or evidence. For example, integration is described as 'a popular concept' often based on unsupported claims made for its effect on 'meaningful learning', citing the equally popular and unsubstantiated 'adult learning theory' which suggests that 'adults' focus on relevance in learning (Wijnen-Meijer et al., 2020). This, of course, could also be said of children (Birbili & Melpomeni, 2008; Zosh et al., 2017). Integration has also been defended in terms of motivation, facilitation of transition to practice, preparation for lifelong learning (Wijnen-Meijer et al., 2020), and simply in terms of advantages and disadvantages (Quintero et al., 2016). The literature about the integrated curriculum in medicine is vast. The claims are many. The range of designs is bewildering in its variety (Atwa & Gouda, 2014; Mathur et al., 2019), and the robust evidence of effect is thin at all levels and in all disciplines (Kreijkes, 2023). It is simply a fashion that many have adopted. And fashion, being based on taste, is difficult to argue with. Nonetheless, critique is required.

The claims made about integration map entirely on to the observations that:

Curriculum ideologies manifest in terms of what might be thought of as values, visions of the future, and venues or forms. This is to say, the curriculum is imbued with processes for valuing assumed choices related to its design, development, and implementation. These choices draw from ideologically based assumptions about the curriculum's basis in political, economic, historical, sociocultural, psychological, and other realities – whether they be discursive or material in effect. (Crowley, 2021)

We can explore this further in relation to Rebecca Gillibrand's experience.

Ideology and Curriculum

We argue in other chapters that choosing a curriculum design is an ideological process:

> A medical school curriculum is a reflection of the relative institutionalised cultural capital (qualifications, educational credentials, values, ideas) of the groups contesting its contents and processes. (Bourdieu, 1986)

Although that argument applies to learning in medical school, Rebecca Gillibrand broadens it out to the effect of the curriculum ideology 'winner' on things that are not specified as curriculum outcomes, such as choice of career specialty. The outcomes are intended, but career choice, or failure to understand the nature and significance of pathology in her case, is an unintended outcome. Similar negative effects on career choice when a specialty is missing from the curriculum have been shown for Family Medicine (Ha et al., 2024). Because such ultimate effects of curriculum are unknown, it has been argued that curriculum heterogeneity is needed, rather than the curriculum uniformity that medical education is pursuing (Grant et al., 2013). When a single approach to curriculum dominates a field, it would be wise to study the reasons for that, and consequences both intended and unintended, as has been done in relation to other levels of education (Shapira et al., 2023). Despite many publications, the effects of curriculum integration are under-researched. Similarly, the nationwide change to a competency-based curriculum in India, as yet, has no comprehensive analysis of the outcome effects of this, either intended or unintended. Instead there are publications about the challenges of implementation which largely and predictably conclude only that more teacher training is required (Gehlawat et al., 2024). What has been said about curriculum decisions at secondary school level in Scotland, could equally apply to medical education around the world:

> There is a pressure on schools to perform in particular ways, and many practices which involve schools striving to meet the demands of the system, rather than the system supporting decision-making grounded in an educational rationale. (Priestley, 2023)

But where does that pressure come from, and why do medical schools comply with it in the face of no evidence of effect and the risk of unintended outcomes? The integrated curriculum in medicine is based on momentum rather than evidence (with over one million publications to date but little evidence of effect), just as the adoption of problem-based learning in medicine has been so often accompanied by the term 'innovative' when it clearly was just attempted replication not innovation (as nearly 150,000 publications suggest—again with little robust evidence of effect). The reason for these fashions brings us back to ideology and power, and curriculum as a political rather than educational statement.

Whatever curriculum is selected, it is a statement of the ideological position of its promoter (Grant et al., 2013). That position might be adopted on the basis of beliefs about teaching or learning, or beliefs that this is 'best practice' somewhere else, or beliefs about positioning their institution either nationally or globally in relation to other institutions. However, in the absence of robust evidence that any particular approach to teaching and learning is generally more effective than any other, it might be reckless to adopt a single educational model. We should not confuse 'best practice' with 'common practice', and perhaps listen to the persuasive arguments that the term 'best practice' and all its unfounded implications should be avoided entirely (Osburn et al., 2011). In a global context, perhaps the almost universal adoption of the integrated curriculum is part of the medical education imperialist project which imposes specific global north practices and ideas not only on all parts of the global north, but also on the global south, facilitating the trade in medical graduates, as we have discussed in Part II of this book. This expansion of ideas and practices has been traced back to the 1970s, just before integrated curricula became popular in medicine (Brown, 1979).

Understanding curriculum choices is limited by lack of evidence for the decisions made to adopt, in this case, the integrated model, and the wide range of arguments put forward to defend such choices which…

> … also pertain to the means by which the curriculum achieves these goals or objectives through the formulation of designed experiences, activities, or other forms of learning opportunities. (Crowley, 2021)

What we have seen in Rebecca Gillibrand's account is that when the choice of integration was made, it did not necessarily take into account the possible effects of that on one aspect of practice: career choice, even though medical schools endeavour to prepare their graduates for the next career stage.

Is Integration Right for the Practice of Medicine? A Contradiction of Theory and Practice

We have argued before that medical education is not a theory-based, academic discipline, but is a practice 'harvesting its theories and ideas from a wide variety of social science, philosophical and methodological disciplines and from experience' (Grant & Grant, 2023).

The original arguments for curriculum integration were set out in relation to primary and secondary education. They focused on learning around real-world problems and '….putting knowledge….. to work in these massive tasks' (Bruner, 1960). This is:

> ...rooted in a view of learning as the continuous integration of new knowledge and experience so as to deepen and broaden our understanding of ourselves and our world. (Beane, 1995)

It could be said correctly, of course, that this construction of memory is the function of learning at all levels. However, we can, and perhaps should, question whether this model of education which was developed for school children, is also appropriate for professional education. To do this, we must take into account the nature of a profession, and the nature of learning for a profession.

The Trajectory of Learning for a Profession: Setting Down and Retrieving Knowledge in Memory

Learning is a process of constructing, using and tuning information in memory. A constructivist approach to learning and teaching would therefore focus on the ways in which that knowledge is laid down and then used and changed (Dennick, 2016). Learners do not, as medical education sometimes erroneously suggests, construct new knowledge. They simply organise and store existing knowledge within their own memory structures (Dong et al., 2021). It is individual memories, sometimes called schemata (Wadsworth, 2004), that are constructed, not new knowledge.

This has implications for curriculum design. If organisation is the basis of learning, then the potential disorganisation of discipline-based knowledge that integration might induce (Bolender et al., 2013) is to be taken seriously. Instead of focusing on how we believe that well-learned and well-used, tuned and pruned knowledge is used by a practitioner, the structure and retrieval of existing knowledge may well be the best basis for structuring knowledge inside the new learners' heads. Such fluent retrieval is the basis of developing expertise, and is best acquired by setting down structured memories and then retrieving them in practice, as happens in 'traditional' medical education when students learn the basic and clinical sciences, and then apply them in the clinical setting (Roediger & Butler, 2011). Through its use in practice, that knowledge will develop and become integrated for each individual. Integration best happens inside the learner's head, not in inside the curriculum. There is a good pedagogical reason for the 'traditional' approach.

Contextualisation Versus Integration

If we accept the rhetoric of adult learning 'theory' that students must see the relevance of what they asked to learn (Knowles, 1984), importantly for Rebecca Gillibrand, contextualisation (rather than integration) of well-structured knowledge, by retrieving and applying it in practice, would be a strong educational approach. And she could argue correctly, that pathology provides a perfect context for the internal integration of basic science and clinical knowledge.

Structure and Memory

Professions are knowledge-based. They are also based in judgement. And the medical profession is based in science. That science is applied in personal, social, political and economic contexts. These features differentiate medicine from learning at the level of primary and even secondary schools, where the rationale for curriculum integration was developed.

The nature of learning for a profession has an important differentiation from many other areas of work and other subjects at university level: the problems that the practice of medicine addresses have no predictable starting point, no set pathway for tackling them (given that history-taking becomes a very fluid process in expert hands), and no predetermined solution. For each clinical problem, the clinician must decide on all of these elements. Unsurprisingly, as clinicians become more and more experienced and retrieve their knowledge to solve clinical problems, their thinking becomes more and more individual (Grant & Marsden, 1987), even though they may come to the same conclusion (or sometimes may not). At the same time, their reservoir of actively used knowledge becomes pruned and tuned to practice, rather than ever increasing. In the hinterland of their memories, they also store extensive knowledge, which includes the basic sciences, which is called on when their more commonly used knowledge does not solve the problem (Grant & Marsden, 1987).

Organising Memory: Structure in Context

To achieve this level of tailored and flexible thinking requires structure. However we view or characterise memory (and learning is all about developing and changing the learner's memory), there is agreement that long-term memory is highly structured and connected, while the limited capacity of short-term memory and working memory are facilitated by ready access to long-term memory, the effectiveness and efficiency of which depend on the structured organisation of different types of knowledge. Given that a clinician needs to retrieve information in response to any clinical problem being addressed, accessibility is best assured by organising knowledge within its own logic, rather than in relation to an external framework that splits that logic. That would suggest that learning basic science as it is, for example, is the most efficient, effective and accessible way of acquiring that building block. As that structured knowledge is used and applied, it will, for each person, gradually change, and develop and enable the speed and fluency of the experienced clinician as compared with the new learner (Grant & Marsden, 1987). While organised and structured memories are the basic building blocks, their tuning and shaping occurs when they are retrieved.

Providing context for the basic and clinical sciences, makes more cognitive sense than splitting up already well-organised knowledge.

This is important for Rebecca Gillibrand; the missing learning and experience of her specialty that she regrets, offers the structure that is needed. The contexts that are required around the structured learning that enables retrieval for current problems, would best be drawn from clinical and laboratory-based specialties. Her specialty, therefore, might be more friendly towards memory structures that are laid down from basic sciences, reinforcing them before being applied to clinical problems. Deconstructing specialties, means deconstructing these relationships between disciplines. That does not help learning, learners, or problem solving.

The key issue is that learning must be seen through two simultaneous lenses: the acquisition of structured knowledge organised around its own logic (not around the logic of its much later expert application, such as problem-based learning might require), and the reinforcement, retrieval and development of that structured knowledge across the trajectory of learning that medical school should organise.

Integration: In Contradiction with Developing Effective Practice

The assumptions underpinning an integrated curriculum are 'intuitive' and 'remain at the grand design level'. Ultimately, a curriculum cannot integrate knowledge; only the learner can do that, inside their own growing memory structures (Prideaux et al., 2013). A variety of ideas have been put forward to defend and promote curriculum integration: for example, constructivism, authentic or situated learning, and transformative learning, but none has robust evidence to support it, and such defences feel like *post hoc* rationalisation rather than reasons for such an approach, and such arguments remain at the level of claims. In parallel with these ideas have been equal changes in fashion for the ways in which curriculum outcomes might be expressed, with equal lack of evidence of effect.

A curriculum must make choices about what is to be taught. In that, we make explicit, but usually implicit, choices about whose knowledge counts and what is worthwhile. The profession in practice, represented by people such as Rebecca Gillibrand, and medical education curriculum theorists seem to be in contradiction with one another. In losing the importance of structured knowledge, perhaps Rebecca Gillibrand's specialty is also suffering from loss of experience of its domains of application. The educational rationale might be in contradiction with the professional reality.

The curriculum is indeed a contested place, where power struggles play themselves out, ideological choices are made, and the consequences of those in practice are not always examined.

References

Atwa, H. S., & Gouda, E. M. (2014). Curriculum integration in medical education: A theoretical review. *Intellectual property rights. Open Access, 2*(2). https://doi.org/10.4172/2375-4516.1000113

Beane, J. A. (1995). *Curriculum integration and the disciplines of knowledge. Service learning, general.* University of Nebraska at Omaha. https://digitalcommons.unomaha.edu/slceslgen/44

Birbili, M., & Melpomeni, T. (2008). Identifying children's interests and planning learning experiences: Challenging some taken-for-granted views. In P. G. Grotewell & Y. R. Burton (Eds.), *Early childhood education: Issues and developments* (pp. 143–156). Nova Science Publishers, Inc.

Bolender, D. L., Ettarh, R., Jerrett, D. P., & Laherty, R. F. (2013). Curriculum integration = course disintegration: What does this mean for anatomy? *Anatomical Sciences Education, 6*(3), 205–208. https://doi.org/10.1002/ase.1320

Bourdieu, P. (1986). The forms of capital. In J. Richardson (Ed.), *Handbook of theory and research for the sociology of education* (pp. 241–258). Greenwood.

Brown, R. E. (1979). Exporting medical education: Professionalism, modernization and imperialism. *Social Science & Medicine. Part A: Medical Psychology & Medical Sociology, 13*, 585–595. https://doi.org/10.1016/0271-7123(79)90101-9

Bruner, J. (1960). *The process of education.* Harvard University Press.

Crowley, C. B. (2021). Curriculum ideologies. In *Oxford research encyclopedia of education.* https://doi.org/10.1093/ACREFORE/9780190264093.013.1033

Dennick, R. (2016). Constructivism: Reflections on twenty five years teaching the constructivist approach in medical education. *International Journal of Medical Education, 7,* 200–205. https://doi.org/10.5116/ijme.5763.de11

Dong, H., Lio, J., Sherer, R., & Jiang, I. (2021). Some learning theories for medical educators. *Medical Science Educator, 31*(3), 1157–1172. https://doi.org/10.1007/s40670-021-01270-6

Drake, S. M., & Reid, J. L. (2020). 21st century competencies in light of the history of integrated curriculum. *Frontiers in Education, 5.* https://doi.org/10.3389/feduc.2020.00122

Gehlawat, M., Thumati, G., Samala, P., Alekhya, C. L., Shailaja, A., & Sharma, A. (2024). Competency-based medical education for Indian undergraduates: Where do we stand? *APIK Journal of Internal Medicine, 12*(1), 7–12. https://doi.org/10.4103/ajim.ajim_161_22

Grant, J., & Grant, L. (2023). Quality and constructed knowledge: Truth, paradigms, and the state of the science. *Medical Education, 57*(1), 23–30. https://doi.org/10.1111/medu.14871

Grant, J., & Marsden, P. (1987). The structure of memorized knowledge in students and clinicians: An explanation for diagnostic expertise. *Medical Education, 21*(2), 92–98. https://doi.org/10.1111/j.1365-2923.1987.tb00672.x

Grant, J., Abdelrahman, M. Y. H., & Zachariah, A. (2013). Curriculum design in context. In K. Walsh (Ed.), *Oxford textbook of medical education* (pp. 13–24). Oxford University Press.

Ha, E., Taskier, M., Anderson, A., Martinez, M. P., & Bazemore, A. W. (2024). Setting the target: Comparing family medicine among US allopathic target schools. *Family Medicine.* https://doi.org/10.22454/FamMed.2024.510377.

Knowles, M. (1984). *The adult learner: A neglected species* (3rd ed.). Gulf Publishing.

Kreijkes, P. (2023). *Differential effects of subject-based and integrated curriculum approaches on students' experiences and outcomes: A review of reviews.* https://www.cambridge.org/

Mathur, M., Mathur, N., & Saiyad, S. (2019). Integrated teaching in medical education: The novel approach. *Journal of Research in Medical Education & Ethics, 9*(3), 165. https://doi.org/10.5958/2231-6728.2019.00030.1

Osburn, J., Caruso, G., & Wolfensberger, W. (2011). The concept of "best practice": A brief overview of its meanings, scope, uses, and shortcomings. *International Journal of Disability, Development and Education, 58*(3), 213–222. https://doi.org/10.1080/1034912X.2011.598387

Prideaux, D., Ash, J., & Cottrell, A. (2013). Integrated learning. In K. Walsh (Ed.), *The Oxford textbook of medical education* (1st ed., pp. 63–733). Oxford University Press.

Priestley, M. (2023, February). *Reduced subject choice under curriculum for excellence is affecting opportunities for young people.* University of Stirling. https://www.stir.ac.uk/news/2023/february-2023-news/curriculum-for-excellence-research-results/

Quintero, G. A., Vergel, J., Arredondo, M., Ariza, M.-C., Gómez, P., & Pinzon-Barrios, A.-M. (2016). Integrated medical curriculum: Advantages and disadvantages. *Journal of Medical Education and Curricular Development, 3,* JMECD.S18920. https://doi.org/10.4137/JMECD.S18920

Roediger, H. L., & Butler, A. C. (2011). The critical role of retrieval practice in long-term retention. *Trends in Cognitive Sciences, 15*(1), 20–27. https://doi.org/10.1016/j.tics.2010.09.003

Shapira, M., Priestley, M., Peace-Hughes, T., Barnett, C., & Ritchie, M. (2023). *Choice, attainment and positive destinations: Exploring the impact of curriculum policy change on young people.* www.nuffieldfoundation.org

Wadsworth, B. J. (2004). *Piaget's theory of cognitive and affective development: Foundations of constructivism.* Longman.

Wijnen-Meijer, M., van den Broek, S., Koens, F., & ten Cate, O. (2020). Vertical integration in medical education: The broader perspective. *BMC Medical Education, 20*(1), 509. https://doi.org/10.1186/s12909-020-02433-6

Zosh, J. N., Hopkins, E. J., Jensen, H., Liu, C., Neale, D., Hirsh-Pasek, K., Solis, S. L., & Whitebread, D. (2017). *Learning through play : A review of the evidence.* LEGO Foundation.

Rebecca Gillibrand is a consultant cellular pathologist and medical examiner working in a district general hospital in North London. Originally a biomedical scientist in histopathology, she joined medical school as a mature student in 1991. Comparing her medical school experience with that of more recent graduates is her particular interest. Her Master's in Health Professions Education dissertation studied changes in selection processes. She enjoys and values her opportunities for teaching students and doctors in training. Developing the local medical examiner service has allowed her to teach, train, and learn from a truly multidisciplinary group from the hospital and wider community.

VI.iii STATEMENT: Managing Medical and Dental Curriculum Reform in a Sub-Saharan Country

E. Oluwabunmi Olapade-Olaopa, Akinyele Adisa, Funmilayo E. Olopade, Babatunde Ademusire, Victor A. Odekunle, Akintunde A. Odukogbe, Adebola O. Ogunbiyi, and Obafunke M. Denloye

A note from the editors: The term sub-Saharan is understood to have racist and colonial origins, not speaking to a geographical division but to a racial one. However, the term is still widely used in the literature and is the choice of the authors.

1 Background

Despite its colonial history, medical instruction in sub-Saharan Africa has always required innovative adaptation of medical education methods to suit the peculiarities of the local teaching and learning environments, and socio-cultural norms.

Medical (and dental) curricula are reviewed infrequently in sub-Saharan Africa due to financial and other resource constraints. The College of Medicine, University of Ibadan (COMUI) therefore took advantage of an institutional development grant from the Bill and Melinda Gates Foundation to undertake a complete review of its 62-year-old traditional MBBS/BDS curriculum inherited from its parent university (the University of London). This 10-year project from 2001–2010, produced an instrument for medical and dental instruction that meets national health needs and global standards.

Competency-based medical education is an outcomes-based model which de-emphasises time-based training and aims to produce health professionals who can practise medicine in accordance with local conditions, to meet local needs. This

---

The authors of this chapter are from the University of Ibadan, Faculties of Medicine, Basic Sciences and Dentistry. They are senior clinicians and academics, medical education specialists and a student.

E. O. Olapade-Olaopa (✉) · A. Adisa · F. E. Olopade · B. Ademusire · V. A. Odekunle ·
A. A. Odukogbe · A. O. Ogunbiyi · O. M. Denloye
College of Medicine, University of Ibadan, Ibadan, Nigeria
e-mail: okeoffa@gmail.com

philosophy of medical education was adopted by the Ibadan Medical and Dental Schools during their curriculum review.

However, curriculum change can only succeed where administrators and faculty are fully committed to its implementation. Revising the medical and dental curriculum in Ibadan was no different. We report here the challenges encountered during the process and the steps taken to overcome them which made the curriculum change successful.

2 Representation on the Curriculum Revision Project

The MBBS/BDS Curriculum Revision Project was initiated by the University administration as part of its institutional strengthening strategy. The Curriculum Revision Committee (CRC) was chaired by the Provost of the College of Medicine with membership from all sections of the College. Whilst most heads of department cooperated with the Committee, some needed to be persuaded to send representatives, and the Vice-Chancellor appointed representatives for others.

3 Implementing the Revised Curriculum: Challenges and Responses

3.1 Establishing the College of Medicine Education Unit

Shortly after the adoption of the revised MBBS curriculum by the University Senate, some members of the CRC were selected to form the College of Medical Education Unit (CMEU) which was established to oversee the process of curriculum change. The unit identified potential challenges facing the implementation process, but some challenges were unexpected. Whilst it was possible to resolve some of the challenges quickly, others took a little longer.

3.2 Effects of Inadequate Preparedness to Implement the Revised Curriculum

Despite concerted efforts made to ensure that all stakeholders were carried along during the curriculum revision process, it was quite a surprise to discover that a significant proportion of the college community appeared unprepared to implement it. The 1-year lag between approval and implementation of the curriculum also resulted in a loss of the momentum achieved during the review process which the CMEU had to contend with during the implementation of the revised curriculum. Major challenges were encountered.

3.3 Faculty Pushback

Although the CMEU was prepared for some resistance from faculty to the curriculum change, the degree and wide-spread nature of the resistance was not expected. This pushback was multifactorial.

Firstly, perhaps the most enduring cause for the resistance of faculty (especially the older ones) to the revised curriculum was a deep-rooted notion that the old curriculum had served the College well for over 60 years and therefore did not need to be revised. The resistance was heightened by the unfamiliarity of a larger than expected proportion of the teaching staff with the revised curriculum. This was due in part to the limited number of awareness programmes and training workshops prior to implementation of the curriculum in the (misplaced) belief that most of the faculty were already familiar with the new teaching and assessment methods having been involved in developing the revised curriculum. This pushback reached its peak in the first four years of the implementation of the revised curriculum during which period the College was running both the old and revised curricula and the teachers had to teach and assess students using both the traditional and CBME methods of instruction.

Secondly, there was initial resistance to the paradigm shift represented by the prioritised learning and assessment methods of the revised curriculum. This was mainly due to the long-held belief that a doctor must know 'almost everything in medicine' which made the concept of 'must know, should know and may know' alien to many teachers. In addition, some teachers were uncomfortable with the introduction of competency-based, problem-solving and formative assessments and the change to an open marking system.

Thirdly, the adjustment of the time allotted to several courses in order to accommodate new courses and the periods of vertical and/or horizontal integration, also met with some resistance from both staff and students, especially in the basic sciences, obstetrics and gynaecology, and dentistry where the clerkship periods had been reduced. Similarly, the increased number of clerkship postings prescribed in the new curriculum increased the number of students rotating through the different disciplines in order to produce well-rounded graduates. This has continued to be a sore point with staff and students mainly because of the feeling that there is not enough time to ensure 'proper' teaching and learning.

3.4 Resolving the Problems

To resolve these challenges, the CMEU solicited the assistance of the College Executive and senior teachers who were supportive of the curriculum revision to advocate for its implementation with the concerned staff and students. This was in addition to the prompt organisation of a series of workshops to familiarise the faculty with the philosophy of the new curriculum and to train them on the new teaching and assessment methods. Other solutions included creating a schedule to evenly distribute faculty engagement with students, the prioritisation of didactic sessions and the use of case-based teaching sessions to create more opportunities for learning. The consensus at the end of the workshops was that we may have been over-burdening the students instead of training them to be competent generalist physicians, as required by law.

Next, the limited understanding of the student body about the implications of the revised curriculum also resulted in a feeling of abandonment and the fear of graduating with an outdated curriculum in the older students, whilst the new entrants felt they were 'guinea pigs' for an untested curriculum. To improve new students' awareness about the curriculum, the College established three orientation programmes which were held at the beginning of the preliminary year, first year preclinical, and first year clinical (White Coat Ceremony), respectively. The College also started a mentoring scheme which allowed students to nominate preferred lecturers as mentors.

4   Other Challenges

4.1   Inadequate Teaching Facilities

In the early phase of implementing the new curriculum, the number of rooms, lecture halls and laboratories available were inadequate for the lectures and practical sessions scheduled, whilst the clinical skills laboratories were also inadequately equipped. The teaching staff, however, responded with ingenious management of the available facilities until additional ones were provided by the College. Several specialties also developed local equivalents to complement imported mannequins and phantom heads in order to ensure adequate skills acquisition by the students.

4.2   Irregular Power Supply, Internet Connectivity

The College installed solar panels and a high-capacity inverter system to provide uninterrupted power supply for the services essential for the implementation of the revised curriculum such as the Library and the information and communications technology networks (the internet, intranet and website). The College intranet was also upgraded to a 10G network with the purchase of additional servers, laying fibreoptic cables and the installation of more wireless connection points across the campus. The College website was overhauled to make it more robust, interactive and user friendly, and able to provide up-to-date information about the College.

4.3   Challenges with Funding: The Health Professionals Training Levy

The cost of training health professionals is high globally but is even higher in sub-Saharan Africa due largely to the additional cost of importing most of the consumables and human replacement equipment (mannequins) used for training. Unfortunately, most publicly owned medical schools in Nigeria have been poorly funded for several years. The paucity of funds reached its peak between 2014 and 2016 and made implementation of the revised curriculum impossible with the centrally regulated tuition fees, due to the ever-rising cost of training.

The College responded to this urgent need to secure funds required to train students by introducing the Health Professional Training Levies (HPTL) in 2017 to cover part of the cost of professional training and examinations. Similar to the process of revising the curriculum, the College management ensured that all stakeholders were carried along in the process of determining the levies for each health professional training course. Despite this, there was an initial resistance by the students and their parents when an additional 30% of the calculated cost of training a student in each discipline was approved by the University Senate, birthing the '#NoTo100K' march that made national news in April 2018. However, after further discussions with the College, University and Executives, the levy was accepted.

With these funds, the College has been able to meet a significant proportion of the costs of the 'essential' training needs which has made it easier to implement the new curriculum. Importantly, the HPTL system included loans and scholarships for deserving medical students who were unable to afford the levies and this initiative was supported by the 'Adopt a Student' scheme which was sourced from corporate and or individual funds. The College also improved its financial processes and accounting standards to ensure a more efficient, effective, and transparent use of all funds collected.

4.4   Disruptions to the Academic Calendar Due to Strike Actions

The 2010 MBBS Curriculum spans a period of 5 years. However, strike actions by the various unions remain the most important cause of disruption to the academic calendar and prolongation of the study period in Nigerian public universities. The College took advantage of the fact that the new curriculum is harmonised within each calendar year of study to reduce the effect of these strike actions by adjusting the academic calendar to regain most of the time lost.

4.5 The COVID19 Pandemic

Before the COVID19 pandemic, teaching and learning at COMUI was almost entirely physical. Like other countries, Nigerian universities were closed for a prolonged period during the pandemic. When the schools were re-opened, the College joined the global trend of adopting online teaching for all lectures and small group teaching sessions, which was relatively easy for our institution because online teaching had already been initiated in 2008. Even though the situation could return to normal, online lectures have remained a key method of learning in the College.

5 Alumni Support

The Ibadan Medical School has always enjoyed alumni support and this has been increased since implementation of the revised curriculum. In most instances, the alumni selected the projects they would support which included the renovation of clinical students' hostels, lecture halls and laboratories, donation of a bus for student transportation, and upgrading the College website and internet connectivity. The alumni also further strengthened their already commendable relationship with the students by increasing their direct support for student-initiated projects focusing on research and mentorship projects.

6 Student-Initiated Responses to Challenges with the Curriculum Change

Even though executives of the University of Ibadan Medical Students' Association (UIMSA) participated in the curriculum review process, the generality of the student body had limited information about the revised curriculum. Therefore, when the implementation of the new curriculum began, UIMSA started several student-led initiatives to complement the efforts of the College administration to manage the curriculum change process.

One of the most important of these initiatives was the UIMSA Presidential Committee on Curriculum Assessment, Research and Development (COMCARD) which studied the students' perception of the curriculum and identified methods to assist the students in adapting to the new methods of teaching and assessment. A 2020 survey by COMCARD confirmed that the knowledge (and hence understanding) of the curriculum amongst students was average and recommended that the orientation programme be extended. In addition, COMCARD identified that not all departments undertook regular formative assessments, and this led UIMSA and some student-led faith organisations to organise mock examinations. They also engaged resident doctors to hold tutorials and practise objective structured clinical examinations (OSCE) and picture test sessions for the students. The association also started a student-mentoring scheme which links students in the pre-clinical classes to student mentors in the clinical classes to complement the efforts of the College mentoring programme with faculty members.

The new curriculum also offered medical students unique opportunities to participate in research by mandating them to submit Term Papers from individual and group research projects. The students capitalised on these opportunities to develop Term Papers into research presentations under the guidance of faculty mentors. This was further enhanced by the cordial relationship between the students and the alumni. Indeed, one alumni set established the College Research and Innovation Hub (CRIH) which was an outlet where students and lecturers can collaborate on research and publish their findings.

A sore point for the students is what they consider to be the partial implementation of the change from the 'closed marking' system of the old curriculum to the 'open marking' system of the new curriculum by their teachers who they perceive still practise the 'closed marking' system and are thus unwilling to give high marks even when deserved. This, they surmise, puts students at a double disadvantage which makes it difficult for them to attain the distinction mark of 80% in the new curriculum (especially in clinical subjects) as opposed to the 70% which was the distinction mark in the old curriculum.

7   Conclusions

Our experience of implementing the transition from a traditional to a CBME curriculum in the University of Ibadan Medical School confirms the assertion that curriculum change can only succeed when the administrators and faculty are fully committed to the process. At the Ibadan Medical and Dental School, the support garnered from all stakeholders and the commitment of those charged with coordinating the implementation and their ability to respond to the various challenges encountered during the process with a combination of diplomacy, tact and innovation, contributed significantly to making the change of benefit to all.

The ranking of the medical school has improved considerably in recent years and the number of students and graduates winning international prizes and awards has increased. Another indication of the success of the transition is the adoption of the curriculum as the template for the National University Commission's 2022 Core Curriculum Minimum Academic Standards for all university undergraduate courses in Nigeria, and by several medical schools across Africa and Asia. The HPTL funding model has also been adopted by several government-owned universities nationwide. We therefore hope that these outcomes will encourage other sub-Saharan medical schools to revise their curriculum periodically.

VI.iii COMMENTARY: Theorising Curriculum Change: Decolonisation, Resistance and Moving the Locus of Control

Janet Grant and Leonard Grant

The account of successful curriculum change in their medical school in Nigeria, given by E. Oluwabunmi Olapade-Olaopa and his colleagues, gives us the opportunity to discuss broader issues: decolonisation, resistance and moving the locus of control. These ideas underpin the work that was conducted to change the curriculum at the University of Ibadan.

The Global Politics of Modernisation

We have seen in other chapters throughout this book, that ideas in medical education tend to originate in the global north, as did competency-based education which medical education itself was relatively late in adopting (Hodge, 2007; ten Cate, 2017). Where those ideas are adopted in the global south (which is itself a term associated with anti-colonial and anti-imperialist movements (Mungwini, 2024)), they are accompanied by contextual and cultural challenges and by the ever-present struggle against the continuation of assumptions about colonial power structures. This introduces a tension between modernisation and the rational and conscious development of each country within its own history and values. In this chapter, we see how one school in Nigeria navigated these contradictions by taking the global north idea of a competency-based curriculum which suited their purposes for change, and consciously using those ideas entirely within the framework of their own context. The authors of this chapter are acutely aware of the colonial influences on their previous curriculum, and the need to fit with their own socio-cultural norms. They describe this succinctly in their statement:

> Despite its colonial history, medical instruction in sub-Saharan Africa has always required innovative adaptation of medical education methods to suit the peculiarities of the local teaching and learning environments, and socio-cultural norms.

After considerable reflection, they chose to implement the currently dominant competency-based medical education model, which they felt would enable them to meet local needs. And they did so with full awareness that this was a model which had to become their own (Olapade-Olaopa et al., 2016; 2024).

So far, this story could be told of many places. But the account given by these authors is unique in this book. It provides insight into the potential for curriculum review to be the site of anti-colonial resistance when a country is expanding away from colonial oversight and is claiming the territory—in this case, a curriculum model—for itself. We have an account of a project that established its own identity and locus, declining offers of assistance from schools in the US and UK who wanted to collaborate. For the leaders of this project, it was important to protect their 'intellectual property rights' over their new curriculum. Being a competency-based curriculum is less important than being a curriculum for a Nigerian school. A competency-based model just happened to work for this purpose.

We can understand from the account, how the authors took control of the process for their purposes. And we can see the managed change that was conducted. This commentary, therefore, can place these within the theoretical frameworks of decolonisation and change management.

Decolonisation from the Key Perspective

The movement to decolonise the curriculum has been widely adopted across higher education in the United Kingdom, not least because of an awareness of its own oppressive colonising history. Although decolonising education had been part of the struggle since the start of colonialism, the specific 'decolonising the curriculum' movement (which started in 2016) was predominantly in Africa, Britain and America. And what we see in the account given by Oluwabunmi Olapade-Olaopa and his colleagues, is part of this drive to decolonise their curriculum, and establish a medical education that is fit for their purposes.

The question of control over education has lasted as long as colonialism itself. Indigenous, First Nations and the people of Africa and Asia in particular, have engaged in contestations over the curriculum since the start of colonisation (Stanek, 2019). Linda Tuhiwai Smith first published "Decolonizing Methodologies" in 1999 (Smith, 2012) and themes of decoloniality and education run through the work of many decolonial scholars (Fanon, 1963; Lugones, 2010; Maldonado-Torres, 2017; Said, 1978; Tuck & Yang, 2012). All of this work links coloniality to power, knowledge and being. Bhambra identifies the university of the global north as a "key site through which colonialism—and colonial knowledge in particular—is produced, consecrated, institutionalised and naturalised" (Bhambra et al., 2018) through which enormous violence has been perpetrated. This history makes the desire of our authors to develop their own curriculum, from within their own context, even more understandable and significant.

More recently, the question of the coloniality of the curriculum has been expressed through the movement to decolonise the curriculum which started in earnest with student protests in South Africa in 2015 and 2016 (Dennis, 2018; Le Grange, 2016) from which developed #RhodesMustFall and #FeesMustFall. In Britain, decolonising the curriculum first gained traction at the University of Oxford in 2015. At the same time, another student-led movement, *Why is my curriculum white?*, started in 2015 by students at University College London (Peters, 2015; Sian, 2019), drew attention to the dominance of white, Eurocentric curriculum material. This particular movement, despite both originating and being predominantly a movement of the global south (especially in Africa), has itself been somewhat colonised. The literature overrepresents the calls from the global north (Oti & Ncayiyana, 2021) thus suggesting that practitioners and educators from the global south have not been involved in these conversations. However, as we see from these authors, whose work predates the *Decolonising the Curriculum* movement, they have no choice but to take action, to develop their curriculum away from and against colonial influence.

Designing the Curriculum

Curriculum design is a relatively limited and consistent field, whereby decisions are made about the overall purpose of the curriculum, how its specific intended achievements will be identified and expressed, how the curriculum will be organised, what educational experiences will be offered, what the assessment system will be, and how the curriculum will be evaluated (Grant, 2019). There is no evidence to guide us about how to conduct each of these stages and elements. The decision to be made is therefore a choice between replication of what others have done or being inspired to find one's own contextual path, using what is helpful from other contexts. Where contexts different from those in which the ideas originated try to replicate an idea, the appropriateness and success of that replication are limited. Others have considered these choices and have concluded that:

> In international development, a one-size-fits-all way of thinking and doing is a recipe for disaster. Of course, principles matter. But success requires seeing things as they are....and finding context-appropriate solutions to problems—not imposing practice from the Global North onto the Global South.
> Nevertheless, it is possible for ideas from the Global North to be adapted and utilised in the Global South in ways that can be helpful. (Bagree, 2024)

Independent use and adaptation are what the authors' account demonstrates in practice, showing that:

> A curriculum is an ideological, social and aspirational statement that should reflect local circumstances and needs. (Grant, 2019)

That reflection is the decolonising process in the site where it is most relevant: in this case, in Nigeria, which had been ruled by the British as a colony from the mid-nineteenth century until 1960 when Nigeria gained independence.

Developing a New Locus of Control

Throughout this book, we have repeatedly stated that the flow of ideas in medical education is from global north to global south. This is true in other fields such as design research where the same variables of inequality are at work: power dynamics and hierarchy, trust, and the acceptance of multiple and contextual truths (Grant & Grant, 2022; Tsekleves et al., 2020). That directional flow is interrupted when the undisputed locus of control is within that site of the change itself. In globalised medical education, we do not often see that locus of control so clearly established as it was in the project described by the authors of this chapter. The control was securely sited within the University of Ibadan, ensuring contextually appropriate curriculum development:

> Curriculum trends are not evidence-based but are social and philosophical. So each country and institution must build its own, on the basis of its own culture, context and needs … But medical education research, which is derivative of educational research as a whole, does not tell us what any curriculum should say. Only a locally owned process made on the basis of negotiation and professional judgement will lead to a relevant curriculum. (Grant et al., 2013)

The origin of the curriculum model in the global north, is not as important as the way in which the chosen design is locally owned and contextually implemented. (Wong, 2011).

The curriculum change process described in this chapter illustrates that an accommodation can be made between the global discourse of curriculum, and the culturalist perspective which demands that context must be the primary consideration (Wong, 2011).

A similar story of tension between visionary modernisation with a global orientation and pragmatic modernisation with a local orientation (Hallsén & Nordin, 2020), or between modernity and cultural tradition, could be told in education at all levels (Johnson, 2018). In many medical schools, especially in low- and middle-income countries:

> There is a constant tension between a vision of education promoted by medical educators, based on contextually non-specific ideas such as those found in the medical education literature, and the sociopolitical foundations and forces that are unique to each country (Segouin & Hodges, 2005).

There is a further tension that the authors of this chapter consciously navigated. In contexts where resources are severely limited, the issue of funding and support might mean acquiring these from external sources, while maintaining the contextual perspective. External funding and collaborations were necessary for the University of Ibadan, given the scale of the changes being managed. In other fields, external funding has had the effect of changing dominant purposes by, for example, requiring demonstrable impacts rather than valuing intrinsic academic merit (Grove, 2017), and decreasing the agency of researchers (Lind et al., 2019). While acquiring external funding was essential, the authors were also aware that:

> …one cannot exclude the fact that because the processes were largely funded externally, external forces may have influenced the changes. (Kiguli-Malwadde et al., 2014)

This is a contradiction that many agencies must navigate (Lind et al., 2019). Being aware of it will decrease its effect.

The Reality of Change

The account presented of a large-scale curriculum change at The College of Medicine, University of Ibadan, is not only an account of developing ownership of an idea, but is also an honest and informative case study in change management. The authors teach us some key lessons.

The approach to change management which the authors describe, is very like the effective research-based model of change in medical education (Gale & Grant, 1997). The key issue, both for decolonisation and for contextual relevance, is that the leaders of the change were part of the institution within which the change would occur. They established the institutional need for change, ensured that they had the power to act, consulted with stakeholders throughout the process, designed the change, consulted widely, and agreed detailed plans. They offered support throughout. But challenges still remained, as they always will, especially in locations where resources are severely constrained (Kiguli-Malwadde et al., 2014). It would be rash to expect change to progress smoothly and to endure in such complex circumstances. The master of the craft is not the one who encounters no problems, but is the one who analyses, addresses and solves those problems through contextual understanding, and continues to provide informed support throughout.

Change managers who are also peers, who are part of the context and culture, are at a distinct advantage, as we have seen in this account. This is so because whenever there is a division between who creates policies and who enacts them, there is an inherent preserve of power (Navarro, 1978) which presents challenges for change managers. That division, in this case study, was minimal.

This detailed account of the progress and challenges of curriculum change, even when well-managed, tells us that change is a difficult process, wherever it occurs. There will always be issues of gain and loss, of ownership, leadership and power (Grant & Gale, 1989). We have read that lack of preparedness and faculty resistance were uppermost on the problem list, closely followed by lack of facilities, infrastructure, funding, strikes, and the disruption of COVID19. Conversely, we have also seen that the support of students (who would, after all, be the main beneficiaries of the change) was a key factor.

In all of this, two essential factors emerge: immersion in the institution in which the change was to occur, and skill in managing that change. Identity of a change as being essentially integral to the institution, and not imported or imposed, are fundamental to success: it is a matter of ownership.

Creating a local, contextual version of the ideas of a global movement, can prove to be rewarding: the global ranking of the authors' medical school considerably increased. But it can also be a problem. The practical issues that the authors and their colleagues had to face often tell us about more than the progress of the idea, as theorists in the politics of curriculum state:

> We believe that context really matters and that understanding of the resources available in specific conditions and circumstances is essential in assessing the possibilities for productive politics in the face of globalising trends and forces (Ozga & Lingard, 2007).

Modernisation and Resistance

In the previous two chapters, we discuss the politics of curriculum design and curriculum change from the point of view of power relationships between different disciplines and between different specialties. In other accounts, the power struggles are located between different groups and sections of society. But in this chapter, the power struggle is between old, colonially imposed but now settled practices, and new global ideas being applied locally. The authors show that '… cultural and social effects of globalisation may foreground and render explicit *local* assumptions and beliefs that were previously hidden or inexplicit'. These may be expressed as a 'collective narrative' asserting cultural and social identity (Ozga & Lingard, 2007).

The authors of this case study, as leaders of the intended change, were acutely aware of the need to take their context and culture into account (Segouin & Hodges, 2005). But even though the authors managed the change in a textbook manner, they were still surprised by this clash of ideas, that manifested itself in what they term 'resistance'. In many examples of change, resistance is an understandable response which does not reflect the value of the change itself, but the worries of those who will have to change.

It has been pointed out that:

> Some of the common causes of resistance include fear of the unknown or only partially understood, fear of becoming unskilled in an area where people were previously skilled (for example, where new teaching methods are introduced), lack of agreement with the need for change, protection of vested interest, poor timing, a threat to security. (Grant & Gale, 1989)

The idea of resistance is an important one. In change processes, it is often thought of as a barrier to be overcome. But 'resistance' contains the elements by which we can analyse the dominant discourse and its relationship to the status quo and to oppositional, emergent or alternative ideas (Williams, 1980). That analysis, in turn, might assist the progress of a managed change by enabling the change leader to address more effectively the design of the project and the consultation around that (Gale & Grant, 1997). To do this, we must regard resistance as rational attachment to the status quo. It is for that reason that the tactics of a change manager, as we have seen, must include consultation, negotiation, explanation, analysis, recognition of problems and support or reward for those who need it (Gale & Grant, 1997).

Resistance is not a sign of poorly managed change. It is simply a part of the ever-changing landscape of education. Ideas about curriculum constantly change, as social ideas and global powerplays change:

> Curriculum is continually contested, and both curriculum policies and practices are not only made, but unmade and remade by numerous official and unofficial education policy-makers and practitioners. (Cornbleth, 2000a)

The account provided in this chapter tells us that CBME, like many other forms of curriculum, can deliver the outcomes required by a community, while the process might not be appreciated by all those who are required to deliver this curriculum. Different stakeholders have different perspectives, and those who 'resist' change may do so for different reasons, each of which is valid in its own terms.

The Politics of Curriculum Change: Globalisation and Colonisation

The account offered by the authors of this chapter, shows that the adoption of a 'global' (global north) idea can be done successfully in the global south, although not without challenges. Their acute awareness of the colonial history helped them in framing their approach and asserting their independence. But the account implies, and its authors suggest, some more fundamental questions about the role of the 'medical education movement', globalisation and colonisation.

The account offered by the authors of this chapter demonstrates a critical pragmatism whereby that 'attention to practice, action, context, and consequence are inextricably theoretical and practical' (Cornbleth, 2000b). Their account is one of local responses to a general curriculum idea. Those responses which have been termed 'resistance' are absolutely rational in their own terms, and are to be expected. In this, we must recognise:

> … the importance of local politics and culture and tradition and the processes of interpretation and struggle involved in translating these generic solutions into practical policies and institutional practices. (Ball, 2007)

These issues highlight the tension between what has been called 'travelling' (supra- and transnational activity) and 'embedded' policy where global policy agendas (in our case, derived from a wider medical education movement) come up against existing priorities and practices at local level (Ozga & Lingard, 2007). The challenge for those in this global movement who are from the global south, to apply ideas to their context and maintain their position in the global movement, is described in this chapter. Their awareness of colonial influence on their previous curriculum, could be mirrored in the global influence on their new one, but their awareness of 'travelling policy' deflected that possibility.

What the authors describe is a very special effort by Africans for Africa, to improve medical instruction on the continent by breaking away from the colonial curriculum they inherited 62 years previously, and by developing a method of medical instruction that was fully homegrown and directed at local health needs. This curriculum, developed in this way has been accepted, wholly or in part, by other medical schools in at least eight countries within Africa and in Asia. It now serves as the template for the recently published Core Curriculum Minimum Academic Standards for all undergraduate curricula in Nigeria.

As one of the authors has written:

> I would counsel against the wholesale adoption of any new system in use elsewhere. …
> each medical school must develop its own curriculum to suit its society and students.
> (Olapade-Olaopa, 2006)

The power of local ownership and leadership, of understanding context and culture is a challenge to the idea and promotion of globalisation.

References

Bagree, S. (2024). Inspiration not replication: Sharing ideas from the Global North to South. *Culturico*. https://culturico.com/2024/03/29/inspiration-not-replication-sharing-ideas-from-the-global-north-to-south/

Ball, S. J. (2007). Big policies/Small world. An introduction to international perspectives in education policy. In B. Lingard & J. Ozga (Eds.), *The RoutledgeFalmer Reader in education policy and politics* (pp. 36–47). Routledge.

Bhambra, G. K., Gebrial, D., & Nişancıoğlu, K. (2018). Introduction: Decolonising the university? In G. K. Bhambra, D. Gebrial, & K. Nişancıoğlu (Eds.), *Decolonising the university*. Pluto Press.

Cornbleth, C. (2000a). National standards and curriculum as cultural containment? In *Curriculum politics, policy, practice. Cases in comparative context* (pp. 211–238). State University of New York Press.

Cornbleth, C. (2000b). Viewpoints. In *Curriculum politics, policy, practice: Cases in comparative context* (pp. 1–20). State University of New York Press.

Dennis, C. A. (2018). Decolonising education: A pedagogical intervention. In G. K. Bhambra, D. Gebrial, & K. Nişancıoğlu (Eds.), *Decolonising the university*. Pluto Press.

Fanon, F. (1963). *The wretched of the earth*. Grove.

Gale, R., & Grant, J. (1997). AMEE Medical Education Guide No. 10: Managing change in a medical context: Guidelines for an action. *Medical Teacher, 19*(4), 239–249.

Grant, J. (2019). Principles of curriculum design. In T. Swanwick, K. Forrest, & B. O'Brien (Eds.), *Understanding medical education: Evidence, theory and practice* (pp. 71–88). Wiley Blackwell.

Grant, J., Abdelrahman, M. Y. H., & Zachariah, A. (2013). Curriculum design in context. In K. Walsh (Ed.), *Oxford textbook of medical education* (pp. 13–24). Oxford University Press.

Grant, J., & Gale, R. (1989). Changing medical education. *Medical Education, 23*(3), 252–257. https://doi.org/10.1111/j.1365-2923.1989.tb01540.x

Grant, J., & Grant, L. (2022). Quality and constructed knowledge: Truth, paradigms, and the state of the science. *Medical Education*. https://doi.org/10.1111/medu.14871

Grove, L. (2017). *The effects of funding policies on academic research* [UCL]. https://eprints.lse.ac.uk/88207/1/Grove_Thesis_2017.pdf

Hallsén, S., & Nordin, A. (2020). Variations on modernisation: Technological development and internationalisation in local Swedish school policy from 1950 to 2000. *Scandinavian Journal of Educational Research, 64*(2), 151–166. https://doi.org/10.1080/00313831.2018.1524396

Hodge, S. (2007). The origins of competency-based training. *Australian Journal of Adult Learning, 47*(2), 179–209.

Johnson, D. (2018). Bhutan: Politics, culture and the modernization of education. In H. Letchamanan & D. Debotri (Eds.), *Education in South Asia and the Indian Ocean Islands* (pp. 69–86). Bloomsbury Academic. https://ora.ox.ac.uk/objects/uuid:a3bad9fe-0483-4f9a-acfe-b40946c0c223/files/rg732d933m

Kiguli-Malwadde, E., Omaswa, F., & Olapade-Olaopa, oluwabunmi, Kiguli, S., Chen, C., Sewankambo, N., Ogunniyi, A., & Mukwaya, S. (2014). Competency-based medical education in two Sub-Saharan African medical schools. *Advances in Medical Education and Practice, 483*. https://doi.org/10.2147/AMEP.S68480

Le Grange, L. (2016). Decolonising the university curriculum. *South African Journal of Higher Education, 30*(2). https://doi.org/10.20853/30-2-709

Lind, J. K., Hernes, H., Pulkkinen, K., & Söderlind, J. (2019). External research funding and authority relations. In R. Pinheiro, L. Geschwind, H. Foss Hansen, & K. Pulkkinen (Eds.), *Reforms, Organizational Change and Performance in Higher Education*. Springer Nature. https://doi.org/10.1007/978-3-030-11738-2_5

Lugones, M. (2010). Toward a decolonial feminism. *Hypatia, 25*(4), 742–759. https://doi.org/10.1111/j.1527-2001.2010.01137.x

Maldonado-Torres, N. (2017). Frantz Fanon and the decolonial turn in psychology: From modern/colonial methods to the decolonial attitude. *South African Journal of Psychology, 47*(4), 432–441. https://doi.org/10.1177/0081246317737918

Mungwini, P. (2024). The global South framework and African philosophy: Epistemologies and struggles for emancipation. *African Identities, 1–16.* https://doi.org/10.1080/1472584 3.2024.2442630

Navarro, V. (1978). Class struggle, the State and medicine: An historical and contemporary analysis of the medical sector in Great Britain. In *Capital & Class* (Vol. Issue 2). https://doi. org/10.1177/030981687900800109

Olapade-Olaopa, E. O. (2006). College of Medicine, University of Ibadan, 2004 College Lecture 'Curriculum change and the College of Medicine, University of Ibadan'. *African Journal of Medicine and Medical Sciences, 35*(3), 395–405.

Olapade-Olaopa, O., Adaramoye, O., Raji, Y., Fasola, A. O., & Olapade, F. (2016). Developing a competency-based medical education curriculum for the core basic medical sciences in an African Medical School. *Advances in Medical Education and Practice, 7*, 389–398. https://doi. org/10.2147/AMEP.S100660

Olapade-Olaopa, E. O., Fasola, A. O., Agunloye, A., Ogunbiyi, A., Odukogbe, A. A., & Ogunniyi, A. O. (2024). Revising a 60-year-old medical and dental curriculum in a medical school in Sub-Saharan Africa. *African Journal of Medicine and Medical Sciences, 53*(1), 21–31.

Oti, S. O., & Ncayiyana, J. (2021). Decolonising global health: Where are the Southern voices? *BMJ Global Health, 6*(7), e006576. https://doi.org/10.1136/bmjgh-2021-006576

Ozga, J., & Lingard, B. (2007). Globalisation, education policy and politics. In B. Lingard & J. Ozga (Eds.), *The RoutledgeFalmer Reader in Education Policy and Politics* (pp. 65–82). Routledge.

Peters, M. A. (2015). Why is my curriculum white? *Educational Philosophy and Theory, 47*(7), 641–646. https://doi.org/10.1080/00131857.2015.1037227

Said, E. (1978). *Orientalism: Western concepts of the Orient.* Pantheon.

Segouin, C., & Hodges, B. (2005). Educating doctors in France and Canada: Are the differences based on evidence or history? *Medical Education, 39*(12), 1205–1212. https://doi. org/10.1111/j.1365-2929.2005.02334.x

Sian, K. P. (2019). *Navigating institutional racism in British universities. Springer International Publishing.* https://doi.org/10.1007/978-3-030-14284-1

Smith, L. T. (2012). *Decolonizing methodologies: Research and indigenous peoples* (2nd ed.). Zed Books.

Stanek, M. B. (2019). Decolonial education and geography: Beyond the 2017 Royal Geographical Society with the Institute of British Geographers annual conference. *Geography Compass, 13*(12). https://doi.org/10.1111/gec3.12472

ten Cate, O. (2017). Competency-based postgraduate medical education: Past, present and future. *GMS Journal for Medical Education, 34*(5) https://pmc.ncbi.nlm.nih.gov/articles/ PMC5704607/pdf/JME-34-69.pdf

Tsekleves, E., Darby, A., Ahorlu, C., Pickup, R., de Souza, D., & Boakye, D. (2020). Challenges and opportunities in conducting and applying design research beyond global north to the global south. In S. Boess, M. Cheung, & R. Cain (Eds.), *Synergy - DRS International Conference 2020, 11-14 August.* https://doi.org/10.21606/drs.2020.145

Tuck, E., & Yang, K. W. (2012). Decolonization is not a metaphor. *Decolonization: Indigeneity, Education & Society, 1*(1) Available at: https://jps.library.utoronto.ca/index.php/des/article/ view/18630

Williams, R. (1980). *Culture and materialism: Selected essays* (Paperback edition). Verso.

Wong, A. K. (2011). Culture in medical education: Comparing a Thai and a Canadian residency programme. *Medical Education, 45*(12), 1209–1219. https://doi.org/10.1111/j.1365-2923 .2011.04059.x

VI.iv STATEMENT: Bedside Teaching: Understanding Which Tails Wag the Dog

Vanessa C. Burch, Savarra Mantzor, and Tonya Arscott-Mills

1 What Is the Problem?

Bedside teaching, which provides an opportunity for practising clinicians to engage in clinical reasoning and problem-solving, is an integral part of undergraduate and postgraduate medical training (Guilbert, 2006; Mokone et al., 2014; Steinert et al., 2006). It offers opportunities for role modelling and the integration and learning of important clinical skills (Peters & Ten Cate, 2013). The sharp decline in bedside teaching in recent decades has been attributed to increasing patient loads, time constraints, and clinical staff who are not trained and do not feel confident to conduct teaching at the bedside (LaCombe, 1997; Nair et al., 1998).

To preserve and sustain the practice of bedside teaching, new teaching approaches have been developed to foster more teacher-learner interaction (Neher et al., 1992; Wolpaw et al., 2003). These approaches have been developed and researched in the global north while implementation in the global south has only been discussed in a limited way (Guilbert, 2006).

The authors of this reflection are clinicians working and teaching at the bedside in South Africa. They each have experience in high-level management and administration roles within universities and medical institutions. They all have substantial experience working and teaching in both the global north and south.

V. C. Burch (✉)
Colleges of Medicine of South Africa, Johannesburg, South Africa
e-mail: Vanessa.Burch@cmsa.co.za

S. Mantzor
Full Circle Health, Pediatrics Residency of Idaho, Boise, ID, USA

T. Arscott-Mills
Department of Pediatrics, Levine Children's Hospital, Wake Forest University School of Medicine, Charlotte, NC, USA

© The Author(s), under exclusive license to Springer Nature Switzerland AG 2026
J. Grant, L. Grant (eds.), *The Contradictions of Medical Education*,
https://doi.org/10.1007/978-3-031-90394-6_21

This chapter explores the challenges we encountered when we introduced a new approach to bedside teaching at a large teaching hospital in the global south. Our insights may contribute to a broader understanding of the controversies that surround this cornerstone of medical education. This approach, referred to as SNAPPS (Wolpaw et al., 2003) involves six steps:

- **S**ummarize history and findings
- **N**arrow differentials
- **A**nalyse differentials
- **P**robe preceptor about uncertainties
- **P**lan management
- **S**elect case-related issues for self-study.

2   Who Are We Talking About?

This reflection considers the trainees and medical staff working and learning in a clinical department in a large global south teaching hospital.

'Trainees' includes all undergraduate medical students and postgraduate doctors. 'Faculty' refers to a wide range of sub-specialist physicians who perform clinical duties and conduct ward rounds.

The 'setting' is an inpatient ward of a clinical department in a large tertiary training hospital. This hospital is home to most undergraduate and postgraduate medical trainees within the country.

'Clinical teaching' primarily occurs at the bedside during ward rounds, supplemented with didactic, classroom-based teaching, problem-based learning, and objective structured clinical mock exams. Ward round teams are comprised of rotating junior and senior medical students, interns, medical officers and residents. Each team is led by one faculty member.

3   What Was Done? The Challenges

During a process of reflection, the department head identified several areas for improvement, including better learner engagement in bedside teaching, standardising the conduct of ward rounds, and improving communication of goals on ward rounds. After a topic-specific review of the literature, we chose a well-studied bedside teaching approach which required more learner engagement and had the potential to address other departmental issues. This approach, while generated in the global north, had been studied and found to be effective in both global north and south clinical settings. While the original research on this model was conducted in an ambulatory setting with medical students, a subsequent review article suggested potential application within the inpatient setting (Pascoe et al., 2015). It will be seen that only after we failed to implement the new system, did we reconsider the literature from our new perspective and found gaps within the literature and how these varied from our findings.

The literature described the approach as relatively easy to learn, requiring only a brief training session of as little as 30–90 min (Fagundes et al., 2020; Wolpaw et al., 2009, 2012). Authors recommended sensitisation prior to clinical encounters, highlighting the need for both teacher and learner engagement in training (Wolpaw et al., 2003). They cautioned that teachers may need to 'coach' learners until the technique has been mastered, so while training for learners may be more extensive, the training for faculty was brief (Wolpaw et al., 2012; Wolpaw et al., 2003). Only one article cautioned that sensitisation within other cultural settings may require more extensive training (Sawanyawisuth et al., 2015), but no articles mentioned any difficulty or resistance to training or uptake of the approach.

We met with significant implementation challenges. While some faculty embraced the new approach and observed a positive effect on learning and teaching on ward rounds, most faculty requested additional training and coaching, feeling that the didactic sessions alone did not prepare them to use the model on busy ward rounds. Faculty experienced a new double burden on their ward rounds of simultaneously teaching medicine *and* implementing a new teaching method, and cited difficulty using it with junior trainees. There was ongoing tension between traditional 'teacher-dominated' ward rounds and poor uptake of the new 'learner-focused' approach. This outcome left us with a critical question: Where did our understanding of the department or planning for the introduction of this bedside teaching innovation fall short?

4   Potential Reasons for Tension

To better understand the tension, we reflected on our actions using the Consolidated Framework for Implementation Research (Damschroder et al., 2022), simplified to a four-part model shown in Fig. 1. This highlights the multiple, nested contextual factors that we encountered in the process of introducing the new approach which did and did not fully fit the norms, values, risks, needs, and workflow of the patient service.

4.1   Training in the New Bedside Teaching Method

Despite claims that the approach is relatively easy to learn and introduce in clinical settings, we found ongoing challenges for both faculty and trainees. While the basic concepts were easily communicated during didactic teaching sessions, ultimately, we found that knowledge of the method was superficial. Participants lacked the necessary skills and confidence to use the method and requested additional training to bridge the gap between theory and application on ward rounds. While faculty reported positively on the perceived helpfulness of the approach to bedside teaching, their use of it was limited. This unanticipated gap resulted in nearly all faculty reverting to a traditional approach to bedside teaching on ward rounds.

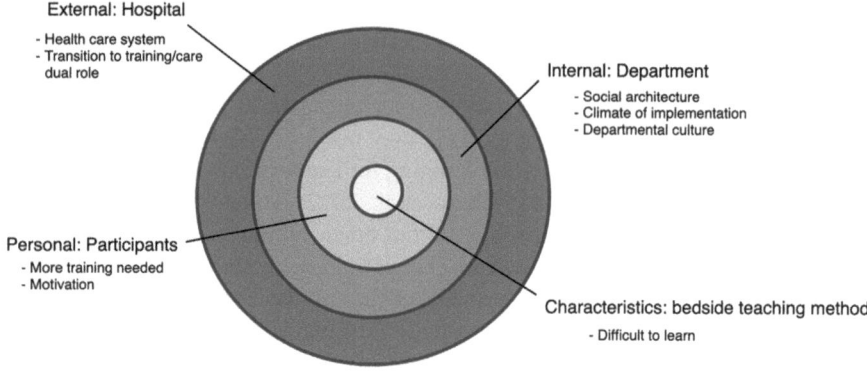

Fig. 1 Contextual factors contributing to bedside teaching tension

4.2 Participants

For faculty members not trained in or using the approach, the most cited reason for their lack of motivation to either learn or use it was competing priorities. It appeared that the effort required to learn and gain confidence in new bedside teaching skills was outweighed by an overall lack of motivation and energy to engage in the implementation process. Those who did use the approach had higher levels of intrinsic motivation to do so.

4.3 Social Architecture of the Department

Historically, the field of medicine is a centralised practice, and so it is not surprising that teachers uphold the longstanding traditions of medicine at the bedside—the senior physician conducting patient rounds with the learner limited to the role of shadowing. The approach we endeavoured to introduce required greater teacher-learner interaction. However, shifting the learner to being a central player in the ward round teaching encounter was just too large a leap. The success of the new approach, in terms of social architecture, could only have been achieved at the level of the faculty, and gaining their commitment was critical. As we saw with the poor faculty orientation attendance rates (in contrast to the excellent trainee attendance), the leverage position of the implementation team within the existing social architecture of the department, was limited by whether we were perceived to be above or below the level of the respective participants.

4.4   Tension for Change

The tension for change varied between faculty and trainees. From a faculty perspective, while there was a general sense that rounds should be more academically focused and have a more standardised approach to teaching, the level of tension was not particularly high. Self-assessment is an unreliable process wherever used (Eva & Regehr, 2005; Gordon, 1991; Kendrick et al., 2021), so unsurprisingly faculty self-evaluation of their own teaching skills was markedly higher than their peer evaluation. Faculty perceived that they were doing a better job at providing clinical teaching than others observed which perhaps partly accounted for poor faculty attendance at training sessions. On the other hand, from a trainee perspective, there was greater tension for change. Prior to implementation, trainees rated the effectiveness of learning and teaching to be low. While trainees' tension for change was greater than that of faculty, they were not able to drive change on ward rounds, limiting their overall influence on the success of the implementation of a new teaching approach.

4.5   Patient Care Versus Teaching

Patient care was clearly a departmental priority, and clinical teaching was largely valued for its potential to have an impact on *future* patient care, but clinical teaching was not viewed to necessarily improve *current* patient care. This created a tension between patient care and teaching, and faculty expressed concerns that spending time teaching could negatively affect patient care. So, of the competing priorities teaching was likely to suffer.

4.6   Culture of Centralised Authority

Due to the heterogeneity of faculty conditions of employment (hospital, local university or affiliated international universities), each faculty member essentially had a different senior to whom they were accountable. This led to a binary staff structure within the department. In turn, authority predominately resided with the most highly ranked senior clinician (i.e., department head), resulting in a model of centralised authority. Making changes within the department was therefore dependent on department head approval and support. But even then, the lack of shared influence and accountability among faculty resulted in less external motivation for behaviour change.

4.7   Culture of Frustration

Trainees described feeling frustrated by frequent challenges and influences within the healthcare system which prevented them from providing optimal patient management or making positive changes within the department. Faculty described low levels of motivation and feeling burnt out by their work in the department. This culture of frustration was aggravated by previously impeded attempts at implementation of other department initiatives, which decreased enthusiasm for new projects in the department.

4.8   Culture of Disorder

There was a sense of disorder within the department. Ward rounds, which started late and were long, negatively affected both learning opportunities and ward work duties. In addition, the structure during the ward rounds was often described as 'a bit hectic'. Frequent interruptions to the ward round were considered standard; for example, looking for a patient's file, attending to a patient emergency, placing an intravenous cannula, or looking up lab results. These frequent interruptions limited opportunities for learning and teaching.

4.9   Hospital

The relatively recent transition of the tertiary hospital into a teaching hospital created tension for faculty and learners to navigate the hospital's new two-fold function: patient care and academic practice. There were ongoing challenges to developing an understanding of and prioritising trainees' clinical learning needs within the historical context of the hospital. For instance, clinical teaching became the assumed role of the practising physician. This assumption created tensions and resulted in physicians feeling unsupported in their new dual role of simultaneously providing patient care and clinical teaching. Perhaps it was assumed by the hospital and the university that clinicians would know how to teach, and that they would seamlessly integrate patient care and academic teaching in a clinical environment. However, this translated into an academically challenging environment filled with tensions between the priorities of practising medicine and teaching the practice of medicine.

5   What Can Be Done?

The challenges we encountered in our attempt to introduce a new bedside teaching approach are likely to be relevant in other settings with similar ambitions. Based on our experience, what would we suggest?

5.1   Awareness of the Social Architecture

Critical review of our practice showed that making a major change on ward rounds is only likely to succeed if the change is aligned with the existing social architecture of the clinical space. Since many clinical training environments are still structured as vertical hierarchies, it is likely that the introduction of a bedside teaching approach which requires greater learner engagement may meet with similar controversies elsewhere. We recommend that this architecture be reviewed and given careful consideration when selecting bedside teaching strategies are being considered for implementation.

5.2   Real-Time Coaching at the Bedside

In addition to didactic sensitisation of faculty and trainees to new bedside teaching methods, real-time coaching to bridge the gap between theory and practice may ensure that new teaching skills are embedded at the bedside.

5.3   Stepwise Introduction

While the didactic portion of faculty and trainee orientation could familiarise participants with all the aspects of the bedside teaching approach, we suggest that bedside coaching be structured so that the approach is learned and practised in incremental steps, focusing on a single step until it is mastered before moving onto the next step.

5.4   Faculty-Trainee Teaching Pairs

Another useful strategy may be a process of assigning faculty-trainee pilot testing dyads to assist in the implementation process and ensure that the roles of faculty in guiding the process and of trainees in thinking through the clinical problem, are well understood. Furthermore, these pilot testing dyads could help identify some of the broader issues relevant to the challenges of implementing new bedside teaching strategies in complex clinical learning environments.

6   Conclusion

Bedside teaching is a cornerstone in the education of medical doctors, and bedside teaching models which aim to enhance learner engagement in the process may be an important step in the right direction. However, our experience shows the necessity of identifying and addressing challenges in the clinical environment in order to maximise opportunities for sustaining the critical practice of bedside teaching.

References

Damschroder, L. J., Reardon, C. M., Opra Widerquist, M. A., & Lowery, J. (2022). Conceptualizing outcomes for use with the Consolidated Framework for Implementation Research (CFIR): The CFIR Outcomes Addendum. *Implementation Science*, *17*(1). https://doi.org/10.1186/S13012-021-01181-5

Eva, K. W., & Regehr, G. (2005). Self-assessment in the health professions: A reformulation and research agenda. *Academic Medicine*, *80*(Supplement), S46–S54. https://doi.org/10.1097/00001888-200510001-00015

Fagundes, E. D. T., Ibiapina, C. C., Alvim, C. G., Fernandes, R. A. F., Carvalho-Filho, M. A., & Brand, P. L. P. (2020). Case presentation methods: A randomized controlled trial of the one-minute preceptor versus SNAPPS in a controlled setting. *Perspectives on Medical Education*, *9*(4), 245–250. https://doi.org/10.1007/S40037-020-00588-Y

Gordon, M. J. (1991). A review of the validity and accuracy of self-assessments in health professions training. *Academic Medicine*, *66*(12), 762–769. https://doi.org/10.1097/00001888-199112000-00012

Guilbert, J.-J. (2006). The World Health report 2006 1 : Working together for health 2. *Education for Health: Change in Learning & Practice*, *19*(3), 385–387. https://doi.org/10.1080/13576280600937911

Kendrick, D. E., Clark, M. J., Fischer, I., Bohnen, J. D., Kim, G. J., & George, B. C. (2021). The reliability of resident self-evaluation of operative performance. *The American Journal of Surgery*, *222*(2), 341–346. https://doi.org/10.1016/j.amjsurg.2020.11.054

LaCombe, M. A. (1997). On bedside teaching. *Annals of Internal Medicine*, *126*(3), 217. https://doi.org/10.7326/0003-4819-126-3-199702010-00007

Mokone, G. G., Kebaetse, M., Wright, J., Kebaetse, M. B., Makgabana-Dintwa, O., Kebaabetswe, P., Badlangana, L., Mogodi, M., Bryant, K., & Nkomazana, O. (2014). Establishing a new medical school: Botswana's experience. *Academic Medicine*, *89*(Supplement), S83–S87. https://doi.org/10.1097/ACM.0000000000000329

Nair, B. R., Coughlan, J., & Hensley, M. (1998). Impediments to bed-side teaching. *Medical Education*, *32*(2), 159–162. https://doi.org/10.1046/j.1365-2923.1998.00185.x

Neher, J. O., Gordon, K. C., Meyer, B., & Stevens, N. (1992). A five-step 'microskills' model of clinical teaching. *The Journal of the American Board of Family Practice*, *5*(4), 419–424.

Pascoe, J. M., Nixon, J., & Lang, V. J. (2015). Maximizing teaching on the wards: Review and application of the One-Minute Preceptor and SNAPPS models. *Journal of Hospital Medicine*, *10*(2), 125–130. https://doi.org/10.1002/jhm.2302

Peters, M., & Ten Cate, O. (2013). Bedside teaching in medical education: A literature review. *Perspectives on Medical Education*, *3*(2), 76–88. https://doi.org/10.1007/S40037-013-0083-Y

Sawanyawisuth, K., Schwartz, A., Wolpaw, T., & Bordage, G. (2015). Expressing clinical reasoning and uncertainties during a Thai internal medicine ambulatory care rotation: Does the SNAPPS technique generalize? *Medical Teacher*, *37*(4), 379–384. https://doi.org/10.310 9/0142159X.2014.947942

Steinert, Y., Mann, K., Centeno, A., Dolmans, D., Spencer, J., Gelula, M., & Prideaux, D. (2006). A systematic review of faculty development initiatives designed to improve teaching effectiveness in medical education: BEME Guide No. 8. *Medical Teacher*, *28*(6), 497–526. https://doi. org/10.1080/01421590600902976

Wolpaw, T., Côté, L., Papp, K. K., & Bordage, G. (2012). Student uncertainties drive teaching during case presentations. *Academic Medicine*, *87*(9), 1210–1217. https://doi.org/10.1097/ ACM.0b013e3182628fa4

Wolpaw, T. M., Wolpaw, D. R., & Papp, K. K. (2003). SNAPPS: A learner-centered model for outpatient education. *Academic Medicine*, *78*(9), 893–898. https://doi. org/10.1097/00001888-200309000-00010

Wolpaw, T., Papp, K. K., & Bordage, G. (2009). Using SNAPPS to facilitate the expression of clinical reasoning and Uncertainties: A randomized comparison group trial. *Academic Medicine*, *84*(4), 517–524. https://doi.org/10.1097/ACM.0b013e31819a8cbf

VI.iv COMMENTARY: Managing Change: Power and Context

Janet Grant and Leonard Grant

The story told by the three authors of this chapter, is a history of challenges in converting ideas into practice. That history tells us that managing change in medical education must be a specific process used to overcome the problems encountered, whether of culture or context.

Drs Burch, Mantzor and Arscott-Mills point out that the new bedside teaching method they wanted to introduce was developed in the global north while they themselves are located in the global south. And although they do suggest that the hierarchical culture in which they work might inhibit learner participation in a process that requires exchange of ideas between learner and teacher, the challenges that they outline could easily occur in the global north too where there may well be equal constraints of resources, habit and opportunity, and similar models of power and influence that can facilitate or inhibit the intended new order.

They have provided a detailed analysis of what happened, and failed to happen, in their context, and have made thoughtful suggestions about how the change might have been better handled. If we locate these within a model of managed change, their experience may be even more generalisable than they suggest.

Power and context matter, as the authors of this chapter show, and respect for power and context is the basis of a well-managed change. The authors of this chapter have analysed and understood these contextual issues, but only as a result of the initial failure of the change they tried to implement. We can recast their analysis and show how it relates to the process of managed change in a medical context.

The Limits of Power and Managing Change

There are different ways of managing change:

> If sufficient power is available and it is felt that it should be used, then it is possible to adopt a directive or coercive style of change management. The gains are speed and integrity of the original idea. The costs are a possibly compliant audience with deep resentments. Lasting change can only be achieved by involving all those affected and accepting long timescales and some dilution of the original concept. (Gale & Grant, 1997)

This recognises that there are different types of power. In the case of this chapter, the department head might have identified a need for change, but if that view is not shared, each teacher's autonomous decisions about practice will always win. Other authors have sought to:

> ...emphasize the subtle and distinctive characteristics of leading professionals that are present to varying degrees within any organization of knowledge workers, where individual autonomy is enshrined within the work processes. (Empson & Langley, 2015)

It is for this reason that models of change management that derive from industry (Kotter, 1996; Schein, 1999) where there is hierarchy and the ability to compel people to comply with decisions, are not appropriate to medicine, academia or a profession, where autonomous behaviour is at the heart of practice. Even in the hierarchical structures that the authors describe (Brown, 2012):

> Staff will not engage in a change effort and the learning that goes with it unless they can personally see that doing so is relevant, desirable, clear, distinctive and, importantly, feasible. (Scott, 2004, quoted in Brown, 2012)

Effective change management might take longer because it is based on negotiation, but it will last longer. Having the vision is one thing, but managing it into place is another, as the authors of this chapter found.

The Culture of the Profession

Many of the challenges that the authors of this chapter encountered derive from the culture of the profession. It did not seem to matter that the proposed change came from the global north, but simply that it did not really fit into their already packed and settled teaching lives. In such circumstances, understanding the culture of the profession underpins successful change. That culture tends to exhibit certain characteristics and styles in the face of change, at least in the UK context (Grant & Gale, 1989):

Professional characteristics and styles	Description
Consultation	Doctors like to be consulted, usually face-to-face, about new ideas, and have their responses taken seriously
Demonstration	Doctors like to see that the innovation has been shown to work elsewhere
Evolution	Doctors prefer gradual evolution to sudden revolution
Ownership	Doctors like to feel that they have ownership of any new idea. They do not like to feel that they are implementing someone else's project
Power to hinder	Doctors rarely oppose innovations directly. They dislike confrontation and prefer to find indirect ways to hamper implementation

Professional characteristics and styles	Description
Commitment	Doctors like to see and feel commitment to a project
Energy and enthusiasm	With commitment goes the need to see energy and enthusiasm for the proposed change
Motives	Doctors like to feel that there are honest and ethical motives for any change

We can see in the account given in this chapter, that some of these were not fully taken into account, and the power of teachers to hinder, or simply to oppose in practice, determined the fate of the project.

Managing Educational Change in the Ward Round

A ward round is an instrument of patient care. It is a place where students witness patient care, or postgraduate trainees play a part which is accountable to their senior clinician. It is a 'complex social process' (Merriman & Freeth, 2022) focused on patient care. Refocusing to its educational function for medical students is, as we have seen, an unequal struggle.

It was not simply a matter of time, but also of style. Clinical teachers were used to the (still probably most common) method of talking through each case around the bedside while the students listened. Increasing pressure on ward-rounds is well-recognised and various attempts to build in structured teaching are reported (Arabshahi et al., 2015; Gray et al., 2020). What seems to emerge is that a working ward round enables a conversation between different healthcare professionals involved in caring for the patient, but adding teaching to that is a challenge and in danger of being relegated in the scramble for time.

Given this, the authors tried to train both teachers and students. Faculty development has become a common approach to managing change in medical education with some challenges in terms of encouraging teacher commitment (Donnelly et al., 2021). It has often tended to be a longitudinal process (Burgess et al., 2019), and more recently has been placed as being in need of partnership at organisational level to sustain effective development (Steinert et al., 2024). The short training for teachers described in this chapter, which was possibly trying to fit in with their available time, was perhaps unlikely to gain commitment.

In their honest analysis of the process of trying to introduce a change in teaching and learning methods, the authors set out practical advice to others about managing such changes. They suggest being aware of the hierarchy of the organisation, coaching teachers and trainees in the new method, rather than just informing them, introducing the change in stages, using trained pairs of teachers and trainees to help others.

Therefore, the authors of this chapter took a 'faculty development' approach to change which has had mixed success when used alone, rather than recognising, at the time, the organisational features which stood in the way of success (Jolly, 2014).

So perhaps we could look at this in another way and fit what the authors of this chapter did into a wider approach to managing change specifically in a medical context.

A Managed Approach to Change: Power to Act

The only research-based change model specifically for medicine has 10 stages that can be passed through at varying speeds. At each stage there is a core activity to be undertaken and options that the change manager has in terms of the tactics employed or the leadership or management style adopted, as follows (Gale & Grant, 1997):

Core activities	Tactical choices and styles
1. Establish the need for or benefit from the change	Lobbying, conjunction of circumstances, consultation, avoid selling solutions
2. Ensure the power to act	Key people, local environment, authority, borrowed power, external power, personal position
3. Design the change	Feasibility, resources, timing, involvement, scale, style, scope, predicting pathways and barriers
4. Consult widely	Appropriateness, leadership, talking and explaining about the changes
5. Publicise widely	Presentation, communication, vision, amending proposals
6. Agree detailed plans	Detailed plans, detailed instructions
7. Implement the plans	Demonstration projects, pathways and barriers, implementation strategy, task mode
8. Provide support	Resistance, maintaining change, overcoming difficulties, objections
9. Modify plans	Compensation, modifications
10. Evaluate outcomes	Evaluation strategy, key result variables

We can see from this, that power within the context is at the heart of the model. It accepts that a medical teacher has the power to act as they choose within their own teaching, as our authors found. The power to act of the change manager is also important: is that power borrowed from a person senior in the hierarchy (as was the case in the account given in this chapter), or does power derive from elsewhere? Is that power personal, positional, reputational, relational, recognised and accepted? Is the position of the leader accepted?

Whether the change envisaged is one created in one part of the globe (the global north, in this case), while attempting implementation in another (the global south, in this case, as is normally the case with changes in medical education), or whether the change, unusually for medical education, has been designed locally, the same issues will arise. Managing change is a political process in that it must understand and contend with power structures. The model of change in medicine does not suggest altering those power structures, but acknowledging and working with them. The power, and power relationships, of physicians have been widely discussed and analysed both in relation to the doctor-patient relationship and in relation to the power relationship between doctors (Bochatay et al., 2021; Hancock, 2018; Nimmon & Stenfors-Hayes, 2016; Saxena et al., 2019; Vanstone & Grierson, 2022). Power is at the heart of the profession and of the organisation: those power structures might not align.

Managing Change Is Managing People

Managing change in medicine must not only take organisational factors into account, but must recognise that change management is an interpersonal process. It must recognise the emotional reactions that those who are required to change might have. That process requires the change manager to establish that there is a need to change, and that the suggested way forward is the right one. Through open stages of negotiation, consultation, planning, implementation, support and adjustment, the purpose is not to change the power relationships, but to work with them to ensure that the power of those who are the focus of the change is used to support it:

> People need help to assume new roles and relationships, they need support and encouragement. (Gale & Grant, 1997)

People do not naturally resist change: they just find ways of not implementing changes that they do not value or that threaten them or their position, and perhaps their self-worth. In such circumstances, medical educators have many ways of not changing, as we have seen, and some of these will be justified and will cause the sort of productive reflection that this chapter has offered. Power and context must be at the heart of that analysis.

References

Arabshahi, K. S., Haghani, F., Bigdeli, S., Omid, A., & Adibi, P. (2015). Challenges of the ward round teaching based on the experiences of medical clinical teachers. *Journal of Research in Medical Sciences, 20*(3), 273–280. http://journals.lww.com/jrms

Bochatay, N., Kuna, Á., Csupor, É., Pintér, J. N., Muller-Juge, V., Hudelson, P., Nendaz, M. R., Csabai, M., Bajwa, N. M., & Kim, S. (2021). The role of power in health care conflict:

Recommendations for shifting toward constructive approaches. *Academic Medicine, 96*(1), 134–141. https://doi.org/10.1097/ACM.0000000000003604

Brown, S. (2012). Managing change in universities: A Sisyphean task? *Quality in Higher Education, 18*(1), 139–146. https://doi.org/10.1080/13538322.2012.663547

Burgess, A., Matar, E., Neuen, B., & Fox, G. J. (2019). A longitudinal faculty development program: Supporting a culture of teaching. *BMC Medical Education, 19*(1), 400. https://doi.org/10.1186/s12909-019-1832-3

Donnelly, J., Ray, A., Lo, M. C., Wardrop, R. M., Ficalora, R., & Amin, A. (2021). Common cause and common purpose: Strategies to increase engagement in faculty development activities. *The American Journal of Medicine, 134*(5), 691–698. https://doi.org/10.1016/j.amjmed.2021.01.002

Empson, L., & Langley, A. (2015). Leadership and professionals: Multiple manifestations of influence in professional service firms. In L. Empson, D. Muzio, J. Broschak, & B. Hinings (Eds.), *The Oxford handbook of professional service firms* (pp. 163–188). Oxford University Press. https://openaccess.city.ac.uk/id/eprint/15427/

Gale, R., & Grant, J. (1997). AMEE medical education guide no.10: Managing change in a medical context: Guidelines for action. *Medical Teacher, 19*(4), 11 (239-249).

Grant, J., & Gale, R. (1989). Changing medical education. *Medical Education, 23*(3), 252–257. https://doi.org/10.1111/j.1365-2923.1989.tb01540.x

Gray, A. Z., Modak, M., Connell, T., & Enright, H. (2020). Structuring ward rounds to enhance education. *The Clinical Teacher, 17*(3), 286–291. https://doi.org/10.1111/tct.13086

Hancock, B. H. (2018). Michel Foucault and the problematics of power: Theorizing DTCA and medicalized subjectivity. *The Journal of Medicine and Philosophy: A Forum for Bioethics and Philosophy of Medicine, 43*(4), 439–468. https://doi.org/10.1093/jmp/jhy010

Jolly, B. (2014). Faculty development for organizational change. In Y. Steinert (Ed.), *Faculty development in the health professions* (pp. 119–137). Springer. https://doi.org/10.1007/978-94-007-7612-8_6

Kotter, J. P. (1996). *Leading change*. Harvard Business School Press.

Merriman, C., & Freeth, D. (2022). Conducting a good ward round: How do leaders do it? *Journal of Evaluation in Clinical Practice, 28*(3), 411–420. https://doi.org/10.1111/jep.13670

Nimmon, L., & Stenfors-Hayes, T. (2016). The "handling" of power in the physician-patient encounter: Perceptions from experienced physicians. *BMC Medical Education, 16*(1), 114. https://doi.org/10.1186/s12909-016-0634-0

Saxena, A., Meschino, D., Hazelton, L., Chan, M.-K., Benrimoh, D. A., Matlow, A., Dath, D., & Busari, J. (2019). Power and physician leadership. *BMJ Leader, 3*(3), 92–98. https://doi.org/10.1136/leader-2019-000139

Schein, E. H. (1999). *The corporate culture survival guide: Sense and nonsense about culture change*. Jossey-Bass Publishers.

Scott, P. (2004, February). *Change matters: Making a difference in higher education*. European Universities Association Leadership Forum. http://www.uws.edu.au/__data/assets/pdf_file/0007/6892/AUQF_04_Paper_Scott.pdf

Steinert, Y., O'Sullivan, P. S., & Irby, D. M. (2024). The role of faculty development in advancing change at the organizational level. *Academic Medicine*. https://doi.org/10.1097/ACM.0000000000005732

Vanstone, M., & Grierson, L. (2022). Thinking about social power and hierarchy in medical education. *Medical Education, 56*(1), 91–97. https://doi.org/10.1111/medu.14659

VI.v STATEMENT: The Importance of First Impressions: Exploring the Hidden Curriculum in Medical Education

Annabel Heybourne

I had completed the end of my first year of medical school. Fantastic! What next? I opened my email to find that my medical school was offering summer research projects to students. Enthused by finishing my exams, I scrolled through the opportunities available and spied one on gender disparities in medical education and the hidden curriculum. I had no idea what the latter was, but the former, as a woman, intrigued me. Within minutes, I had emailed the supervisor and applied for the project. Later that day I found that the hidden curriculum project was mine. My initial feelings were a mixture of excitement and, overwhelmingly, confusion. There were two (main) issues:

 (i) I had never heard of the hidden curriculum; and
(ii) I had never participated in research.

In this essay, I will examine my introduction to medical education research, including the topic of the hidden curriculum and the crucial support of my supervisor.

1 The Hidden Curriculum Project

The hidden curriculum may be thought of as one aspect of the non-formal curriculum (i.e. it is not included in the written and enacted curriculum) and sources of this include:

  (i) the physical organisation of the learning environment
 (ii) how things are said vs. what is said
(iii) what is assessed vs. what learners are formally told is important

A. Heybourne (✉)
University Hospitals Southampton, UK
e-mail: annieheybourne@gmail.com

J. Grant, L. Grant (eds.), *The Contradictions of Medical Education*,
https://doi.org/10.1007/978-3-031-90394-6_22

(iv) physical gestures
 (v) peers and 'corridor conversations'
(vi) how tutors who are role models act around patients/staff/each other (Chan & Pawlina, 2015).

The research project was to explore if and how the hidden curriculum contributed to undergraduate medical education.

Within a month, the project was accepted and we had been granted ethical approval by the medical school committee to proceed. Over the following month, I interviewed 16 students and six members of staff, transcribed these verbatim and used a computer programme to undertake thematic analysis. I then formally wrote up this work and submitted an abstract to the medical school, to demonstrate the work I did over the summer.

A few months later, I received a letter stating that I had won an award at the medical school for the Best Student Research Project. I was very pleased and a little surprised. I was presented with the award at the medical school awards ceremony, and later presented my work at the medical school research conference. I went on to co-author a paper which was published (Brown et al., 2020).

2   The Supervisor

On reflection, a phrase all medical students dread, this success was a result of one very crucial aspect: my supervisor. From the moment I joined her team, she took me under her wing and guided me through each research hurdle (and there were quite a few!). I will always be incredibly thankful for this positive and supportive introduction to research.

My supervisor knew I was a novice and provided ample face-to-face meetings to answer my multitude of questions. Her guidance allowed me to optimise the time I was allocated to undertake the research, whilst involving me in crucial aspects of the research process. This facilitated simple but crucial aspects of my research journey, from responding to queries via email to practising my oral presentation before a conference. Ultimately, it gave me a positive insight into research, and has shaped my approach and opinion of medical research. It has motivated me to continually get involved with research projects, and laid a great foundation for me to build on.

Medical schools often assist students to find opportunities to help with research projects, and this often is initiated by pairing them up with a supervisor. Unfortunately, whoever you are paired with is sometimes luck of the draw. I had heard many horror stories from my medical student colleagues, where they had not heard from their supervisor for months, despite reaching out on multiple occasions. A good supervisor is crucial, irrespective of your experience with research, but particularly when introducing medical students to the world of research, as it can be quite daunting. As with a lot of things, the role model you receive in an area of medicine often governs whether you enjoy or loathe it—and this is a perfect example of the role of the hidden curriculum in medical education. My positive experience of medical education research, mainly due to a fantastic supervisor, was an example of the hidden curriculum acting as a force for good.

3   The Hidden Curriculum and My Medical Education

For medical students, the world of research remains a little elusive. Medical schools are incorporating research into the curriculum; for instance, we were taught about the hierarchy of evidence, the importance of evidence-based medicine and ultimately how to appraise research, and this was built on each year during medical school. However, we are not taught to critically examine the teaching techniques we are exposed to, including whether these are evidence-based. We were often asked to provide feedback about teaching sessions, but often did not see this being truly considered.

This is not the only time I have noticed the impact of the hidden curriculum, both good and bad, on my medical education. As students, we are taught by numerous healthcare professionals and the attitude of the teacher, to the students and the subject matter, often influenced how the teaching session went.

Role models have also contributed to developing my professional identity. Observing doctors on ward rounds, including how they communicate with patients and members of the multidisciplinary team, has enabled me to identify what works well, and what works less well, and incorporate these aspects into my professional persona. Furthermore, resident doctors on the wards often taught helpful tips and tricks for practical and communication skills that are not taught in medical school; they taught the practicalities of being a doctor.

My favourite conversations on placement are often with seasoned doctors discussing real-world medicine; by this, I do not mean the knowledge that we are assessed on at the end of each year, but all the 'stuff' that no one really talks about. For instance, whilst with an anaesthetist in theatre, we spoke for 20 minutes about the perceived versus actual risk of anaesthetics, the safety measures put in place to reduce human error, and issues about raising concerns in the NHS. There are so many conversations that happen on placement which are not part of our formal curriculum but which are equally as important to professional development.

4   The Hidden Curriculum: Exposing Differences

Contrary to all this, the hidden curriculum can present challenges for a medical student. For instance, we are told that certain specialities, for instance cardiology and respiratory, will be examined 'more' in written exams, compared with the other specialities, such as Ear, Nose and Throat. This ultimately guided and influenced how much teaching time we received in certain subjects, as well as how much time medical students allocate to revising different areas of medicine. As medical students, we often faced contradictions between what was formally taught versus what is practical and clinically useful. Medical school teaches us the tick-box examination, but in practice many of the steps are skipped over or performed in a different manner.

The General Medical Council (GMC) lists the requirements for medical students' undergraduate curricula, but does not include skills which are fundamental to being a foundation doctor including writing a discharge letter and ordering investigations (Nunez-Mulder, 2019). The hidden curriculum has been described as the 'unofficial rules' for surviving medical school (Davies, 2017) that are delivered through the learning environment.

The contradictions between what is taught and what is observed can cause frustration and tension for medical students. It may also cause a loss of enthusiasm, reduced morale, and cynicism (Davies, 2017). The project I undertook identified these inconsistencies observed between medical school and placement, and that there is a constant struggle of weighing up what is important to focus on as a student.

The hidden curriculum can also result in professional dilemmas for medical students and therefore may result in distress (Davies, 2017). Similarly, those I interviewed identified that the hidden curriculum played a role in their personal and professional development. The British Medical Journal (BMJ) launched a podcast called *The Sharp Scratch*, which aims to help prepare medical students and newly qualified doctors with their version of the hidden curriculum, including 'tips for success and wellbeing' and 'healthcare culture' (Nunez-Mulder, 2019). The hidden curriculum includes the environment where you work or study and therefore can end up teaching resident doctors' unsafe practices or assist in maintaining harmful cultures (Nunez-Mulder, 2019).

5   Examining the Hidden Curriculum

The hidden curriculum is clearly a crucial part of medical education and it has received a lot of attention in medical education research. Like many, I was previously unaware of the term. However, when I broke the term down, and brought the hidden curriculum out into the open, the staff and students that I interviewed recognised the role it had in medical undergraduate education and could provide clear examples of the hidden curriculum in action. To paraphrase, according to these individuals, it is what makes us able to deal, or in some cases not cope, with the practicalities of being healthcare professionals. Despite its negative connotations, the hidden curriculum, when brought out in the open, can be a force for change (Nunez-Mulder, 2019). One method of bringing the hidden curriculum out into the open, that was suggested by participants in the project, could be to encourage medical students to talk and reflect on their experiences of the hidden curriculum and medical education.

6 Medical Education Research

The hidden curriculum project I was involved in opened my eyes to the world of medical education; I naively did not realise this was an area of research, despite its clear importance. Medical education and medical education research are gaining momentum. This has been helped by the increased availability of medical education and research intercalated degrees (a chance for students to take a year out of medical school and attain a Bachelor's or Master's degree) and the growing popularity of clinical teaching fellowship jobs for qualified doctors. Although having never experienced either of these opportunities, I personally think it is incredibly useful to have teaching experience as a medical student and resident doctor. As a student, I rely on ad-hoc teaching from doctors on each ward I am attached to, and teaching experience is almost unavoidable if you wish to apply for any sort of speciality training post-graduation.

Medical education research enables students to analyse the current curriculum (both informal and formal), question what successfully educates the doctors of tomorrow, and challenge the current system. Getting involved with this research enables medical students to feel empowered and, as the ones currently receiving education, they are often the best people to incorporate into research, both as participants and researchers. I became involved with medical education fairly early on in my medical school journey which has led me to get involved as a participant in other projects, and enabled me to formulate my own research projects. It has ultimately shaped my personal and professional identity, and it was all down to a good first experience of research.

References

Brown, M. E. L., Coker, O., Heybourne, A., & Finn, G. M. (2020). Exploring the hidden curriculum's impact on medical students: Professionalism, identity formation and the need for transparency. *Medical Science Educator, 30*(3), 1107–1121. https://doi.org/10.1007/s40670-020-01021-z

Chan, L. K., & Pawlina, W. (Eds.). (2015). *Teaching anatomy.* Springer International Publishing. https://doi.org/10.1007/978-3-319-08930-0

Davies, M. (2017). The risks of following the informal and hidden curriculums. *British Medical Journal,* j3287. https://doi.org/10.1136/sbmj.j3287

Nunez-Mulder, L. (2019). Sharp scratch: Shining a light on the hidden medical curriculum. *British Medical Journal,* l2223. https://doi.org/10.1136/bmj.l2223

VI.v COMMENTARY: The Hidden Curriculum, the Reproduction of Social Order and Development of Critical Consciousness

Janet Grant and Leonard Grant

Curriculum has been theorised in countless ways, for example as 'intended', 'envisioned', 'enacted', 'on paper', 'stated, 'experienced', formal', informal', and 'hidden'. In addition, there is another ever-expanding raft of terms that are used to describe the design approach that a curriculum takes: 'contextual', 'modular', 'spiral', 'integrated'. As many as 120 such definitions, the result of a 'human construct', have been claimed (Mitchell, 2016). Regardless of how a curriculum is described, it has limits:

> A curriculum is an aspirational statement: not a predictor of reality but a reflection of values, beliefs, intentions and hopes…. Translation into practice will be limited by a variety of factors (Grant et al., 2013, p. 14).

Those factors, at a minimum, will concern resources, ideologies, management, cultures, contexts, personal and professional values, what has been termed in relation to secondary school education, the 'agency' and 'autonomy' of teachers to interpret the curriculum as part of their professional practice (Erss, 2018), relationships, skills and understanding, and the degree of alignment of understanding between curriculum developers and those who must enact it.

It is clear, from all these uncontrolled variables, that there will be aspects of education and training that people inaccurately call the 'hidden curriculum', a term adopted from writings about secondary school classrooms. These variables have been classified as structural, educational, cultural and social (Sarikhani et al., 2020). Annabel Heybourne's reflection on the experience of entering medical education research illustrates that the frequently cited 'hidden' curriculum is not hidden at all, just not written down, often because some things simply cannot be identified, defined, written or controlled. This phenomenon has been defined as a:

> …set of influences that function at the level of organisational structure and culture (Hafferty & O'Donnell, 2014)

'Influences', clearly, are difficult to observe, but their effects are not.

Studies have been made of this phenomenon at the levels of undergraduate and postgraduate medical education, and continuing professional development (Bennett et al., 2004; Boer & Daelmans, 2020; Brown et al., 2020; Lempp & Seale, 2004; Mahood, 2011). The hidden curriculum has been blamed for loss of empathy in students (Howick et al., 2023), although it has been argued that such effects can be mitigated if students are made aware of the hidden curriculum (Neve & Collett, 2018). Annabel Heybourne's own research shows that it contributes to the development of professional identity (Brown et al., 2020) while she also identifies factors such as supervisor behaviour as part of that hidden curriculum. The contradictions and tensions of what is said and what is done have been discussed:

We teach that family medicine and whole-person care are critical, but the hidden curriculum continues to denigrate family medicine and glorify specialization (Mahood, 2011)

The hidden curriculum is most often portrayed as something that is in contradiction to the formal curriculum (that which exists 'on paper') and that it is a negative influence upon that curriculum (Balboni et al., 2015; Lawrence et al., 2018; Lee et al., 2023; Martimianakis et al., 2015; Mawdsley & Willis, 2023). The hidden curriculum is found in the experiences that students have when in education, rather than the stated objectives of the planned curriculum (Grant et al., 2013). It 'transforms and organises institutions in ways that reinforce and legitimise asymmetrical power relationships' (Zaidi et al., 2021). The written or intended curriculum is often constructed as something that is always improving and always more suitable for the future, thus the hidden curriculum holds medicine in the past, and certainly in the present. However, as we can see from Annabel Heybourne's account; not all aspects of what is experienced are negative and not all parts of the intended curriculum are positive.

Is Experience Hidden?

What is clear is that no part of the learner's experience is actually hidden—but some of that experience is not written down in the curriculum document for a number of reasons. Firstly, some knowledge is tacit, acquired and internalised individually through application, practice and experience, such that 'we can know more than we can tell' (Polanyi, 1966), and so more than can be written down in a curriculum document or described as a curriculum outcome, that nonetheless informs teaching. Secondly, the curriculum in practice is enacted by people who come to that with their own agency and interpretation (Choppin, 2011; Deng, 2011; Shkedi, 1998). That enactment cannot be monitored. So if any part of a curriculum is hidden, it is not hidden from teachers and learners, it is hidden from those who originate and perhaps manage but do not implement the written curriculum.

Annabel Heybourne examines this in her own experience, from the point of view of a researcher and a postgraduate doctor. This elegant juxtaposition illustrates the case that all education and training occur with many levels of meaning. This is especially so where learning is occurring in the real world, as part of actual practice, as much of medical education is. In Annabel Heybourne's case, that real world was also the process of undertaking a supervised research project. In doing so, she experienced the very thing that she was researching: the hidden curriculum which for her, consisted of the supportive, guiding and educative behaviours of her supervisor. And those, in turn, depended on the personal and professional qualities of that person, and probably on her perceptions, time and motivation, and many other things that we cannot and do not know.

In this, we see that the hidden curriculum is not hidden at all, in practice. It is simply not describable, or predictable. It is the part of education that a curriculum on paper or what the author calls the formal curriculum, cannot articulate.

The Quest for Curriculum Control and Universal Truth

Annabel Heybourne's account of her development as an educational researcher illuminates the hopeless quest for control of the curriculum. The myriad publications that analyse the hidden curriculum in so many ways, imply that things might be better if we could actually define and control this aspect of the educational process: in which case, of course, it would become part of the formal 'curriculum on paper' (Coles & Gale, 1985). Annabel Heybourne suggests that if students discuss and reflect on their experiences of the hidden curriculum, it can be a force for change.

Education is a human, interactive process. As such, it cannot be fully controlled:

> …the most powerful learning experiences cannot be planned; they occur serendipitously. These impromptu learning experiences allow students to expand their horizons and become empathic, conscious global citizens. Although when and how these experiences occur cannot be controlled, teachers can capitalize on them and maximize their learning benefits by providing students with freedom to explore, opportunities to reflect, and tools to further understand their experiences (Jefferies & Nguyen, 2014).

Paulo Freire would argue that the purpose of education is to develop this 'critical consciousness' derived from thinking about and then changing the real world (Freire, 1997). Building on this, others went on to develop ideas of experiential learning:

> … whereby the learner encounters multiple and often contradictory perspectives from interacting with the environment, leading him/her to refine original beliefs and develop new ones (Jefferies & Nguyen, 2014).

Such experiential learning has been called informal, unplanned, incidental, impromptu (Jefferies & Nguyen, 2014) and perhaps we can see it as the hidden curriculum. Whichever it is, it is important and unavoidable.

Annabel Heybourne points to the confusion experienced by students who witness inappropriate role models. It has been claimed that such role models can themselves cause inappropriate and unethical behaviours in learners, while, on the other hand, 'so-called anti-models may represent a valuable experience for students, as it could serve as an effective mechanism of social learning' (Mileder et al., 2014). The development of critical thought must encompass a range of positive and negative experiences. But we must be cautious. It has been shown that negative role models can have a positive effect on learning, depending on culture and purpose. In collectivist cultures, negative role models may motivate people more than in individualist cultures where positive role models are more effective (Lockwood et al., 2002):

> Perhaps this is why negative role models have not been focussed on in the literature since Lockwood's work, because western, liberal society is seen to lean towards individualism

and positive goal-setting, so positive role models would show the more significant effect (Coppell, 2020).

As we have argued in many commentary chapters, there are few universal truths in education, even in the effect of the 'hidden' curriculum which is acknowledged to be affected by cultural context, even though the published literature has not yet properly addressed this issue (Sarikhani et al., 2020).

This imbalance of cultural focus brings us to the politics of the hidden curriculum.

The Politics of the Hidden Curriculum

Having acknowledged that there is a part of any educational process that is inevitable and important but not written into the formal curriculum and its outcomes, we must ask where this comes from, and what its messages are. Curriculum, whether hidden or not, is not immune from society, its values and relationships. For many writers, the 'hidden' curriculum guides the socialisation of the learner. In medical education, that socialisation is into the profession, and into its educational roles, just as Annabel Heybourne notices and learns from the behaviours of her supervisor. It has been argued that:

> … education is preparation for future market evaluation and the process of commodification through which capitalism assesses human value and worth (Hill et al., 2009).

We can translate this into the professional medical employment market determining the worth of graduates for purposes of, for example, matching graduates to speciality training places. It has been said that:

> What was once the hidden curriculum of many universities…has now become an open and much celebrated policy of both public and private higher education (Giroux, 2009).

We can see this in offshore (and other) medical schools, for example, which deliberately prepare students to sit the United States Medical Licensing Examination (USMLE) (Morgan et al., 2017) rather than purporting to prepare graduates for the local healthcare economy while the clear 'hidden' curriculum expresses otherwise.

Giroux, a leading theorist about the hidden curriculum, considered its derivation in wider society, advocating in relation to the 'covert and overt role of schooling':

> …a theoretical foundation that acknowledges the dialectical interplay of social interest, political power, and economic power, on the one hand, and school knowledge and practices on the other (Giroux, 1981, p. 284).

Medical education tends to think of the hidden curriculum in relation to the demonstration of professional practices and values, but the wider educational literature sees this phenomenon differently:

> I use the term to refer to those non-academic but educationally significant consequences of schooling that occur systematically but are not made explicit at any level of the public rationales for education. It refers broadly to the social control function of schooling (Vallance, 1973).

This is understood in three ways: Traditionally, the hidden curriculum is seen as transmitting the existing structures and values of society, averting critique; a more liberal interpretation focuses on the ways in which meaning is negotiated in the classroom intentionally and consciously through interpersonal interactions; a more radical approach analyses the political role of the hidden curriculum in the classroom which reflects the power relationships of wider society.

Giroux rejects these interpretations as failing to '…provide the theoretical elements necessary to develop a critical pedagogy based on a concern with cultural struggles in the schools' (Giroux, 1981). In this view, while we can see that the hidden curriculum can reinforce the positive values and behaviours that Annabel Heybourne describes in her supervisor, it can also transmit the values of a dominant, and even alien, ideology to the possible detriment of the learner. So with both existing and new educational practices and processes (especially if they are imported from another culture and context), paying attention to the hidden curriculum is an essential activity, because:

> …any pedagogical approach to curriculum and course development in the schools that ignores the existence of the hidden curriculum runs the risk of being incomplete as well as insignificant. (Giroux, 1978)

Although the hidden curriculum is commonly portrayed as separate and in tension with the formal curriculum, the formal and hidden curricula exist in relation to one another and to hegemonic ideology. In attempting to separate the parts of the curriculum and to study them separately, the ways in which they are co-constitutive are overlooked.

Annabel Heybourne shows that the hidden curriculum is not really hidden at all—but even then, it can be ignored in plain sight.

References

Balboni, M. J., Bandini, J., Mitchell, C., Epstein-Peterson, Z. D., Amobi, A., Cahill, J., Enzinger, A. C., Peteet, J., & Balboni, T. (2015). Religion, spirituality, and the hidden curriculum: Medical student and faculty reflections. *Journal of Pain and Symptom Management, 50*(4), 507–515. https://doi.org/10.1016/j.jpainsymman.2015.04.020

Bennett, N., Lockyer, J., Mann, K., Batty, H., LaForet, K., Rethans, J.-J., & Silver, I. (2004). Hidden curriculum in continuing medical education. *Journal of Continuing Education in the Health Professions, 24*(3), 145–152. https://doi.org/10.1002/chp.1340240305

Boer, C., & Daelmans, H. E. M. (2020). Team up with the hidden curriculum in medical teaching. *British Journal of Anaesthesia, 124*(3), e52–e54. https://doi.org/10.1016/j.bja.2019.12.031

Brown, M. E. L., Coker, O., Heybourne, A., & Finn, G. M. (2020). Exploring the hidden curriculum's impact on medical students: Professionalism, identity formation and the need for transparency. *Medical Science Educator, 30*(3), 1107–1121. https://doi.org/10.1007/s40670-020-01021-z

Choppin, J. (2011). Learned adaptations: Teachers' understanding and use of curriculum resources. *Journal of Mathematics Teacher Education, 14*(5), 331–353. https://doi.org/10.1007/s10857-011-9170-3

Coles, C. R., & Gale, G. J. (1985). Curriculum evaluation in medical and health-care education. *Medical Education, 19*(5), 405–422. https://doi.org/10.1111/j.1365-2923.1985.tb01345.x

Coppell, R. (2020). Revisiting the concept of the anti-role-model for social learning theory in UK education. *Research Ideas and Outcomes, 6.* https://doi.org/10.3897/rio.6.e60683

Deng, Z. (2011). Revisiting curriculum potential. *Curriculum Inquiry, 41*(5), 538–559. https://doi.org/10.1111/j.1467-873X.2011.00563.x

Erss, M. (2018). 'Complete freedom to choose within limits' – Teachers' views of curricular autonomy, agency and control in Estonia, Finland and Germany. *The Curriculum Journal, 29*(2), 238–256. https://doi.org/10.1080/09585176.2018.1445514

Freire, P. (1997). *Pedagogy of the oppressed.* Continuum.

Giroux, H. A. (1978). Developing educational programs: Overcoming the hidden curriculum. *The Clearing House: A Journal of Educational Strategies, Issues and Ideas, 52*(4), 148–151. https://doi.org/10.1080/00098655.1978.10113565

Giroux, H. A. (1981). Schooling and the myth of objectivity: Stalking the politics of the hidden curriculum. *McGill Journal of Education, 16*(3), 282–304.

Giroux, H. A. (2009). Neoliberalism, youth, and the leasing of higher education. In D. Hill & R. Kumar (Eds.), *Global neoliberalism and education and its consequences.* Routledge.

Grant, J., Abdelrahman, M. Y. H., & Zachariah, A. (2013). Curriculum design in context. In K. Walsh (Ed.), *Oxford textbook of medical education* (pp. 13–24). Oxford University Press.

Hafferty, F. W., & O'Donnell, J. F. (Eds.). (2014). *The hidden curriculum in health professional education.* Dartmouth College Press.

Hill, D., Greaves, N. M., & Maisuria, A. (2009). Education, inequality and neoliberal capitalism. A classical Marxist analysis. In D. Hill & R. Kumar (Eds.), *Global neoliberalism and education and its consequences.* Routledge.

Howick, J., Dudko, M., Feng, S. N., Ahmed, A. A., Alluri, N., Nockels, K., Winter, R., & Holland, R. (2023). Why might medical student empathy change throughout medical school? A systematic review and thematic synthesis of qualitative studies. *BMC Medical Education, 23*(1), 270. https://doi.org/10.1186/s12909-023-04165-9

Jefferies, J., & Nguyen, A.-M. (2014). Impromptu learning: Unplanned occurrences, intended outcomes. *International Journal of Teaching and Learning in Higher Education, 26*(2), 182–192. http://www.isetl.org/ijtlhe/

Lawrence, C., Mhlaba, T., Stewart, K. A., Moletsane, R., Gaede, B., & Moshabela, M. (2018). The hidden curricula of medical education: A scoping review. *Academic Medicine, 93*(4), 648–656. https://doi.org/10.1097/ACM.0000000000002004

Lee, C. A., Wilkinson, T. J., Timmermans, J. A., Ali, A. N., & Anakin, M. G. (2023). Revealing the impact of the hidden curriculum on faculty teaching: A qualitative study. *Medical Education, 57*(8), 761–769. https://doi.org/10.1111/medu.15026

Lempp, H., & Seale, C. (2004). The hidden curriculum in undergraduate medical education: Qualitative study of medical students' perceptions of teaching. *BMJ, 329*(7469), 770–773. https://doi.org/10.1136/bmj.329.7469.770

Lockwood, P., Jordan, C. H., & Kunda, Z. (2002). Motivation by positive or negative role models: Regulatory focus determines who will best inspire us. *Journal of Personality and Social Psychology, 83*(4), 854–864. https://doi.org/10.1037/0022-3514.83.4.854

Mahood, S. C. (2011). Medical education: Beware the hidden curriculum. *Canadian Family Physician, 57*(9), 983–985.

Martimianakis, M. A. (Tina), Michalec, B., Lam, J., Cartmill, C., Taylor, J. S., & Hafferty, F. W. (2015). Humanism, the hidden curriculum, and educational reform. *Academic Medicine, 90*, S5–S13. https://doi.org/10.1097/ACM.0000000000000894

Mawdsley, A., & Willis, S. C. (2023). Hetero- and cisnormativity – UK pharmacy education as a queer opponent. *Medical Education, 57*(6), 574–586. https://doi.org/10.1111/medu.15018

Mileder, L. P., Schmidt, A., & Dimai, H. P. (2014). Clinicians should be aware of their responsibilities as role models: A case report on the impact of poor role modeling. *Medical Education Online, 19*(1), 23479. https://doi.org/10.3402/meo.v19.23479

Mitchell, B. (2016). Understanding curriculum. *Asian Journal of Humanities and Social Studies*, 2321–2799. https://www.ajouronline.com/

Morgan, J., Crooks, V. A., Sampson, C. J., & Snyder, J. (2017). "Location is surprisingly a lot more important than you think": A critical thematic analysis of push and pull factor messaging used on Caribbean offshore medical school websites. *BMC Medical Education, 17*(1), 99. https://doi.org/10.1186/s12909-017-0936-x

Neve, H., & Collett, T. (2018). Empowering students with the hidden curriculum. *The Clinical Teacher, 15*(6), 494–499. https://doi.org/10.1111/tct.12736

Polanyi, M. (1966). *The tacit dimension*. Doubleday.

Sarikhani, Y., Shojaei, P., Rafiee, M., & Delavari, S. (2020). Analyzing the interaction of main components of hidden curriculum in medical education using interpretive structural modeling method. *BMC Medical Education, 20*(1), 176. https://doi.org/10.1186/s12909-020-02094-5

Shkedi, A. (1998). Can the curriculum guide both emancipate and educate teachers? *Curriculum Inquiry, 28*(2), 209–229. https://doi.org/10.1111/0362-6784.00085

Vallance, E. (1973). Hiding the hidden curriculum: An interpretation of the language of justification in nineteenth-century educational reform. *Curriculum Theory Network, 4*, 5–21.

Zaidi, Z., Partman, I. M., Whitehead, C. R., Kuper, A., & Wyatt, T. R. (2021). Contending with our racial past in medical education: A Foucauldian perspective. *Teaching and Learning in Medicine, 33*(4), 453–462. https://doi.org/10.1080/10401334.2021.1945929

Annabel Heybourne   has been involved with medical education and research since the end of her first year at Hull York Medical School, teaching medical students, undertaking quality improvement projects, and conducting research. Annabel wrote this examination of her experience of the hidden curriculum during her fourth year of medical school. She hopes to combine an academic and clinical career in surgery.

CONCLUSIONS: The Politics and Contradictions of Medical Education

Leonard Grant and Janet Grant

This book has illustrated and analysed the power and politics of medical education, just as a social scientist would analyse the power and politics of any other aspect of society and social practice. We have presented accounts of practice, each with its accompanying commentary and analysis. We gave the authors no guidance on what they might write about. We simply asked that they might reflect on an issue that was of current concern to them. To that extent, we have a book that describes the lived experience of 35 people learning or working in medical education in 11 different countries in four different continents. The overlapping concerns that they describe attest to the problematical globalisation of medical education. We organised the authors' accounts into six groups which addressed:

- Culture and context
- Globalisation and its problems
- Negotiating identities in medical education and medicine
- Managing the system, the profession and the business of medical education
- Medical education and the workplace
- The power and politics of curriculum.

At the outset, we might have imagined that some of the popular themes in medical education research and practice such as workplace-based assessment, equity, diversity and inclusion, physician wellbeing and burnout, interprofessional collaboration, accreditation, regulation, stakeholder input, and social accountability (Eady & Moreau, 2024), might have featured. But they did not. Neither did they present issues

L. Grant
School of Medicine, University of Liverpool, Liverpool, UK
e-mail: leonard.grant@liverpool.ac.uk

J. Grant (✉)
Centre for Medical Education in Context (CenMEDIC), Hampton, UK
e-mail: janet@cenmedic.net

J. Grant, L. Grant (eds.), *The Contradictions of Medical Education*,
https://doi.org/10.1007/978-3-031-90394-6_23

concerning the development of their actual healthcare services, on which medical education depends, for which medical education exists, but over which medical education itself has little control. These are not the issues that concern these authors in practice. Although if asked to speak about them, they undoubtedly could.

Having grouped and discussed the authors' accounts, we observed that there are five overarching, all-pervasive themes:

- The unclear status of medical education
- Culture and context
- Neoliberalism, globalisation, standards and market forces in medicine
- The business of medical education and the profession
- The power and the politics in a post-colonial era.

We now gather together and end with these overarching themes.

1 The Unclear Status of Medical Education

It seems unlikely that anyone enters medical school or university with the intention of becoming a medical educationalist. The journey into medical education is often serendipitous, as we can see in chapter III.i "The Road Not Taken: Transitioning to Full-Time Medical Education Research from Clinical Practice as a Junior Doctor" and chapter III.ii "Finding the Centre of My Venn: Navigating Experiences of Identity Challenge as a Medical Student". Or the medical education journey may just be a sideline to the main job of being a doctor or a non-medical academic, as is the case with many of our authors. It seems likely that all clinician medical educators originally intended to practise as doctors but found that their working conditions or culture, or perhaps chance or interest, forced a reconsideration.

Although medical education has been added to the UK government medical careers page (NHS, n.d.), there is no clearly defined pathway for medical education in Britain, since, as in most other countries, medical education is not a recognised academic discipline that has its own undergraduate, postgraduate and career routes, nor its own entry or exit qualifications. Despite its plethora of Master's degrees and doctoral programmes, and its departments inside medical schools, it remains as an instrumental practice that:

> …takes strength from being an applied discipline, not a pure one, harvesting its theories and ideas from a wide variety of social science, philosophical and methodological disciplines and from experience (Grant & Grant, 2023).

Because of this, individuals are often reliant on their own personal determination and chance opportunities. The struggle with identity—'If I am not a doctor then what am I?' (in chapter III.i "The Road Not Taken: Transitioning to Full-Time Medical Education Research from Clinical Practice as a Junior Doctor")—is not helped by this lack of subject identity and career structure. Medical education faces ongoing contradictions as it tries to establish its place in the academic and medical landscape.

The authors in this book are full-time clinicians, part-time clinicians, ex-clinicians, and non-clinicians. They are employed as doctors, trainers, researchers, academics, managers, or educational developers, working in government, public and private education and healthcare, and professional organisations. Some have medical education 'qualifications', some do not. It is because of this lack of settled structure and identity of medical education, that the chapters in this book and the reflections of their authors are so important—they are the authentic voices of medical education practitioners, telling their own stories from their own experience of medical education. So this first theme is one that depicts individuality within a broad, inchoate field that might never develop into anything more defined and consistent: which would be a strength in terms of the second overarching theme.

2   Culture and Context

Despite medical education's global pretensions, each national medical education system has its own historical and cultural character. This is social science and so:

> There is a constant tension between a vision of education promoted by medical educators, based on contextually non-specific ideas such as those found in the medical education literature, and the sociopolitical foundations and forces that are unique to each country. (Segouin & Hodges, 2005)

2.1   Global Forces and Local Contexts

Much of this book has an explicit focus on global forces and local contexts in medical education. The centrality of cultural imperialism in medical education is illustrated, whereby practices and standards from global north countries, particularly the US and Britain, are adopted or imposed globally without primary consideration of local contexts and cultures. This process occurs through various mechanisms, including international accreditation, faculty development programmes, and the pressure to compete in global rankings. We have seen how these dynamics play out in various contexts—from global south countries dealing with neocolonial and postcolonial influences, to developed nations negotiating their relationship with perhaps alien dominant educational models. We question whether global standardisation is compatible with the need to develop cultural identity and function in relation to local healthcare systems.

Throughout our commentaries, the importance of context and culture in relation to global trends is examined. This constantly reflects:

> Tension between 'travelling' and 'embedded' policy. The former refers to supra- and transnational agency activity…, embedded policy is to be found in *local* spaces…where global policy agendas come up against existing priorities and practices. (Ozga & Lingard, 2007)

As we explored in our commentary on chapter I.i "Socio-cultural Contexts and Medical Education: Tales from Four Continents", medical education should not be considered homogeneous or divorced from its context. We have discussed the influence of the US and Britain on global medical education in our commentary on chapter I.ii "Glocalisation of Medical Education: Impact and Challenges" and medical education imperialism (Bleakley et al., 2008) in our commentary on chapter II.iii "Greater Than the Sum: International Partnerships in Medical Education". Emulating what works in one setting may not be the best thing to do in a different setting. Thorough study of our own particular conditions is a prerequisite for any change we are considering. But what of the other themes, how do they also shape the context of medical education and the tension between global and local?

3   Neoliberalism, Globalisation, Standards, and Market Forces in Medicine

Throughout our commentaries, we have argued, as others have (Navarro, 2007), that neoliberalism (espoused by global north governments and international institutions for many decades) has had great, and often negative, effects on medicine and medical education (in our commentary on chapter V.iii "Training During the Real Work of After-Admitting Ward Rounds"). The main relevant tenets of neoliberalism are that:

- the state should reduce its interventions in social and economic activities
- financial and labour markets should be deregulated
- borders and barriers to the mobility of goods and labour should be eliminated.

In medicine, however, to facilitate the movement of medical labour, this is contradictorily accompanied by efforts to set and impose 'global' (generally meaning 'global north') standards or working methods. We can see the effects of these in the globalisation of medical education, and the trade in trained doctors (from global south to global north) that is increasingly being enabled under the guise of international accreditation. In this, a contradiction is created between globalisation (otherwise described as medical education imperialism, reflecting the attempt to transcend borders and barriers to the trade in medical graduates) and the imperative to address local healthcare training needs.

Neoliberalisation of trade therefore affects medical training, causing more focus on measurable outcomes (proving the quality of the commodity) and market-driven approaches. Since the buyer's market is in the global north, the qualities that 'sellers' must aspire to are those of the global north, perhaps in the guise of imported global north methods and USMLE pass rates:

> The theory of globalization coincides with several elements from the theory of modernization. One aspect is that both theories suggest that the main direction of development should be that which was undertaken by the United States and Europe. (Uzomah & Folorunso, 2020)

In medical education, it is undoubtedly true that all new ideas derive from the global north and tend to be taken up by or imposed on the global south, whether or not they suit the culture and context. So:

> …wealthy countries superimpose their political ideals and core values on the less wealthy and under-developed countries as paradigms. (Uzomah & Folorunso, 2020)

3.1 Standards and Standardisation in Neoliberal Policies

Of course, the rhetoric and the practice of neoliberal policies are different. To make open borders and transnational trade (such as the migration of doctors) work, apparent deregulation (often called 'contextualisation' in medical education) has had, contradictorily, to be accompanied by global standards. We see this in the efforts towards international standardisation by organisations such as the World Health Organisation and the para-regulatory World Federation for Medical Education, whose first foray into international accreditation facilitated the migration of doctors to the US (Rashid et al., 2021). Responses to the pressures of the global market in health professionals, draw our attention to the 'contradictory imperatives of globalisation'(Weisz & Nannestad, 2021), and its mutually antagonistic yet simultaneous ideas of standardisation and local diversity (Bleakley et al., 2008).

It has been suggested that standardisation (as argued against in chapter II.ii "Standardisation: The Root of the Flat Curve") and its quality assurance mechanisms (such as international recognition of medical education organisations), are actually an important device for neoliberalism (Rasco, 2020), for a continuing focus on the global north as the standards setter, and so for the continuing, some might say exploitative, medical migration that disadvantages global south countries.

Others have been concerned about this trend from a different point of view:

> The concepts of standardisation and regulation have … become culturally synonymous with 'education'. … through this apparent conformity with the culturally dominant ideologies of modernisation and neoliberalism, a new hegemony is being created…, changing the nature of medical education towards industrial training, rather than meeting the wider vocational demands for independent and critical practitioners. (Park, 2012).

The mechanisms of neoliberalism and globalisation have not gone unnoticed:

> For many African and Asian scholars, globalization is a modern-day neo-colonization scheme and conspiracy. (Uzomah & Folorunso, 2020)

The forces of globalisation and standardisation, referred to as homogenising forces and processes (Ozga & Lingard, 2007), were illustrated in this book where authors described struggling to develop local, contextual educational processes and practices while feeling constrained by the geopolitics of medical education.

We explored the contradictions between local needs and global standards, suggesting that successful change requires careful navigation between these various forces. This is unlikely to be something that can be achieved by one person, but requires a collective effort of educators, managers, practitioners and patients.

3.2 Neoliberalism and the Global Market

The impact on medical education systems of those neoliberal policies which empha-sise deregulation, globalisation, and market forces is felt keenly. We see this in Brazil's rapid expansion of private medical schools (chapter IV.iii "Medical Education in Brazil: Context and Challenges"). We are also concerned, as we have been in other themes, about influences from the global north encroaching in unwanted ways on others' educational systems. Mechanisms such as international partnerships and global accreditation systems often create tensions with local con-texts and needs, further complicated by economic disparities. In response, we can explore how to build meaningful personal partnerships across these divides (chapter II.iii "Greater Than the Sum: International Partnerships in Medical Education"), finding ways to mitigate and manage inherent power imbalances. But at all levels, neoliberal approaches may have affected professional autonomy and identity in medicine, leading to increased standardisation and regulatory control which has the potential to undermine professional values (chapter II.ii "Standardisation: The Root of the Flat Curve").

Perhaps this is simply an element of the global economy:

> … nearly every corner of the world is rapidly becoming an integral part of the global eco-nomic system… dominated by large transnational corporations … These transnational cor-porations have the support and protection of the dominant forces in the regulation of international finance and trade, such as the International Monetary Fund, the World Bank, the World Trade Organization, and governments of strong countries such as the United States, Britain, and Japan … (Uzomah & Folorunso, 2020, p. 98)

Perhaps we can add global medical education organisations to this list.

The chapters written by those practising in the global south tell again and again of the pressures they face from globalisation and adopting methods from the global north. The US and UK are the beneficiaries of workforce migration from, in particu-lar, India and Pakistan (OECD, 2019), and increasingly from Africa (Duvivier et al., 2017). No wonder that medical schools in these countries are 'fast and fashionable' in adopting teaching and assessment methods designed for and relevant to the global north (chapter II.i "The 'Fast and Fashionable' Syndrome"). The market pressure to do so is almost unavoidable. And yet, each one of our authors, in their own way, is resisting.

4   The Business of Medical Education and the Profession

We might have expected that some authors would address directly the very many ways in which money is made from medical education, that money usually moving from global south to global north. None did address this directly, but the ideas threaded through many chapters.

We can see that the logic of business is making its way firmly into medical education and that the drivers of business (profit, extraction of resources in the form of medical graduates, and monopolisation in, for example, international accreditation of regulatory agencies) may be at odds with education which, at its core, is about sharing and developing knowledge.

While there is a market and trade in medical graduates, there are also industrial qualities in the production of that commodity. In chapter III.i "The Road Not Taken: Transitioning to Full-Time Medical Education Research from Clinical Practice as a Junior Doctor", it is clear that the working conditions of medicine in Britain made staying in the profession untenable for our contributors, despite many years of industrial action and protest (Baldwin, 2023; Katharine Garratt, 2024). Doctors in Britain do experience distress over unmanageable workloads and constraints on their ability to provide adequate care (Beech et al., 2023; Khan, 2023a, b; Matheson et al., 2020). These conditions are not accidental, but are related to deliberate decisions to increasingly privatise and underfund healthcare in Britain (Powell & Miller, 2016), so worsening patient outcomes (Goodair, 2024; Goodair et al., 2024). Population health is declining in Britain and fiscal austerity has been shown to increase the prevalence of multi-morbidity (Stokes et al., 2022). This is their context of learning to practise, or teaching, medicine. Medical education itself has little moderating effect on this decline.

When neoliberalism is the dominant political and economic philosophy, it is perhaps to be expected that the language of business makes its way into medical education. We discussed in Part IV the increasing presence of leadership and management in medical education. This area has its history in business and the military (Bass & Bass, 2008) which, we might imagine, are a long way from the profession of medicine. In relation to the management and uses of medical education, we see the dangers of turning medical education into a business that marginalises the profession or uses medical education as a commodity to sell for profit, rather than an academic and professional endeavour. We have explored the range of interests, from profit, to global influence, to the profession, that are present in medical education. Although there may be a desire for co-operation, some interests will triumph over others and perhaps it is those with the deepest pockets, or perhaps which can evoke post-colonial sentiment, which prevail.

The management of medical education is a complicated endeavour. The interplay between management, professional identity and institutional power creates various tensions between different groups—particularly academics, administrators and clinicians in management roles. There are shifting dynamics; professional hierarchies can be challenged by management requirements which leads to conflict between professional autonomy and organisational control.

We are experiencing a shift from professional bureaucracy to professional business. However, there has never been a time when medical institutions did not have to balance multiple competing demands; implementing change in medical institutions has always required careful navigation of interests, resource constraints and cultural factors. A recurrent thread in this theme is, yet again, the question of professional identity—how do medical professionals navigate dual roles as clinicians and managers, as colleagues and profit-makers or fund-raisers, and how does this affect institutional dynamics and decision-making processes?

5   The Power and the Politics in a Post-Colonial Era

Although professions do tend to be concerned about how new generations are educated and trained (there are, for example, professors of legal education and chemistry education), medicine is singular in the extent to which this concern has become an institutionalised undertaking in its own right. We might wonder why the cleverest learners in any society, who have succeeded in entering one of its most competitive courses of study, need to have so much effort put into how they might be helped to be taught and to learn.

But perhaps it is not primarily about helping people to teach and learn at all.

5.1   Enabling Medical Migration Is a Political Choice

We have put forward the radical view that medical education as big business plays a large part in terms of:

• the trade in cheaply produced doctors exported from the global south to the global north (requiring acceptable production processes, quality-stamped by fee-charging para-regulatory 'global' organisations that actually represent global north values and practices)
• the profit to be made from private medical education (or, indeed, the competitive advantages to be sought among publicly funded institutions)
• the commodification of medical education and the selling of its components in consultancies, curricula, and teaching and learning methods.

A wish to improve healthcare might be part of the argument, and this can happen when medical education focuses on improving performance on tasks (McGaghie et al., 2024). However, although a well-educated workforce is a fundamental condition for improvement, if the healthcare service itself is inadequate or inaccessible, then medical education alone can have little effect. Compounding this, medical migration is ever increasing, facilitated by globalised medical education itself.

5.2   Engaging with the Healthcare Service or Not, Is a Political Choice

We might imagine that UK medical schools produce well-trained graduates (despite not having dedicated medical education departments), but these well-trained medical graduates are not always able to find postgraduate training posts (which are obligatory for career progression). Doctors are increasingly dissatisfied with their working conditions and the barriers they experience to offering the care they have been trained to deliver, resulting in 15 percent of all doctors taking steps to leave the NHS. More than one third of UK doctors in training are choosing not to proceed (Armitage, 2023). Their medical education is usually of high quality, but that is of limited effect on patient care under the conditions of the healthcare service itself. So where medical education does not engage with the state of actual healthcare services which can directly change the health of the people, or is happy to facilitate medical migration from poorer to richer countries, we should reflect on what the potentially powerful medical education movement, which tends to focus on what happens in medical school, is actually intending to achieve. The power in relation to improving the health of the people, is with the service, not with medical education.

If medical education does not align itself with the state of the healthcare service, then its achievements for the care of populations will be limited, regardless of any claims it makes. Medicine, and so medical education, are inevitably political undertakings, because they have a key social function. That political role can be engaged with or ignored. It is there, nonetheless.

5.3   The Social and Political in Medical Education

Medical education has been criticised for being 'politicised' in its advocacy of social justice and 'communal' or 'collaborative' methods of learning which, of course, derive from the politics of socialism following Russian learning psychologists such as Alexander Luria, rather than the individualistic politics of 'Protestant-Capitalism' (Bleakley, 2020). Education is a social science and as such cannot avoid also being a political science. In advocating any practice in medical education, we are taking a political view. Almost any of the learning methods that have a title ending in '-based' will have a politically left-wing identity, being structured on group work or co-operative learning. And while doctors themselves, at least in the UK and US, tend to have left-leaning or politically moderate views (Mandeville et al., 2018; Patel et al., 2024), the picture is less clear elsewhere. At all levels, a political analysis of medical education reveals many tensions and contradictions.

6   Politics, Power and Contradictions in Medical Education

Having thought about the themes that run through all Parts of this book, we should
try to understand how they are interrelated and co-constitutive. Medical education
does not exist in silos; these themes constantly interact to shape the field. Everything
is always changing and developing in response to such tensions and contradictions
(Lauesen, 2020; Mao Zedong, 1937). The accounts of our authors show the complexity of medical education, the unclear identity of medical education itself, its
internal and international contradictions, and the post-colonial global forces of
power and politics that drive the content and practice of this field at every level.

Politics describes power relations:

> Power, Foucault (Foucault, 1970) pointed out, resides not only in individuals and groups
> but also and perhaps more importantly in social organizations, institutions, and systems.
> (Cornbleth, 1990)

We can read the politics of medical education as the tension between control and
autonomy, particularly as it manifests between global standardisation and regulation and the local context (Rashid et al., 2023; Rashid & Grant, 2024). This fundamental tension, a contradiction that often arises from medicine being increasingly
driven by the pursuit of value (Montori, 2019), appears in multiple forms throughout our authors' reflections. *On the professional level*, there are tensions between
individual practice and standardised competencies, and between professional values
and market-driven approaches. *On the educational level*, there are tensions between
standardised curricula and contextual learning needs, and between competency-
based education and apprenticeship models (Brightwell & Grant, 2013). *On the
global level*, the all-pervasive tensions are between global north and global south.
And *at the institutional level*, tensions arise between academic freedom and managerial control, and between educational quality and business imperatives. But
fundamentally:

> We believe that context really matters and that understanding of the resources available in
> specific conditions and circumstances is essential in assessing the possibilities for produc-
> tive politics in the face of globalising trends and forces. (Ozga & Lingard, 2007)

In the end, the power within the politics must find a different balance.

Nothing in this book suggests that the tensions revealed are easily resolved or
resolvable. In the absence of a political analysis, medical education might believe
that international regulation, or advocating new methods of teaching and learning,
or a new curriculum style or content are politically neutral events. But they are not.
They reflect deep contradictions in how medical education is conceived, delivered,
managed and influenced in an increasingly globalised world where the balance of
power is currently in favour of the global north.

We commend and support all the authors in this book who are struggling to preserve local, contextual and professional autonomy in medical education. A political
view might help.

References

Armitage, R. (2023). Junior doctors leaving the NHS: What would it mean for general practice? *The British Journal of General Practice, 73*(728), 126–127. https://doi.org/10.3399/bjgp23X732189

Baldwin, A. (2023). The history of industrial action in the NHS. *The Bulletin of the Royal College of Surgeons of England, 105*(4), 158–160. https://doi.org/10.1308/rcsbull.2023.61

Bass, B. M., & Bass, R. (2008). *The Bass handbook of leadership: Theory, research, and managerial applications* (4th ed.). Free Press.

Beech, J., Fraser, C., Gardner, T., Buzelli, L., Williamson, S., & Alderwick, H. (2023). Stressed and overworked: What the Commonwealth Fund's 2022 International Health Policy Survey of primary care physicians in 10 countries means for the UK. https://doi.org/10.37829/HF-2023-P12.

Bleakley, A. (2020). Embracing the collective through medical education. *Advances in Health Sciences Education, 25*(5), 1177–1189. https://doi.org/10.1007/s10459-020-10005-y

Bleakley, A., Brice, J., & Bligh, J. (2008). Thinking the post-colonial in medical education. *Medical Education, 42*(3), 266–270. https://doi.org/10.1111/j.1365-2923.2007.02991.x

Brightwell, A., & Grant, J. (2013). Competency-based training: Who benefits? *Postgraduate Medical Journal, 89*(1048), 107–110. https://doi.org/10.1136/postgradmedj-2012-130881

Cornbleth, C. (1990). *Curriculum in context.* Falmer.

Duvivier, R. J., Burch, V. C., & Boulet, J. R. (2017). A comparison of physician emigration from Africa to the United States of America between 2005 and 2015. *Human Resources for Health, 15*(1), 41. https://doi.org/10.1186/s12960-017-0217-0

Eady, K., & Moreau, K. A. (2024). A medical education research library: Key research topics and associated experts. *Medical Education Online, 29*(1). https://doi.org/10.1080/1087298 1.2024.2302233

Foucault, M. (1970). *The order of things: An archaeology of the human sciences.* Pantheon.

Garratt, K.. (2024). *NHS industrial action in England.* https://commonslibrary.parliament.uk/research-briefings/cbp-9775/

Goodair, B. (2024). Still safe? In *Still in their hands? An evaluation of NHS privatisation in England since 2010.* University of Oxford.

Goodair, B., Bach-Mortensen, A. M., & Reeves, A. (2024). 'Two sides of the same coin'? A longitudinal analysis evaluating whether financial austerity accelerated NHS privatisation in England 2013–2020. *BMJ Public Health, 2*(1), e000964. https://doi.org/10.1136/bmjph-2024-000964

Grant, J., & Grant, L. (2023). Quality and constructed knowledge: Truth, paradigms, and the state of the science. *Medical Education, 57*(1), 23–30. https://doi.org/10.1111/medu.14871

Khan, N. (2023a). Is there a shelf with spare GPs coming to the rescue? *British Journal of General Practice, 73*(732), 312–313. https://doi.org/10.3399/bjgp23X733329

Khan, N. (2023b). Put a cap on it: Safe workload levels in general practice. *British Journal of General Practice, 73*(728), 122–123. https://doi.org/10.3399/bjgp23X732165

Lauesen, T. (2020). *The principal contradiction.* Kersplebedeb.

Mandeville, K. L., Satherley, R.-M., Hall, J. A., Sutaria, S., Willott, C., Yarrow, K., Mohan, K., Wolfe, I., & Devakumar, D. (2018). Political views of doctors in the UK: A cross-sectional study. *Journal of Epidemiology and Community Health, 72*(10), 880–887. https://doi.org/10.1136/jech-2018-210801

Matheson, J., Patterson, J., & Neilson, L. (2020). *Tackling causes and consequences of health inequalities: A practical guide.* CRC Press.

McGaghie, W. C., Barsuk, J. H., Wayne, D. B., & Issenberg, S. B. (2024). Powerful medical education improves health care quality and return on investment. *Medical Teacher, 46*(1), 46–58. https://doi.org/10.1080/0142159X.2023.2276038

Montori, V. M. (2019). Turning away from industrial health care toward careful and kind care. *Academic Medicine, 94*(6), 768–770. https://doi.org/10.1097/ACM.0000000000002534

Navarro, V. (2007). Neoliberalism as a class ideology; or, the political causes of the growth of inequalities. *International Journal of Health Services, 37*(1), 47–62. https://doi.org/10.2190/AP65-X154-4513-R520

NHS. (n.d.). *Medical education | Health Careers*. Retrieved December 9, 2024, from https://www.healthcareers.nhs.uk/explore-roles/doctors/career-opportunities-doctors/alternative-roles-doctors/medical-education

OECD. (2019). *Recent trends in international migration of doctors, nurses and medical students*. https://doi.org/10.1787/5571ef48-en

Ozga, J., & Lingard, B. (2007). Globalisation, education policy and politics. In B. Lingard & J. Ozga (Eds.), *The RoutledgeFalmer reader in education policy and politics* (pp. 65–82). Routledge.

Park, S. (2012). The industrialisation of medical education? Exploring neoliberal influences within tomorrow's doctors policy 2009. In M. Lall (Ed.), *Policy, discourse and rhetoric. Educational futures rethinking theory and practice* (Vol. 52, pp. 121–140). SensePublishers. https://doi.org/10.1007/978-94-6091-817-9_7

Patel, M., Lyons, G., Fitzgibbon, K., & Webb, B. C. (2024). The doctor vote: Interactions between political ideological preferences and healthcare reform strategies among U.S. physicians. *Health Policy OPEN, 7*, 100123. https://doi.org/10.1016/j.hpopen.2024.100123

Powell, M., & Miller, R. (2016). Seventy years of privatizing the British National Health Service? *Social Policy & Administration, 50*(1), 99–118. https://doi.org/10.1111/spol.12161

Rasco, A. (2020). Standardization in education, a device of neoliberalism. *Journal for Critical Education Policy Studies, 18*(2). https://www.researchgate.net/profile/Jose-Felix-Angulo-Rasco/publication/344498137_Standardization_in_education_a_device_of_Neoliberalism/links/5f7cab62299bf1b53e12fe80/Standardization-in-education-a-device-of-Neoliberalism.pdf

Rashid, M. A., & Grant, J. (2024). Power and place: Uncovering the politics of global medical education. *Medical Education, 58*(8), 930–938. https://doi.org/10.1111/medu.15459

Rashid, M. A., Smith, V., Tackett, S., Arfeen, Z., & Mughal, F. (2021). What will it mean for me? Perceptions of the ECFMG 2023 accreditation requirement from an online forum. *Journal of Medical Regulation, 107*(2), 49–56. https://doi.org/10.30770/2572-1852-107.2.49

Rashid, M. A., Ali, S. M., & Dharanipragada, K. (2023). Decolonising medical education regulation: A global view. *BMJ Global Health, 8*(6), e011622. https://doi.org/10.1136/bmjgh-2022-011622

Segouin, C., & Hodges, B. (2005). Educating doctors in France and Canada: Are the differences based on evidence or history? *Medical Education, 39*(12), 1205–1212. https://doi.org/10.1111/j.1365-2929.2005.02334.x

Stokes, J., Bower, P., Guthrie, B., Mercer, S. W., Rice, N., Ryan, A. M., & Sutton, M. (2022). Cuts to local government spending, multimorbidity and health-related quality of life: A longitudinal ecological study in England. *The Lancet Regional Health – Europe, 19*, 100436. https://doi.org/10.1016/j.lanepe.2022.100436

Uzomah, M., & Folorunso, P. O. (2020). Globalization: An inexorable phenomenal force. *International Journal of Humanities and Innovation (IJHI), 3*(2), 92–100.

Weisz, G., & Nannestad, B. (2021). The World Health Organization and the global standardization of medical training, a history. *Globalization and Health, 17*, 96. https://doi.org/10.1186/s12992-021-00733-0

Zedong, M. (1937). *On practice*. https://www.marxists.org/reference/archive/mao/selected-works/volume-1/mswv1_16.htm

Leonard Grant, MChem(Oxon), MSc, PhD is an early career academic interested in the political economy of work as a determinant of health. Leonard's PhD thesis used a dialectical materialist methodology to consider the workplace as part of the postgraduate General Practice curriculum. From 2013 to 2024, Leonard was the Academic Course Manager for the FAIMER/Keele MHPE in Assessment and Accreditation where he managed the educational process for hundreds of students, taught Research Methods and wrote on distance and distributed learning. Leonard has developed and taught a new Public Health MSc at the University of Winchester, and is currently Lecturer in Medical Education in the University of Liverpool School of Medicine where he is also Programme Director for a new PGCert in Clinical Education.

Janet Grant PhD, FBPsS, FRCGP[Hon], FRCP[Hon], MRCR [Hon], ARSM is a chartered educational psychologist and Honorary Professor in University College London Medical School. She is the Academic Director of CenMEDIC (the Centre for Medical Education in Context) and Emerita Professor of Education in Medicine at the UK Open University. She was the first non-clinical Lecturer in Medical Education in the world, being appointed at King's College Hospital Medical School, London in 1972. For most of her academic life, Janet has conducted policy research in medical education for the UK government and professional medical and regulatory bodies. Her interests are in policy research, regulation, educational development, continuing professional development and curriculum. She has worked in many countries and with international organisations around the world, and has written extensively on contextual relevance in these topics. Janet has been a regulator in both postgraduate medical education and legal education.

MIX
Papier aus verantwortungsvollen Quellen
Paper from responsible sources
FSC® C105338

If you have any concerns about our products,
you can contact us on
ProductSafety@springernature.com

In case Publisher is established outside the EU,
the EU authorized representative is:
Springer Nature Customer Service Center GmbH
Europaplatz 3, 69115 Heidelberg, Germany

Printed by Libri Plureos GmbH
in Hamburg, Germany